Core of the YOGA SŪTRAS

By the same author:

Light on Prāṇāyāma
Light on Yoga
The Concise Light on Yoga
Light on the Yoga Sūtras of Patañjali
The Tree of Yoga

B.K.S. IYENGAR

The World's Most Respected Yoga Teacher

Core of the YOGA SŪTRAS

The Definitive Guide to the Philosophy of Yoga

HARPER thorsons

HarperThorsons
An imprint of HarperCollins*Publishers*
77–85 Fulham Palace Road,
Hammersmith, London W6 8JB

www.harpercollins.co.uk

HARPER™ thorsons

and HarperThorsons are trademarks
of HarperCollins*Publishers* Ltd

First published by HarperThorsons 2012

1 3 5 7 9 10 8 6 4 2

B.K.S. Iyengar asserts the moral right to be
identified as the author of this work

A catalogue record of this book is available
from the British Library

ISBN 978-0-00- 792126-3

Printed and bound in Great Britain by
Clays Ltd, St Ives plc

My mother in 1956

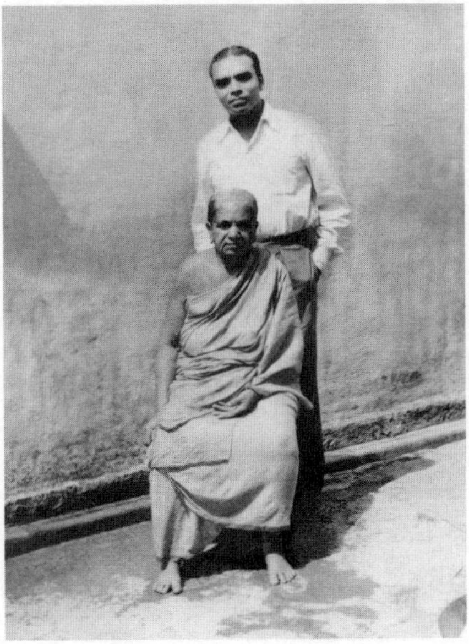

Dedicated to my father,
Bellur Krishnamachar,
and particularly to my mother,
Seshamma

Invocation

ॐ

॥श्रीमत् पतञ्जलि महामुनये नमः॥
योगेन चित्तस्य पदेन वाचां
मलं शरीरस्यच वैद्यकेन ।
योऽपाकरोत् तं प्रवरं मुनीनां
पतञ्जलिं प्राञ्जलिरानतोऽस्मि ॥
आबाहु पुरुषाकारं
शङ्खचक्रासि धारिणम् ।
सहस्र शिरसं श्वेतं
प्रणमामि पतञ्जलिम् ॥

yogena cittasya padena vācāṁ
malaṁ śarīrasya ca vaidyakena /
yo'pākarot taṁ pravaraṁ munīnāṁ
patañjaliṁ prāñjalir ānato'smi
ābāhu puruṣākāraṁ śaṅkha-cakra-asi-dhāriṇaṁ
sahasra-śirasaṁ śvetaṁ praṇamāmi patañjaliṁ //

Let us bow before the noblest of sages, Patañjali, who presented yoga for the serenity of the mind, grammar for clarity of words and medicine for keeping the body clean.

Let us prostrate before Patañjali, an incarnation of Ādiśeṣa crowned with a thousand heads, whose upper body represents the human form with four hands, holding a conch (*śaṅkha*) and disc (*cakra*) in two arms and the sword of knowledge (*asi*) in the third, and gracing the yoga *sādhakas* with the fourth.

Invocation of Sage Vyāsa

ॐ

यस्त्यक्त्वा रूपमाद्यं प्रभवति जगतोऽनेकधाऽनुग्रहाय ।
प्रक्षीणक्लेशराशिर्विषमविषधरोऽनेकवक्त्रः सुभोगी ।
सर्वज्ञान प्रसूतिर्भुजगपरिकरः प्रीतये यस्य नित्यम् ।
देवोऽहीशः स वोऽव्यात्सितविमलतनुर्योगदो योगयुक्तः॥

Yas tyaktvā rūpam ādyaṁ prabhavati jagato'nekadhā anugrahāya
Prakṣīṇa-kleśa-rāśir viṣama-viṣadharo'neka-vaktrāḥ subhogī //
Sarva-jñāna-prasūtir bhujaga-parikaraḥ prītaye yasya nityaṁ /
Devo'hīṣaḥ sa vo'vyāt sita-vimala-tanur yoga-do yoga-yuktaḥ //

Let us prostrate before Lord Ādiśeṣa, who manifested as Patañjali to grace the human race with correct word, work and wisdom.

Let us salute Ādiśeṣa of the myriad serpent heads and mouths carrying noxious poisons who descended as Patañjali, discarding the poisons to eradicate ignorance and vanquish sorrow.

Let us pay our obeisance to him, repository of all knowledge, amidst His attendant retinue.

Let us pray to the Lord whose primordial form shines with pure and white effulgence, pristine in body, a master of yoga who bestows on us his *yaugika* light of wisdom in order to enable us to rest in the house of the immortal Universal Self.

Contents

Foreword by the Dalai Lama **xix**

Preface by Honourable Shri Murli Manohar Joshi (MP) **xxi**

Acknowledgements **xxxi**

Prologue **xxxiii**

***Yoga Pīṭhikā* – Introduction** **1**

I ***Yoga Paraṁparā* – *Yaugika* Lineage** **11**

II ***Yoga Dharma* – The Concept of Yoga** **13**

III ***Janma Mṛtyu Cakra* – The Wheel of Birth and Death** **20**

IV ***Sṛṣṭikartā* – *Ādi Puruṣa* or *Īśvara*** **27**

V ***Sṛṣṭikrama* – The Structure of the Universe** **32**

1. *Puruṣa* (Ātman) 32
2. *Ahaṁ-ākāra* 33
3. *Viśva Caitanya Śakti* 33
4. *Guṇas* 34
5. *Prakṛti* 37

6. The Conjunction between *Puruṣa* and *Prakṛti* 38
7. *Citta* (Consciousness) 42

VI *Puruṣa* – Seer 44

VII *Citta Svabhāva* – The Natural State of Consciousness 50

1. *Ahaṁkāra* (I-maker), a Mirror of the Seer and the Seen 51
2. *Buddhi* (Wisdom, Intelligence) 53
3. *Manas* (Mind) 56
4. *Kūṭastha Citta* (Big 'I') 59
5. *Pariṇāma Citta* (Small 'i') 59
6. *Citta Nirūpaṇa* (Representation or Definition of *Citta*) 64

VIII *Citta Lakṣaṇa* – Characteristics of Consciousness 66
1. *Citta Bhūmi* 68
2. *Citta Lakṣaṇa* 69

IX *Citta Śreṇi* – Stages of Consciousness 72
1. *Vyutthāna Citta* and *Nirodha Citta* 73
2. *Śānta Citta* 75
3. *Ekāgra Citta* 75
4. *Chidra Citta* 75
5. *Nirmāṇa Citta* 76
6. *Divya Citta* (*Paripakva Citta*) 77

X *Kleśa*, *Vṛtti* and *Antarāya* – Afflictions, Fluctuations and Impediments 78
1. *Vṛttis* 83
2. *Saṁskāra Vṛtti* 86
3. *Anukūla* and *Pratikūla Vṛtti* 87
4. *Anukūla Vṛtti* 87

5. *Pratikūla Vṛtti* 93

6. *Nava Antarāya* – Nine Types of Impediments 94

XI *Citta Parivartana* through Yoga – Transformation of *Citta* through Yoga 98

XII Sādhanā Krama – Method of Practice 106

1. *Sādhanā Krama* 109

2. *Sādhanā Kriyā* 111

3. *Tapas* 113

4. *Svādhyāya* 114

5. *Īśvara Praṇidhāna* 115

6. *Sādhanā Stambha* (Pillars for *Sādhaka* and *Sādhanā*) 120

XIII *Adhaḥpatana Rekhā* in *Sādhanā* – The Razor Edge of Yoga 121

1. *The Precipice* 126

XIV *Aṣṭāṅga Yoga Prayoga, Tathā Pariṇāma* – The Application of *Aṣṭāṅga Yoga* and Its Effects 127

1. *Śarīra Śarīrī Bhāva* 127

2. *Kośas* of the Body 128

3. *Bahiraṅga* and *Antaraṅga Saṁyama* 134

4. Effects of *Saṁyamas* 139

5. Application of Yoga 143

6. *Yama* 144

7. Effects of *Yama* 145

8. *Niyama* 146

9. Effects of *Niyama* 147

10. *Āsana* 147

11. How Should an *Āsana* Be Done? 148

12. Effects of *Āsanas* 153
13. Differences between *Āsana* and *Dhyāna* 155
14. *Prāṇāyāma* 155
15. Effects of *Prāṇāyāma* 157
16. *Vāyu* 160
17. *Cakras* 162
18. *Pratyāhāra* 164
19. Effects of *Pratyāhāra* 166
20. *Dhāraṇā* 166
21. Definition of *Dhāraṇā* 167
22. Effects of *Dhāraṇā* 168
23. *Dhyāna* 168
24. Effects of *Dhyāna* 169
25. *Antarātman* Aspect of Yoga 171
26. *Samādhi* or *Samāpatti* 171
27. Effects of *Samādhi* 172
28. *Antaraṅga Samādhi* 173
29. *Virāma Pratyaya* 175
30. Effects of *Virāma Pratyaya* 175
31. Cautions to *Sādhakas* on *Samādhi* 176
32. *Samādhi Phala* 177
33. *Nirbīja Samādhi* 177
34. *Yogaphala* (Effects of *Aṣṭāṅga* Yoga) 178
35. *Prakṛti Puruṣa Jaya* 181
   a) *Bhūta jaya* – mastery over the elements 181
   b) *Tanmātra jaya* – mastery over the infrastructural qualities of the elements 182
   c) *Śarīra jaya* – mastery over the body 182

d) *Indriya jaya* – mastery over the organs of action and senses of perception 182
e) *Manojaya* – mastery over the mind and consciousness 182
f) Realising the seer 183
g) *Ātmajaya* – sight of the seer 183

XV *Samādhi-Kaivalya Bheda* – The Difference between *Samādhi* and *Kaivalya* 185

Glossary of *Saṅskṛta* Words 189
Appendix I – Patañjali's *Yoga Sūtras* 231
Appendix II – Alphabetical Index of the *Sūtras* 259
Index 269

THE DALAI LAMA

FOREWORD

I have met Shri B. K. S. Iyengar and was touched by his scholarship and understanding of the relationship between the mind and the body.

In conversation with him, it seems there are many terms in common between Yoga and Buddhism, although their connotation may be different. In the Buddhist tradition, for example, we also use the term Yoga. In the Vajrayana tradition, in particular, it refers to the utilization of physical energy as part of the meditation practice, recognizing that the movement of the mind and the body are intricately connected. It is explained that purifying and channeling our physical energies has a place in the practice of training and disciplining the mind. We believe that our actions (karma) and the disturbing emotions (klesha) that give rise to them propel us into the cycle of suffering, but that by realizing the natural purity of the mind we can gain complete freedom from that suffering. This is why training and disciplining the mind is so important.

All our religious and spiritual traditions believe in the innate goodness of human beings. Different religions exist to develop and strengthen this quality. Since human beings naturally possess diverse mental dispositions and interests, it is inevitable that different religious traditions emphasize different philosophies and modes of practice. This diversity is actually a source of enrichment. Because of the astounding variety of human beings' intellectual and emotional dispositions, we require a variety of spiritual traditions and practices to meet our various needs. The most important thing is practice in daily life that is how we can gradually get to know the true value of whatever teaching we follow.

What we need is a good heart, a disciplined mind and a healthy body. We will not transform ourselves merely by making wishes, but through working hard over a long period of time. Seeing how energetic he is at the age of 93 and his approach towards his students is an inspiration to all.

This book presents the tradition of Yoga as taught by the great Indian master Patanjali interpreted for our times by a great contemporary teacher. May Shri Iyengar continue to live long in good health.

August 4, 2011

Preface

Yoga is the most wonderful gift from India to humankind. It is as much a philosophy as a science, as well as being an art. yoga is the perfect embodiment of Satyam, Shivam and Sundaram. According to Hindu tradition, yoga is as old as human civilisation. Vedic Rishis had from the earliest times known yoga and considered it as a supra-human revelation (a *puruṣeya*). *Pāñcarātra*, a Vedic text, says that yoga is a divine subject and is as old as Creation. However, yoga is neither faith nor superstition; it is a subject with a well-defined philosophy, grammar and goal, and epitomises India's spirituality.

Sages in India have always looked to the Vedas for the origin of what we now call as the yogic tradition. The term 'yoga' can be found in the *Ṛgveda*, but the present-day technical connotation of yoga has taken a long journey. As a spiritual discipline, the term 'yoga' appeared (probably for the first time) in the *Taittīrya* Upanishad, which dates from the sixth century BCE. That yoga was practised in India during the Indus Valley Civilisation (3300–1300 BCE) has been established by archaeological findings. Terracotta figurines in yogic *āsana*s have been found in the excavations from Harappa and Mohenjo-daro. A limestone statuette of a priest from Mohenjo-daro is undoubtedly in a meditative pose (*dhyāna*). Thus India has known and practised yoga for several millennia. Several Western scholars have attempted to trace the origin of yoga but almost all of them have not gone beyond speculation – primarily, because of their lack of knowledge of Vedic Sanskrit; and secondly, because of their poor understanding of the contents, meanings and the wisdom of various Vedic texts. However, scholars like Swami Dayananda Saraswati and Maharshi Aurobindo, and yoga masters like Paramhansa Yogananda have spoken about the deep philosophical content of the Vedic literature and the antiquity of the yogic tradition. A closer scrutiny of the Jain and Buddhist literature reveals that even these non-Vedic traditions have strong Vedic roots and accept yoga as a discipline that has been practised from antiquity.

From the *Ṛgveda* to Ahirbudhnya Samhita and *Taittīrya* Upanishad, the concept of yoga has evolved considerably. The Samhita defines yoga as the union between the individual soul and the cosmic or Universal Soul. It is a *saṁyoga* yoga, which is predominantly spiritual. This definition is deficient, as it does not take into account other aspects of human personality and contemplates that the *jīvātman* (the individual soul) should be completely devoted to *paramātman* (God, the supreme soul). Any serious student interested in exploring the evolution of yoga, from a mere concept in Veda to a fully fledged discipline as propounded by Patañjali, finds that such an exercise is not easy. However, no science or discipline, particularly one like yoga, can achieve perfection in a small span of time. Much research and experimentation must have been undertaken to build its philosophical base and theories, as well as its methodology. As in the process of science, theories are developed and experiments performed, and the results lead to further refinement of the theories; so too the ancient sages must have undertaken serious experimentation for refining yoga as a system.

It may be recognised that the Vedas themselves do not mention specific yoga postures or *āsana*s and so these postures are not described by Patañjali in the *Yoga Sūtra*s written after a gap of few millennia. The numerous postures prevalent today must have been the result of the innovations of the sages, who probably practised and experimented with a view to redefining and refining the yogic system. The present state of the yogic system is the result of the *tapasya* of ancient sages over the millennia.

Dr B.K.S. Iyengar is himself a shining example of this *tapasya.* He was initiated to yoga by a great scholar and master in yoga at the young age of 15, and since then, over a period of about eight decades, he has been teaching, practising and unravelling the secrets of yoga. His whole life is of a *Sādhaka* completely dedicated to yoga, resulting in the transformation of his physical, psychological, intellectual and spiritual frame. It is interesting to note that Yogacharya Iyengar was not initially trained in the classical philosophical literature of yoga, but as he has himself said, his keen observation of the deep reflexes gradually resulted in an intuitive understanding of the subject. He explains, 'in my practice I annointed my body and mind with knowledge, which soaked deep into all the layers of the self, enabling me to be aware of my own presence, and kindling an awareness in my tendons, fibres, muscles, joints, nerves and cells.'

It is easy to comprehend that the flowering of the tree of yoga from the tiny seed in the *Ṛgveda* is the result of personal experiences repeated and shared by the sages over a long period of history. During his studies of the various commentaries on the *Yoga Sūtra*s and also other related texts, Dr Iyengar found that most of them suffered from contradictions and were influenced by a particular school of philosophy. His own experiences did not conform to what was indicated in those texts. Further, the commentaries did not offer any satisfactory method for practical adaptation. Having realised the limitations of the existing literature on yoga, Dr Iyengar decided to undertake a comparative and critical study of the *Yoga Sūtra*s on the one hand and of the *Haṭhayoga Pradīpikā*, *Śrīmad Bhagavad Gītā* and Upanishads on the other.

Not being satisfied only with a theoretical knowledge of yoga, Dr Iyengar went for practical experience as well. In his own words, 'In my *sādhanā*, my body, mind, intelligence and awareness became a laboratory for experience. I tried to do a comparative and analytical study of the *Sūtra*s with *Haṭhayoga Pradīpikā*, *Bhagavad Gītā* and *Yoga Upaniṣads*. This helped me gradually to grasp the essence of the *Yoga Sūtras* of Patañjali.' *Light on Yoga* was published in 1966 and *Light on the Yoga Sūtras of Patañjali* in 1993, but the relentless researcher in Dr Iyengar did not stop there. Even at the ripe age of 93 years, he continues on his quest for a deeper and fuller understanding of the Patañjali *Yoga Sūtras*.

In the two decades since the publication of *Light on the Yoga Sūtras of Patañjali*, Dr Iyengar in his *sādhanā* has experienced a total transformation of his being. As a true yogi he experiences his self expanding and merging in vastness. In his own words, 'Thus in my practice I found myself closely connected to the *Yoga Sūtras*, and I began to feel their values featuring directly in my *sādhanā*.'

These experiences led Dr Iyengar towards a better understanding of the *Yoga Sūtras* and also suggested the need to reconsider his earlier work, along with a fresh look on Patañjali's presentation. This book, *Core of the Yoga Sūtras*, is based on the yogic experiences of the great Sadhaka Yogacharya Dr B. K. S. Iyengar, and it reveals the heart of the *sūtras* in a new light. It unravels the hidden core aspects of *Pātañjala Sūtras* and provides a better understanding of the discipline of yoga. The importance of this seminal work lies in the fact that it is based on the personal yogic experiences of the author and his understanding of the interconnections between the *Yoga Sūtras* during the *sādhanā*, and is expressed by a highly illuminated mind and equally evolved soul.

Dr Iyengar emphasises that the yogic *sādhanā* leads to the transformation of a *sādhaka* from the natural (*prakṛta*) or unrefined state to a refined (*saṁskṛta*) state. Ordinarily a person remains in a state where he instinctively responds to the forces of nature (*prakṛti*) and is governed by the law of Karma; the yoga *sādhanā* leads him to act according to the law of *Dharma*. This transformation does not come from outside forces but by drawing from within what is already present. Just as the real teacher illuminates the mind of a student and makes him feel that knowledge comes not from somewhere outside but from within, so also the guru makes a *sādhaka* realise that he has to learn from within. How this can be achieved needs a very clear understanding of both the philosophy and the practical aspects of yoga. In this work, Dr Iyengar has explained in very lucid and simple language how the *Pātañjala Sūtra*s can promote this learning form within and achieve a state where the *sādhaka* (self) merges with the Self – where, in other words, the difference between the seer and the seen vanishes.

The author has already provided a perfectly logical interpretation of the *Yoga Sūtra*s, which is concise and can be easily comprehended even by a person not acquainted with the classical texts on yoga and the terse commentaries on the *Yoga Sūtra*s. In this new work the interconnections and linkages in the *Yoga Sūtra*s have been arranged in such a manner that their hidden meanings can be easily comprehended. The author has discovered/experienced these interconnections and linkages during his own yoga *sādhanā*, and these will motivate a *sādhaka* to further understand and explore them. In the spirit of a true researcher, Dr Iyengar does not claim this work to be the last word on the interpretation of the *Yoga Sūtra*s but rather hopes that these efforts (*anusādhana*) to further refine the de-codifying and re-codifying of the *Sūtra*s will continue.

Core of the Yoga Sūtras consists of two parts. The first part deals with the translation of the aphorisms based on the author's personal experiences and the existing commentaries. The second part of the treatise deals with the author's arrangement of the *Sūtras* along with a comparison with other texts and the author's interpretation of various concepts that are generally difficult to comprehend. Dr Iyengar argues that the *Yoga Sūtra*s have four chapters and each represents the four *āśrama*s and four *puruṣārtha*s (aims of life). The parallels drawn between the four *varna*s, four *āśrama*s, and four *puruṣārtha*s and the four chapters (*pāda*s) of the *Pātañjala Yoga Sūtra*s is a unique feature of this treatise. This is perhaps the first ever attempt to establish a correlation between the social structure of yoga and its spiritual framework.

It must be recognised that yoga practice has generally been considered to be highly internal, completely unrelated with the external. This practice, or *sādhanā*, is an individual effort whereas the *varṇa*, *āśrama* (*brahmacarya*, *gṛhastha*, *vanaprastha* and *saṅnyāsa*) and *puruṣārthas* (*dharma artha*, *kāma* and *mokṣa*) are related to societal systems and structures. Dr Iyengar has argued that the *jīvātman* (individual) can merge in to *paramātman* through the preparation of the body, mind, intellect and soul as propounded by the *Yoga Sūtras*, but the process also requires a social structure to facilitate such a journey. However, he also makes it clear that the *varṇas* (*brāhmaṇa*, *kṣatriya*, *vaiśya* and *śūdra*) have faded and only the *āśramas* and the *puruṣārtha* are currently in vogue.

In no way is Dr Iyengar arguing for retaining out-of-date social structures. He is only suggesting that a spiritual journey of an individual is facilitated if there is a favourable social environment for such a course. In other words, a symbiotic relation between a yogic *sādhaka* and the environment is desirable. The yogi is not alienated from society or the material world but rather considers it as a necessary instrument to prepare himself for seeking freedom from bondage. In fact, the body is the supporter of consciousness.

The concept of consciousness has baffled most modern scientists trained with a reductionist or mechanistic world view. But Dr Iyengar has dealt with this subject with great felicity. Starting from the natural state of consciousness and describing its characteristics and its transformation, the author describes for us the transformation of consciousness through yoga. As a connecting link between the ten organs (*indriyas*) and the intelligence and consciousness, the mind has to play multiple roles. Dr Iyengar goes on to describe 35 facets of mind, which demonstrate its capabilities to function in different roles. Starting from the biological mind, moving to the temporal mind and finally reaching the stage of the yogic or divine mind, the list also includes confused, wandering, split and attentive minds. If mind, the connecting agent between intelligence and consciousness, becomes multiple, the *citta* (consciousness) also becomes multiple.

Dr Iyengar further points out that *buddhi manas* and *vijñāna manas* are two extremely delicate means of analysis, which a *sādhaka* must apply constantly in gauging his evolution and escaping from the pitfalls on the path of the yogic journey. As and when the mind is controlled and does not waver, and yogic practices cleanse the senses of perception, the mind reaches the state of divine or yogic mind. Then the *citta* too does not waver and becomes a fit instrument to experience the sight of *puruṣa* (*ātmā-darśana*).

Dr Iyengar has defined the term *Kutastha chitta* as absolute consciousness. It is the seer-I (*ahaṁ-ākāra* or 'I am') and the term *pariṇāma citta*, as the state of consciousness that fluctuates due to the wavering of mind, is the ego. In order to have a clear vision of 'I', the *pariṇāma citta* must be disciplined. Dr Iyengar has shown that the process of achieving self-restraint can be understood through the correct performance of *prāṇāyāma*.

In further discussion of the *āsanas*, Dr Iyengar explains the true meaning of *sthiram sukham āsanam*. He argues that the *āsanas* are performed primarily in a state where the limbs of the body are guided by the *citta*, but then the *sādhaka* must make efforts to seek a situation so that the *pariṇāma citta* aligns with the *kūṭastha-citta*. It is only when such an alignment takes place that the sadhaka experiences a state of *sthiram sukham āsanam*. There are no impediments, no afflictions, no wavering of the mind, and a complete harmony is established between the body, intelligence and consciousness. In this condition there is a uniform flow of intelligence all over the body and the *pariṇāma citta* is unwavering and the mirror is quite clear to reflect the true image of I (*puruṣa*). The secrets of the *Yoga Sūtra*s have been clearly unravelled in this treatise and one has to recognise that Dr Iyengar has in all probability attained the state where his consciousness has come close to experiencing the cosmic consciousness, when the true meanings of yoga and the *Yoga Sūtra*s were revealed to him. I most respectfully salute this great *sādhaka-Yogirāj* for his brilliant and groundbreaking exposition of an extremely difficult subject.

It would be interesting to compare the experiences of Dr Iyengar with those of Western thinkers. During the last decade much literature has been published about the Western approach to transcendental experience. This tends to categorise yogic experiences as a mystic phenomenon. The authors of *Why God Won't Go Away* have argued that the conclusions of the mystics are clear: God (the ultimate Reality) is by his nature unknowable. He is not an objective fact, or an actual being; he is, in fact, being itself, the absolute, undifferentiated oneness that is the ground of all existence. When we understand this truth, the mystics claim, all religions connect us to this deeper, divine power. If we fail to understand it and we cling to the comforting images of a personal, knowable God – a God who exists entirely apart from the rest of creation as a distinct, individual being – we diminish the ultimate realness of God and reduce his divinity to the stature of the small, 'deaf idol'.

Mystics further claim that the true nature of God can be known only through a direct mystical encounter. Evelyn Underhill writing in *The Essentials of Mysticism* explains that 'Mysticism, in its pure form, is the science of ultimates, the science of union with the Absolute and nothing else,' and that 'the mystic is the person who attains this union, not the person who talks about it. Not to know about, but to Be, is the mark of the real initiate.'

Dr Beatrice Bruteau argues in the preface to *The Mystic Heart*, by Wayne Teasdale, that mysticism may provide the world with its last, best hope for a happier future, by allowing us to overcome the greed, mistrust and self-protective fears that have led to so many centuries of suffering and strife: 'Consider that domination, greed, cruelty, violence, and all our other ills arise from a sense of insufficient and insecure being.'

According to Bruteau, mysticism allows us to transcend these egotistical fears. The awareness of mystical wholeness shows us that we are not so fundamentally alienated from one another and that, in fact, we do have all the being we need to be happy. When the appreciation of this mystical oneness rises to the surface, Bruteau says, 'our motives, feelings, and actions turn from withdrawal, suspicion, rejection, hostility, and domination to openness, trust, inclusion, nurturance, and communion.'

'This oneness – this freedom from alienation and insecurity – is the sure foundation for a better world,' she says. 'It means that we will try to help each other rather than hurt each other.' This oneness takes us towards a state of unification with those whom we had considered as 'others'.

The transforming power of these unitary states is what makes mysticism our most practical and effective hope for improving human behaviour, she believes. 'If we could arrange energy from within, if we more often nurtured our companions and promoted their well-being, we would suffer much less. Rearranging energy from within is what mysticism does.' Generations may pass before human society is ready for such transforming ideas, but it is intriguing to know that if such a time should arrive, the brain will be ready, possessing the machinery it needs to make those ideas real.

The question of why we humans have always longed to connect with something larger than ourselves, and why consciousness inevitably involves us in a spiritual quest, has been answered by two neurologists, Andrew Newberg and Eugene D'Acuily, in their brilliantly researched treatise *Why God Won't Go Away*. And the answer is simple and scientifically precise: the religious impulse is rooted in the biology of the brain. In experiments, they found that intensely focused spiritual contemplation triggers an alteration in the activity of the brain, which leads us to perceive transcendent religious experiences as solid and tangibly real. Their inescapable conclusion is that God is hardwired into the human brain. The authors further argue that if Absolute Unitary Being is real, then God – in all the ways humans have personified him in order to know him – can only be a metaphor. But metaphors are not meaningless, they do not point to nothing. What gives the metaphor of God its enduring meaning is the very fact that it is rooted in something that is experienced as unconditionally real.

Newberg and D'Acuily conclude their findings by observing:

> 'The neurobiological roots of spiritual transcendence show that Absolute Unitary Being is a plausible, even probable possibility. Of all the surprises our theory [the religious impulse is rooted in the biology of the brain] has to offer – that myths are driven by biological compulsion, that rituals are intuitively shaped to

trigger unitary states, that mystics are, after all, not necessarily crazy, and that all religions are branches of the same spiritual tree – the fact that this ultimate unitary state can be rationally supported intrigues us the most. The realness of Absolute Unitary Being is not conclusive proof that a higher God exists but it makes a strong case that there is more to human existence than sheer material existence. Our minds are drawn by the intuition of this deeper reality, this utter sense of oneness, where suffering vanishes and all desires are at peace. As long as our brains are arranged the way they are, as long as our minds are capable of sensing this deeper reality, spirituality will continue to shape the human experience, and God, however we define that majestic, mysterious concept, will not go away.'

Whatever Western scholars says about mysticism and whatever these two neuroscientists have concluded about the present structure of the human mind–body complex and its capability of sensing deeper reality and spirituality, Dr Iyengar shows in this book that the ancient Indian sages had understood the same phenomena at the very dawn of civilisation. His book establishes beyond doubt that the human mind–body–consciousness complex has been designed to be a fit instrument for experiencing Cosmic consciousness and that yoga practised in the prescribed manner is the golden path leading to that stage of ecstatic experience where ego ('I am this or that') merges in the absolute that is 'I am'. At this stage the ego melts down and submerges in the vastness. The book is free from any religious bias and does not require any God as the creator. It has a universal appeal and will stand as a real guide for serious *sādhaka*s of yoga. In fact, it is Patañjali reinvented. Dr Iyengar will be remembered as perhaps the best commentator on the *Yoga Sūtra*s of Patañjali.

Murli Manohar Joshi
New Delhi
27 September 2011

Acknowledgements

I wish to express my gratitude to my daughter, Geeta S. Iyengar, and my thanks to Stephanie Quirk, Uma Dhavale, Patxi Lizardi, Faeq Biria and other senior students for their encouragement, support and care in reading the entire manuscript, which was re-written several times to quell their doubts and questions. I am particularly grateful to John Evans for his editorial guidance.

Prologue

I offer reverential respects with my body, senses, mind, intelligence and conscientiousness to Maharṣi Patañjali, Vyāsa-muni, Vācaspati Miśra, Bhoja Rāja, Vijñāna Bhikṣu and all other commentators on the *Yoga Sūtra*s, as well as the great yoga masters by whose grace I was progressively led from arrogant ignorance towards humbleness and knowledge. Both knowledge and wisdom dawned on me after years of *sādhanā* with indelible experiences to live in the divine present.

I am neither a *Saṅskṛta* scholar nor a philosopher. I am purely someone who has been an ardent student of yoga for nearly 80 years, totally involved in the *sādhanā*, exploring its depth to understand the beauty and majesty of this vast ocean of *yaugika* knowledge and its wisdom in tracing the core of the being or the spiritual heart – the soul.

My long, reverential practice not only burnt away all types of physical and mental impediments, but made me face all obstacles that came in the way of my *sādhanā*, kindling the flame of *yaugika* wisdom.

I had a great master in yoga, Śrī Tirumalai Krishnamacharya, who was highly qualified in all the six *darśana*s. He initiated me into yoga at the age of 15. Maybe on account of that young age, I never had the privilege of his theoretical tuition or access to his storehouse of knowledge, which was filled to capacity in him.

I was bedridden from birth with influenza, followed by malaria, typhoid and tuberculosis, so it was for my health that my brother-in-law, my *guru*, initiated me into yoga. Though I questioned him many times on the finer aspects of yoga, he avoided or ignored my queries. Perhaps this was because I was schooled in institutions where *Sanskṛta* was not taught to the students, or it may have been that he considered my age a bar for delving deeper into the subject of yoga. Whatever knowledge I gained through his public lectures was the basis on which I built up a career, as my *gurujī*[1] sent me within two years of beginning training to teach at Dharwar (Karnataka) and Pune (Maharashtra), India.

This job that was thrust upon me turned out to be a God-given opportunity. I was compelled to commit myself to the subject in my personal life as well as in practice.

As I was left to tread this path unsupported, I had to bear the formidable load of practising, teaching and exploring the principles of yoga. I had a big disadvantage due to my impaired physical health and mental growth, both the result of dire poverty. Hence, this was not an easy task; I was a novice both in theory and practice.

To gain some knowledge, I had to depend on my own practice as well as a watchful observation of the presentation of *āsana*s by the students, noticing their actions and reflexes, which were reflected in both their physical set-up and mental make-up.

It was impossible for me to get help from scholars in Pune because I did not know a word of the local language, and there was no one acquainted with the subject. The salary I was drawing was just sufficient to meet my basic needs, so I could not afford to buy any books for study. I was also under contract to teach for all hours of the day. Though I had accepted the orders of my guru to go to Dharwar and Pune to teach, yoga also became vital for my survival. Exhausted, I used to practise the *āsana*s, to be fit the next day to

1 A *guru* is one who eradicates darkness in his pupils and brings illumination. The *guru* is addressed as *gurujī*, acknowledging respect and reverence.

continue. It was only after 12 years of practice and teaching that I committed myself to yoga.

I began practising with reverence, to study my own body and mind in those rare moments when they were co-operating; usually there was a tug-of-war between them. Despite many restless and negative thoughts, I persisted and pursued my *sādhanā*, and this began to transform my physical and mental framework, bringing positive thoughts and hopes. I began to observe the deep reflexes of my practices, and penetrate my inner self, which enthused me and brought me further understanding.

My practice roused my instinctive reflex actions, which remain sharp even now in spite of my advanced age. They are innate responses to natural tendencies (*sahaja-pravṛtti* or *svabhāva-pravṛtti*). I began correlating and transforming these natural tendencies that occurred in my *sādhanā* with my own reflexive, intuitive thoughts (*svayaṁ prakāśa*, or intuitive light), to achieve right and ever-lasting experiential feelings.

In Hindu temples, the priests anoint and rub oil upon the idols as part of religious ceremonies. So in my practice I annointed my body and mind with knowledge, which soaked deep into all the layers of the self, enabling me to be aware of my own presence, and kindling an awareness in my tendons, fibres, muscles, joints, nerves and cells.

I began to visit the Pune library, which was open to the public, free of charge. When occasion permitted, I sat for hours to study, but the *yaugika* books in the library were very few.

As I did not have any background on the subject, I found it extremely hard to grasp what was written. My education had been poor, and the language expressed in the books was too academic, beyond what my raw, ruffled and restless mind and intellect could grasp.

Despite all these set-backs, I look back now and feel that this was my good fortune, that I could not learn the *Yoga Sūtras* in a formal or traditional way. Whenever I referred to the *Yoga Sūtras*, they appeared to be too terse to understand because they are condensed, coded and succinct. After years of total involvement and absorption in my *sādhanā*, without reference to the *Yoga Sūtras*, but with the aid of the *Haṭhayoga Pradīpikā* and the chapters of the *Bhagavad Gītā* where Lord Krishna deals with the practice of yoga, I began to gain some basic knowledge. Then I began to read translated commentaries on the *Yoga Sūtras*.

In the light of the knowledge and experience that I had gained through my own practice (*sādhanānubhava*), I saw the shortcomings of the authors and the manifold contradictions in their works. This encouraged me to study the *Yoga Sūtras* carefully on my own along with the classical commentaries, keeping in mind the experiences (*bhāvanā*) of my own *sādhanā*. I found that the explanations and commentaries were academic and scholarly and mostly influenced by the respective *vedāntika* schools of thought of the commentators. Though these commentaries offered me an overall view of the philosophy of yoga, their practical applications appeared quite limited.

In my *sādhanā*, my body, mind, intelligence and awareness became a laboratory for experience. I tried to do a comparative and analytical study of the *Sūtras* with *Haṭhayoga Pradīpikā*, *Bhagavad Gītā* and *Yoga Upaniṣads*. This helped me gradually to grasp the essence of the *Yoga Sūtras* of Patañjali.

Patañjali's masterpiece must be looked at as a compendium of the entire spiritual and literary heritage of classical India. Though it is not a *śruti* (revelation) like the *vedas* and classical music, it conveys the essence and the depth of the sacred scriptures. This masterful composition of the *Yoga Sūtras*, with its beautiful rhythm, is usually considered as literature, specifically a *kāvya* (poem), whereas it may easily be considered as a synthesis of all *smṛti* (remembered literature), the *itihāsa* (*Mahābhārata* and *Śrīmad Rāmāyaṇa*), and all major (*mahā-*) and minor (*upa-*) *purāṇas*.

The last *śloka* of Chapter III of *Bhagavad Gītā*[1] says that the Self is superior to the intelligence and the ego (the small self). As such,

---

1 *evaṁ buddheḥ paraṁ buddhvā saṁstabhyātmānam ātmanā /*
jahi śatruṁ mahābāho kāmarūpaṁ durāsadam // (*B. G.*, III.43) – Thus knowing him who is beyond intelligence, steadying the (lower) self by the Self, smite, O mighty armed (arjuna), the enemy in the form of desire, so hard to get at!

Krishna advises Arjuna to control the ego and steady the movements of the mind by cultivating indifference to lust, anger, greed, infatuation and envy. By the grace of the invisible hands of destiny and by my *sādhanā*, I was able to gain control over my shortcomings in the early stages of my practice, and to keep an open mind that enabled me to learn.

I must emphasise that my experience and belief both lead me to suggest that students of yoga must read and study *Bhagavad Gītā* thoroughly before undertaking the study of *Pātañjala Yoga Sūtra*s.

HarperCollins, London, published my book *Light on the Yoga Sūtras of Patañjali* in 1993. Now in the light of my experience and the wisdom I have gained since then, I am attempting a new offering, in which I have considered the hidden links inside the text in order to unveil the core meaning, or heart, that is implied in the *sūtra*s. In accordance with this core meaning, I have re-evaluated, re-arranged, re-composed and re-strung the *Yoga Sūtra*s. My purpose is to make *yaugika* scholars understand the in-depth philosophy and interconnection of the *sūtra*s better. I also want to provide an educational tool for students of yoga and Indian philosophy, to help them grasp the meaning of the *sūtra*s and learn how to put them into practice so that they may experience the fruits of yoga faster than I did.

This work is based on a meticulous study of the *Yoga Upaniṣad*s with a close assessment of the *sūtra*s. Though I am a fervent student of yoga, I must admit humbly that any error is solely mine and reflects neither on my *guru* nor on other exponents of yoga.

'To err is human.' Knowledge is infinite and eternal, but the human mind's thoughts lie in the field of the finite. The infinite is hidden in the finite, and the finite is hidden in the infinite. In my *sādhanā* I tried to explore finite within the infinite body. This helped me to understand the *Yoga Sūtra*s with clarity. As I mentioned above, the knowledge I absorbed along with an awareness of the self (*jīvātman*), gave me the courage to undertake this work.

Each day, the moment I begin my *sādhanā*, my entire being is transformed into a fresh state of mind. My mind extends and expands to the vastness. It is in that inner limitless space that I begin to work, trying various ways and means. Thus in my practice I found myself closely connected to the *Yoga Sūtra*s, and I began to feel their values featuring directly in my *sādhanā*.

These experiences helped me to write my previous book, *Light on the Yoga Sūtras of Patañjali*,[1] in which I found interconnections among the *sūtra*s, laying out a detailed synoptic table[2] and a thematic key to the *sūtras*.[3] In the first volume of *Aṣṭadaḷa Yogamālā* I made a first attempt to rearrange the *sūtra*s thematically, offering a ready reference.[4]

My almost 80 years of uninterrupted practice has formed the basis for me to reconsider my own previous work on the *sūtra*s as well as to re-study Patañjali's presentation.

Almost 20 years after the publication of *Light on the Yoga Sūtras of Patañjali*, and 10 years after the first volume of *Aṣṭadaḷa Yogamālā*, my reflections and my practice have led me to present a re-systematised structure of the *sūtra*s. I came to the conclusion that de-codifying and re-arranging the *sūtra*s go hand in hand, and each one helps to better approach the other.

As the physical heart is the core of our span of life, so too are the *Yoga Sūtra*s the core from which to trace *hṛd* – the spiritual heart, the seed of consciousness or the seat of the soul – so that each one of us resides in the soul. I am offering this new arrangement of the *sūtra*s because thousands and thousands of people now practise yoga seriously and try to delve deeper and deeper into its subtle aspects. I am sure that this presentation will offer new, inexperienced practitioners a way in and will guide them towards further penetration.

I have arranged the *sūtra*s so that the practitioner understands them easily and is thus encouraged to explore further via my reflections.

---

1 See *Light on the Yoga Sūtras of Patañjali*, Appendix II: Interconnection of *sūtras*.

2 *Id.*, Appendix I: A thematic key to the *Yoga Sūtra*s.

3 *Id.*, Yoga in a nutshell.

4 *Aṣṭadaḷa Yogamālā*, vol. 1, pp. 266–282, Allied Publishers, New Delhi, 2008.

Patañjali established and fixed the yoga system once and for ever. The book you have in your hands is, therefore, a re-arrangement of the *sūtras* and concepts of *Pātañjala Sūtra*, and aims to shed a better light on the hidden aspects and untold links present in his text.

I am expressing with courage and enthusiasm my innermost experiences through the core of the *Yoga Sūtras* so that readers may perfect their *sādhanā* to feel and savour fully the nectar of the essential life force – the Core of the Being, the spiritual heart. This is why I call the *Yoga Sūtras* the core or heart of the *sādhanā*.

Sage Vyāsa stipulates in his commentary on *sūtra* I.1, that a distracted consciousness is not fit to reach the zenith of yoga. I will feel that my immense debt towards my invisible guru has been partly repaid if my humble attempt helps each and every student of yoga and seeker of Truth, regardless of their individual physical, intellectual, psychological and spiritual make-up, to experience and to walk on a firm and sure ground towards the realisation of the Self.

It is a great honour and privilege for me that H.H. Dalai Lama has written a Foreword, and that the Honourable Shri Murli Manohar Joshi (Member of Parliament, India), has written a Preface for this work.

I am also delighted to express my sense of gratitude to HarperCollins in presenting the *Core of the Yoga Sūtras*, and inspiring both yoga practitioners and the public worldwide.

B.K.S. Iyengar
Pune
6 March 2012

Yoga Pīṭhikā – Introduction

Pātañjala Yoga Sūtra is the most authoritative and oldest available text on the subject of yoga in detail. At the very beginning of the first chapter, the great seer defines yoga as the cessation of waves and movements (*vṛtti*) of consciousness. Interestingly, at the very beginning of the following chapter, he talks about the effects of *kriyā yoga* on afflictions (*kleśa*s). I have often thought about the parallels between *vṛtti*s and *kleśa*s.

By a close assessment of *vṛtti*s and *kleśa*s, we can easily come to the conclusion that *vṛtti*s, or mental fluctuations, are connected to the subtle body (*sūkṣma śarīra* or *antaraṅga śarīra*). But *kleśa*s are more related to the gross, or external, body (*bahiraṅga śarīra*) or the body of action (*kārya śarīra*), which create a volcanic turbulence in *sūkṣma śarīra*. The restrained state of consciousness (*citta nirodha*) makes one experience the tranquil and peaceful state of the *citta* when there are no *vṛtti*s and no *kleśa*s in these two sheaths of the self.

*Kleśa*s are somatic, psychic, somatopsychic or psychosomatic, and affect the causal body (*kāraṇa śarīra*). They affect the causal body – the self – directly (*kṛta*), by inducement (*kārita*) or by abetment (*anumodita*). They make us suffer as they revolve around possessions and belongings (*parigraha*), reflecting our fear of death (*abhiniveśa*). This fear of death, or attachment to life, is instinctive and taunts one and all.

Kleśas are somatically dormant and the way to eradicate them is *tapas* or the path of action (*karma mārga*). Though *vṛttis* exist on the psychological level, they get intermingled with *kleśas*. These have to be conquered by *svādhyāya* or *jñāna* (study of oneself, from the cells to the self and from the self to the cells). One realises the *kāraṇa śarīra* or the self (*jīvātman*) only when *kleśas* and *vṛttis* stop revolving. Stopping the *vṛttis* helps the individual to surrender to God (*Īśvara praṇidhāna*). Thus, the causal, the subtle and the gross bodies are brought under control through *tapas, svādhyāya* and *Īśvara praṇidhāna*. These three ways constitute the *tridaṇḍa* of *yaugika sādhanā*.

Kleśa nivṛtti (the involution of afflictions) develops from *tapas*. *Vṛtti nirodha* (restraint of modification) develops from *svādhyāya*, while *antaḥkaraṇa śuddhi* (sanctity and purity of the conscience – *dharmendriya*) develops through *Īśvara praṇidhāna*. The *tridaṇḍa* of yoga *sādhanā* is meant to understand the interconnections between body, mind, intelligence and self. Accurate methodical practice results in the disassociation of the self from the body and mind.

We have hundreds of muscles and joints along with five organs of action, five senses of perception, five *vāyus* and five *upavāyus*, mind, intelligence, I-maker, consciousness, conscience, self with form (*sākārātman*) and Self without form (*nirākārātman*). Through the medium of yoga *sādhanā*, we learn to use these tools, so that they co-ordinate and co-operate, until the mind cultivates both the external organs and internal organs to experience balance, harmony and concord between the Self and the agents of the Self. This is *samānatā* of the pure consciousness.

The Self is essentially *nirākāra*. The difference between *nirākāra puruṣa* and *sākāra puruṣa* is that this *nirākāra puruṣa* is indestructible, imperishable and immeasurable. He neither destroys, nor can be destroyed. He is birthless and deathless, without beginning or end. He cannot be wounded by weapons, burned by fire, moistened by water or blown away by the wind. He cannot be divided, burnt, dissolved or dried up. He is beyond 'I' or 'me' or 'mine'. He is 'Thou' beyond 'I', untouched by the power of the elements.

When the *nirākāra puruṣa* changes into *sākāra puruṣa* or the I-ness, he is called *jīvātman* or the individual self (small self). This *sākāra puruṣa*, or *jīvātman*, comes under the influence of *viśva-caitanya-śakti* or *prāṇa* and the powers of the elements. He who is with form is enshrined in the human body and renders the capacity of motion and sensation – *jīva* means influence of life force, and *ātman* means the self. Hence *jīvātman* is the self that has connection with *pañca bhūta*s and *pañca prāṇa*s.

According to the *aupaniṣadika* terminology, the Self remains as a *kūṭastha citta*. When the same *nirākāra* Self takes the *sākāra* form as I-ness, it determines the activities of *pariṇāma citta*.

***vitarka-vicāra-ānanda-asmitārūpa-anugamāt saṁpra-jñātaḥ* (I.17)**

The practice of yoga develops four types of *samādhi:* these are self-analysis, synthesis, bliss, and the experience of a Pure Being.

Vitarka and *vicāra* are the expressions of the self, *pariṇāma citta*. *Ānanda* nullifies the formful state of the Self and *asmitā* is *kūṭastha citta*, which is beyond the influence of *kāraṇa*, *sūkṣma* and *kārya śarīra*. *Kūṭastha citta*, or the formless self, when the same nirākāra self takes the form as 'I-ness', as *sākāra citta* he determines the activities of life as *pariṇāma citta*.

***maitrī-karuṇā-muditā-upēkṣāṇāṁ sukha-duḥkha-puṇya-apuṇya-viṣayāṇāṁ bhāva-nātaḥ-citta-prasādanam* (I.33)**

Through cultivation of friendliness, compassion, joy, and indifference to pleasure and pain, virtue and vice, consciousness becomes favourably disposed, serene and benevolent.

Maitrī and *karuṇā* represent *pariṇāma citta. Muditā* nullifies and transforms the *pariṇāma citta* and *upekṣā* makes the *pariṇāma citta* indifferent so that this *pariṇāma citta* becomes *kūṭastha citta* and experiences the pure state of Being.

I found that the four chapters (*pādas*) of the *Yoga Sūtras* have their own parallels in the structure of the four *varṇas*, four *āśramas* and four aims of life (*puruṣārthas*). Nowadays the *varṇas* (*brāhmaṇa*, *kṣatriya*, *vaiśya*, *śūdra*) have faded, but *āśramas* and aims of life are still in vogue.

Here I have to stress that consciousness is an evolution of the *varṇas* and that the *varṇas* must be considered as a hierarchy of consciousness, representing its four levels.

Cāturvarṇyaṁ mayā sṛṣṭaṁ guṇakarma-vibhāgaśaḥ / Tasya kartāram api māṁ viddhy akartāram avyayam // (Bhagavad Gītā,* IV.13*)	The fourfold order was created by me according to the divisions of quality and work. Though I am its creator, know me to be incapable of action or change.

Lord Krishna explains that the creation of classes reflects the quality of ones's work (*guṇa karma*). I feel Patañjali deals in the same way with four classes of consciousness in practitioners according to their interest in life as well as the *sādhanā*.

He explains *guṇa karma citta* (quality of actions according to consciousness) as *kleśa citta karma*, *manovṛtti citta karma*, *nirodha citta karma* and *divya citta karma*.

Kleśa citta karma exists mainly in somatic afflictions that affect the psyche of the person. On the *kleśas* and the tolerance to bear the afflictions, Patañjali suggests gaining control by *tatra sthitau yatnaḥ abhyāsaḥ* (I.13) – practice. This practice is laborious, hence it can be attributed to the *śūdra* or labour class.

Sa tu dīrghakāla nairantarya satkāra āsevitaḥ dṛḍhabhūmiḥ **(I.14)**	This leads to stability in body and mind and helps in gaining control of *manovṛtti citta*. Besides acting on *kleśas*, it may tempt one to seek a benefit, which is nothing less than *vaiśya* – a state of mind seeking to attain wealth.

Tatpratiṣedhārtham ekatattva-abhyāsaḥ (I.32) leads towards the martial qualities (*kṣatriya* class) to remove all defects in one's *sādhanā* in order to reach a state above one's peers or colleagues. This state of *sādhanā* is nothing less than *nirodha citta vṛtti karmas*.

The highest and noblest quality of the *divya citta karma* makes one free from taints, and its practice takes the form of *nimittaṁ aprayojakaṁ prakṛtīnāṁ varaṇabhedaḥ tu tataḥ kṣetrikavat* (IV.3). The *sādhaka* practises just for the sake of experiencing the divine state of consciousness (*divya citta*). In this state he develops the *brāhmaṇika* mind to live in the state of purity, experiencing not only the state of cosmic consciousness but also the sight of the Self. Living in the flame of Self's light makes him *tataḥ kleśa karma nivṛttiḥ* (IV.30), when he will not act in any way that creates disturbances or turbulences within himself or among his family, society or community.

This is how yoga acts as a means to lift the *citta* from *kleśa citta* to *divya citta*.

In one word, if the *sūtras* I.13–14[1] convey the idea of stable and continuous effort from the third and fourth *varṇa*, the *sūtra* I.32[2] is more related to the single-minded effort of the second *varṇa*. An important part of *Vibhūti Pāda* also deals with the attainments of the second *varṇa*, whereas the *Kaivalya Pāda* reveals the effort required for final emancipation and absolute freedom, pointing us towards *vidyāvinayasaṁpanne* (being equipped with the humility of True Knowledge):

Vidyāvinayasa-ṁpanne brāhmaṇe gavi hastini / śuni cai'va śvapāke ca paṇḍitāḥ samadaršinaḥ // (B. G., V.18)

Sages see with an equal eye a learned and humble Brahmin, a cow, an elephant or even a dog or an outcast.

---

1 *tatra sthitau yatnaḥ abhyāsaḥ* (I.13) – Practice is an effort to still the mind's fluctuations in order to silence consciousness.

sa tu dīrghakāla-nairantarya-satkāra-āsevitaḥ dṛḍhabhūmiḥ (I.14) – Long, uninterrupted, alert practice is the firm foundation for stabilising consciousness.

2 *tatpratiṣedhārtham ekatattva-abhyāsaḥ* (I.32) – Single-minded effort is the only way to overcome the defects in one's own self.

The *āśramas* are *brahmacaryāśrama*, *gṛhasthāśrama*, *vānaprasthāśrama* and *sannyāsāśrama*. According to the *Vedas*, the human span of life is said to be 100 years, so each *āśrama* is said to be of 25 years. In *brahmacaryāśrama*, the youth is made to learn and earn knowledge on both spiritual and worldly planes, and then to use this knowledge in the best way to live. After acquiring material and spiritual wisdom, the youth is allowed to marry to become a householder (*gṛhasthāśrama*), to learn humane qualities, to serve those who need help and then ensure that his progeny are educated. After having children and living as a family man or woman, a person begins to learn to cultivate non-attachment (*vānaprasthāśrama*), and when non-attachment is transformed into detachment and renunciation he or she loses all attachment to the world and becomes attached only to *Īśvara* – God. This is *sannyāsāśrama*.

Similarly, the four aims, or *puruṣārtha*s, of life are *dharma*, *artha*, *kāma* and *mokṣa*.

The *Yoga Sūtra*s have four chapters, each one representing respectively the four *āśrama*s and the four aims of life.

The *Samādhi Pāda* as the *dharma* of the *puruṣārtha*s represents student-hood (*brahmacaryāśrama*). *Dharma* means religiousness in *sādhanā* and indicates a righteous duty. *Dharma* is what sustains and supports a person towards the realisation of the *puruṣa*. In this chapter, the study of science and philosophy as well as right discipline in the form of '*anuśāsanam*' is explained. *Anuśāsanam* means to think correctly and act from within the frame of *yama* and *niyama*, which is explained in *Sādhana Pāda*.

The second chapter (*Sādhana Pāda*) is on the purpose of life (*artha*) with the means for living (*gṛhasthāśrama*). It explains in detail the 'how and whys' of our means and purposes in practice (*artha*) as the frame within which we should live. It places this understanding and practice within the codes of conduct of yoga.

Vibhūti Pāda concerns itself with the gaining of supernatural powers. 'Power' means the *puruṣārtha* of *kāma*. One must remain indifferent to these powers, for they tempt one to fall from spiritual grace. Hence, non-attachment towards supernatural powers must be practised by a householder, to transcend sensual desire and reach the higher aspects of love. This is *vānaprasthāśrama*, the third stage of life, and is the preparation for the fourth stage.

The last chapter (*Kaivalya Pāda*) speaks about *mokṣa*, the fourth stage of *sannyāsāśrama*. This guides the *sādhaka* to detach from the infatuation of powers. *Kaivalya* means aloneness. In this state, intelligence shines like a full moon. It shows ways to earn freedom from infatuations (*moha*) and to reach the final freedom, the *mokṣa*. Then the accomplished *sādhaka* lives in *satyam* (truth), *śivam* (eternal) and *sundaram* (beauty of life).

Having drawn parallels between the four *puruṣārtha*s and the four chapters, I must add that Patañjali conveys also the idea of a zenith in *kaivalya* in the form of the natural, pure *Īśvara praṇidhāna*.

The four *pāda*s also represent respectively four types of action, namely *karma*, *vikarma*, *sukarma* and *akarma*. *Karma* stands for general actions or performances. *Vikarma* means actions with pleasant motivations. *Sukarma* means good actions with auspicious motivations whereas *akarma* stands for actions that are totally free from expectations of reactions and rewards. *Akarma* is the most skilful action performed totally and effortlessly.

In the same way, the *pāda*s may stand for *jñāna*, *vijñāna*, *sujñāna* and *prajñāna*. If *jñāna* is just knowledge on objects, *vijñāna* is scientific enquiry, *sujñāna* is the acquisition of auspicious spiritual knowledge and *prajñāna* is the pinnacle of experiential illuminative wisdom.

It is also possible that the four chapters relate to the states of *sālokya*, *sāmīpya*, *sārūpya* and *sāyujya*. *Sālokya* is a means to feel the kingdom of God through *Samādhi Pāda*; *sāmīpya* is the closeness or proximity to God in *sādhanā*; *sārūpya*, assuming God as natural through the wealth (*vibhūti*) of yoga, which comes as a natural phenomenon; and *sāyujya* is when one lives in awareness, extending and expanding without a feeling of self, then merging

	Samādhi Pāda	***Sādhana Pāda***	***Vibhūti Pāda***	***Kaivalya Pāda***
Four types of actions	*Karma:* general actions	*Vikarma:* actions with pleasant motivations	*Sukarma:* good actions with auspicious motivations	*Akarma:* actions free from expectations of reactions or rewards
Four types of knowledge	*Jñāna:* knowledge of objects	*Vijñāna:* scientific enquiry	*Sujñāna:* acquisition of auspicious spiritual knowledge	*Prajñāna:* pinnacle of experiential illuminative wisdom
States of relationship to God	*Sālokya:* feeling God	*Sāmīpya:* closeness or proximity to God	*Sārūpya:* embraces and encompases God once free from the wealth of yoga (supernatural powers)	*Sāyujya:* living in awareness without the feel of the Self and mingling with God
Guidance in the *nivṛtti mārga*	*Paripakva karma:* Ripe action	*Para jñāna:* Knowledge beyond the boundaries of discrimination	*Parā bhakti:* Utter devotion	*Śaraṇāgati:* Culminating in total surrender

and finally uniting with God. This is the ultimate union of the Self with the divine – *Īśvara*.

Thus the *Yoga Sūtra*s guide the *sādhaka*s through ripe action (*paripakva karma*), knowledge beyond the boundaries of discrimination (*para jñāna*) and utter devotion (*parā bhakti*) towards the completion of total surrender (*śaraṇāgati*).

My approach may seem excessive, but I felt that someone had to take the initiative. This is an attempt to offer a condensed and compact guide so that readers may grasp the objective views subjectively on *vedānta*, as *pratyakṣa pramāṇa*, which is without doubt the direct path for the Sight of the Soul (*ātmadarśana*), and proceed through a systematic evolution from the first suggested choice of *sādhanā* in *'Īśvara-praṇidhānāt vā'* (*Y. S.*, I.23) towards the untold, full *'Īśvara-praṇidhāna'*, which follows naturally and spontaneously as a fifth aim of *sādhanā* (*Īśvaradarśana*).

This is the fifth *puruṣārtha*, the culminating point of the spiritual quest, where the teachings of Lord Patañjali and Śrī Rāmānujācārya meet.

I

Yoga Paraṁparā – *Yaugika* Lineage

According to tradition, yoga has existed from time immemorial. The *Mahābhārata* explains that yoga was revealed when Brahmā created the world:

***hiraṇya garbha yogasya proktā nanyā purātanaḥ* (*Mahābhārata*)**	Yoga came from the embryo of Brahmā, the Creator, who rose up from the navel of Viṣṇu – and none other's. Brahmā himself came out of Viṣṇu and hence the first preceptor of yoga is Viṣṇu, who imparted it to Brahmā.

According to *Bhagavad Gītā*, yoga exists from time immemorial.

***sa evā'yaṁ mayā te'dya yogaḥ proktaḥ purātanaḥ / bhakto'si me sakhā ce'ti rahasyaṁ hy etad uttamam //* (B. G., IV.3)**	Lord Krishna says to Arjuna, 'This same fundamental secret of ancient yoga has been today told to you by me; for you are my devotee and my friend.'

Patañjali uses the word *anuśāsanam* at the very beginning of the text. The prefix *'anu'* means 'traditionally followed', indicating that yoga came from the mouth of Brahmā and exists from the time of the *Vedas*.

It is said that one should ask neither the origin of a *ṛṣi* (sage) nor the source of a river, and this also holds good for *Veda* and *Vedānta*. As it is said that yoga came from Brahmā through the *mūla puruṣa*, Śrī Viṣṇu, yoga has existed since the universe existed.

The beauty of yoga is that it is meant for the evolution of the entire human race. Yoga is *sarva bhauma*, universal. It brings out the instinctive weaknesses of a man or a woman, and offers ways to overcome (*see Y. S.*, II.1)[1] intellectual, emotional and instinctive defects (*see Y. S.*, II.3).[2]

Undoubtedly, God and nature, along with the pleasures of the material world and the spiritual kingdom, existed before humans could realise their own potential. Humans are endowed with intelligence and the power of discernment. With this intelligence, words were evolved. With words came the concept of God, nature, *dharma* (science of duty with right justice and merit), and yoga in order to distinguish the differences between pleasures of the senses and spiritual delight.

With words, each person began to interpret the worldly joys and sought emancipation according to his or her individual mental calibre. Later, humans became prey to worldly pleasures, forgetting the permanent bliss. This created the motivation for people to reconsider the pairings of good and evil, virtue and vice, the ethical and unethical, and the moral and immoral.

Then, they had the idea of using yoga as a way to practise *dharma* for gaining back their original state of well-being.

To reach both intellectual and spiritual development, ways were found by the ancient sages to develop a balanced mind by associating and uniting the body with the mind and the mind with the self through the performance of righteous duty (*dharma*) and yoga.

---

1 *tapaḥ-svādhyāya-īśvarapraṇidhānāni kriyāyogaḥ* (II.1) – Burning zeal in practice, self-study and study of scriptures, and surrender to God are the acts of yoga.

2 *avidyā-asmitā-rāga-dveṣa-abhiniveśāḥ kleśāḥ* (II.3) – If ignorance and ego are intellectual defects, rāga and dveṣa are emotional defects while *abhiniveśa* is an instinctive defect.

II

Yoga Dharma – The Concept of Yoga

Conscientiousness is the key for our growth. It is *antaḥkaraṇa*, the field of *dharma*, or *dharmendriya*. A Vedic adage states that '*Dharmo rakṣati rakṣitaḥ*'. *Dharma*, as the art and science of duty, protects one who follows the path of righteousness. Similarly, I say, '*Yogo rakṣati rakṣitaḥ*', meaning that yoga protects those who practise and live dynamically in it.

The first and foremost explanation of *yoga dharma* is found in *Ahirbudhnya Saṁhitā*. According to this text (I.15), *saṁyoga yoga ityukto jīvātmaparamātmanaḥ* // : The union of the individual soul with the Universal Soul is said to be yoga.

Yoga is no less than *citta staṃbha vṛtti*, or the stable state of consciousness, like the *prāṇa staṃbha vṛtti* explained by Patañjali while dealing with *prāṇāyāma*. The stable state of consciousness explains the suspension of breath after the in-breath or out-breath in *prāṇāyāma yaugika* practice. It is nothing but a suspension or pause in the movements of thought waves.

samaṁ kāyaśirogrīvaṁ dhārayann acalaṁ sthiraḥ / saṁprekṣya nāsikāgraṁ svaṁ diśaścā'navalokayan // (B. G., VI.13)

See what Lord Krishna says in the *Bhagavad Gītā*. Taking the centre body as a plumb line, He wants us to hold the right and left sides of the body evenly with a determined effort. He advises us to keep the centre of the crown of the head, centre of the throat and centre of the perineum in one line, and learn to adjust and bring the sides of the body parallel to each other. As the body is held stable through *yaugika* practice, *citta staṃbha vṛtti* or *cittavṛtti nirodha* occurs. Fix the gaze on the tip of the nose. This non-movement of the eyes pacifies and quietens the brain, stabilising the mind and consciousness. If the eyes flicker, the brain (*mastiṣka*), mind (*manas*) and consciousness (*citta*) also flicker and are perturbed.

Therefore, looking at the tip of the nose is just a method shown for '*citta staṃbha vṛtti*'. Steady eyes with restfulness release stress from the brain and stabilise the mind to be attentive to its means and goal.

Again Lord Krishna defines yoga:

yogasthaḥ kuru karmāṇi saṅgaṁ tyaktvā dhanaṁjaya / siddhyasiddhyoḥ samo bhūtvā samatvam yoga ucyate // (B. G., II.48)

With a non-attached mind to success and failure, follow the *yaugika* discipline with zeal and passion and/or intense enthusiasm for the self (*jīvātman*) to remain passive and pensive. This gives one an even temperament in all circumstances. Hence Lord Krishna says that yoga is a way to maintain an even temper in one's word, work and thought. This attitude of cultivating oneness in word, work and wisdom helps one to reach the goal of uniting the self with the Self.

buddhiyukto jahātī'ha ubhe sukṛtaduṣkṛte / tasmād yogāya yujyasva yogaḥ karmasu kauśalam // (B. G., II.50)

With the quality of skilfulness (*yukti*) in intelligence, devote yourself to yoga, endowed with equanimity for all good and evil actions as well as thoughts, renouncing the fruit of all actions. By this, you will be freed from the bondage of obstacles and afflictions and experience the state of auspicious beatitude (*sundaram*). In this state, there is no *śukla* (white), *kṛṣṇa* (black) or mixed (white and black) *karma*, but pure *karma* free from these three states (*Y. S.*, IV.7).[1]

He adds:

1 *karma aśukla akṛṣṇam yoginaḥ trividham itareṣām* (IV.7) – A yogi's actions are neither white nor black. The actions of others are of three kinds – white, black or grey.

taṁ vidyād duḥkha--saṁyoga-viyogaṁ yogasaṁjñitam / sa niścayena yoktavyo yogo'nirviṇṇacetasā // (B. G., VI.23)

The meaning of yoga is to restrain oneself from all bonds of pain and sorrow. Hence, yoga must be resolutely practised with a determined mind.

Yoga has to be practised without distress, anxiety or fear, so that one can reach the zenith in yoga.

According to Patañjali, yoga is a discipline. This is indicated by the very first *sūtra*, wherein Patañjali explains that the discipline of yoga has been followed from time immemorial without interruption, maintaining its lineage.

***atha yogānuśāsanam* (I.1)**

The text begins expressing auspiciousness and reverence by the word *'atha'*. This term stands for benediction (*maṅgalāśāsana*) for the subject as well as for the *gurus*. It is a prayer. It also suggests beginning yoga with a disciplined frame of mind.

***yogaḥ citta-vṛtti--nirodhaḥ* // (I.2)**

Consciousness is affected more often by emotional upheavals than by intellectual deficiencies. Yoga begins with the mind, as this is the part of *citta* that comes into contact with the objects and creates the feelings. Yoga is a mental discipline for restraining the fluctuations of thoughts, so that consciousness (*citta*) is kept in an unoscillated, steady and stable state (*staṃbha vṛtti*).

It is a course of conduct for gaining a steady state of *citta*.

Coordinating the intellect of the head with the intelligence of the heart achieves integration (*saṁyama*) between the two. I believe that yoga is the union (*saṁyoga*) of these two branches of intelligence. Though Patañjali does not say this explicitly, I feel that this union – of the intellect of the head with the intelligence of the heart – does take place through yoga *sādhanā*. This integration makes consciousness spread in the body from the inner layer of the skin up to the seat of the soul (*citta prasādanam*), just as water spreads evenly across any surface. This, for me, is yoga.

***vitarka-vicāra- -ānanda-asmitārūpa- -anugamāt saṁpra-jñātaḥ* (I.17)**	The brain has four biological lobes, and the great sage explains these four lobes on the intellectual level. These are analysis or argumentation (*vitarka*); logical insight that creates synthesis (*vicāra*); the seat of joy (*ānanda*); and the seat of the self (*asmitā*).

The seat of *vitarka* or the analytical brain is on the left side, whereas that of the reasoning brain is on the right. Between these two lobes, there is a space. We can conceptualise this space as the mind, which connects the two brains. When these two functions of the brain co-ordinate, there arises right synthesis, leading to correct judgement. From this judgement, one experiences a state of bliss (*ānanda*), nullifying the divisions of the brain as well as the feeling of the 'I'. As the feeling of 'I' fades, a pure state of just 'beingness' is felt without any expression. This is *asmitā*, the illuminative *sāttvika* state of experiencing the distinguished pure self.

Patañjali similarly has dealt with the four biological chambers of the heart as four facets of emotional intelligence.

***maitrī-karuṇā- -muditā-upēkṣāṇāṁ sukha-duḥkha- -puṇya-apuṇya- -viṣayāṇāṁ bhāva-nātaḥ-citta- -prasādanam* (I.33)**	Patañjali indicates in *Y. S.*, III.35, '*hṛdaye cittasaṁvit*', that the spiritual heart is the seat of consciousness. As such the four chambers of the heart are physiological, psychological, mental and spiritual. The emotional divisions that correspond to these four chambers of the heart are friendliness (*maitrī*); compassion (*karuṇā*); gladness (*muditā*) and indifference (*upekṣā*) towards pleasure and pain, virtue and vice; through experience (*ānubhāvika*). These have to be harmonised.

These two *sūtras* opened up my thoughts, enabling me to understand the necessity for balance, harmony and concord between the intellect of the head and the intelligence of the heart.

Patañjali explains four types of actions with reference to the four lobes of the brain and four chambers of the heart[1]. When one is free

1 *karma aśukla-akṛṣṇam yoginaḥ trividham itareṣām* (IV.7) – A yogi's actions are neither white nor black. The actions of others are of three kinds, white, black or grey.

from the three types of *karmas* tinged black, white or grey, this is the sign of a balanced mind.

The *sūtras* I.17 and I.33 imply that yoga is a practice designed to steady the intellect and bring it into harmony with the stable, emotional intelligence of the heart. Indeed, the meaning and the feeling (*artha* and *bhāvanā*) of yoga are revealed.

tīvrasaṁvegānām āsannaḥ **(I.21)**

mṛdu-madhya--adhimātratvāt tataḥ api viśeṣaḥ **(I.22)**

[1]These four divisions of the head and heart probably led Patañjali to consider four types of *sādhakas* according to their progressive growth on the intellectual and emotional level.[2]

We find the same classification of *sādhakas* in *Haṭhayoga Pradīpikā* (IV.69–76) and *Śiva Saṁhitā* (III.33–81) with a different terminology. These are seen in the table overleaf.

Perhaps these gradations are there due to the effects of herbs, incantations, past *karmas* affecting birth, and a burning passion to reach perfection, or profound absorption.

janma-auṣadhi--mantra-tapaḥ--samādhi-jāḥ siddhayaḥ **(IV.1)**

Probably *janma* and *auṣadhi*[3] represent the mild *sādhaka*, *mantra* the moderate, *tapaḥ* the dedicated and ardent, while *samādhijāḥ* stands for intensely vehement *sādhakas*.

The standard of the *sādhakas* may be inferred from the cause. These might change and transform the capability of the *sādhaka*. Obviously these *sādhakas* take from *prakṛti* the required energy to progress further in their *yaugika sādhanā*.

jāti-antara-pariṇā-maḥ prakṛti-āpūrāt **(IV.2)**

According to the standard of the *sādhanā*, nature's energy flows marginally or abundantly.

---

1 (I.21) – For one who is sharp and extremely vehement in practice, the goal is instant.

2 (I.22) – For those whose practices are mild, average or intense, it becomes time-bound.

3 Divine powers are the results of birth, herbs, incantations, self-discipline and meditation.

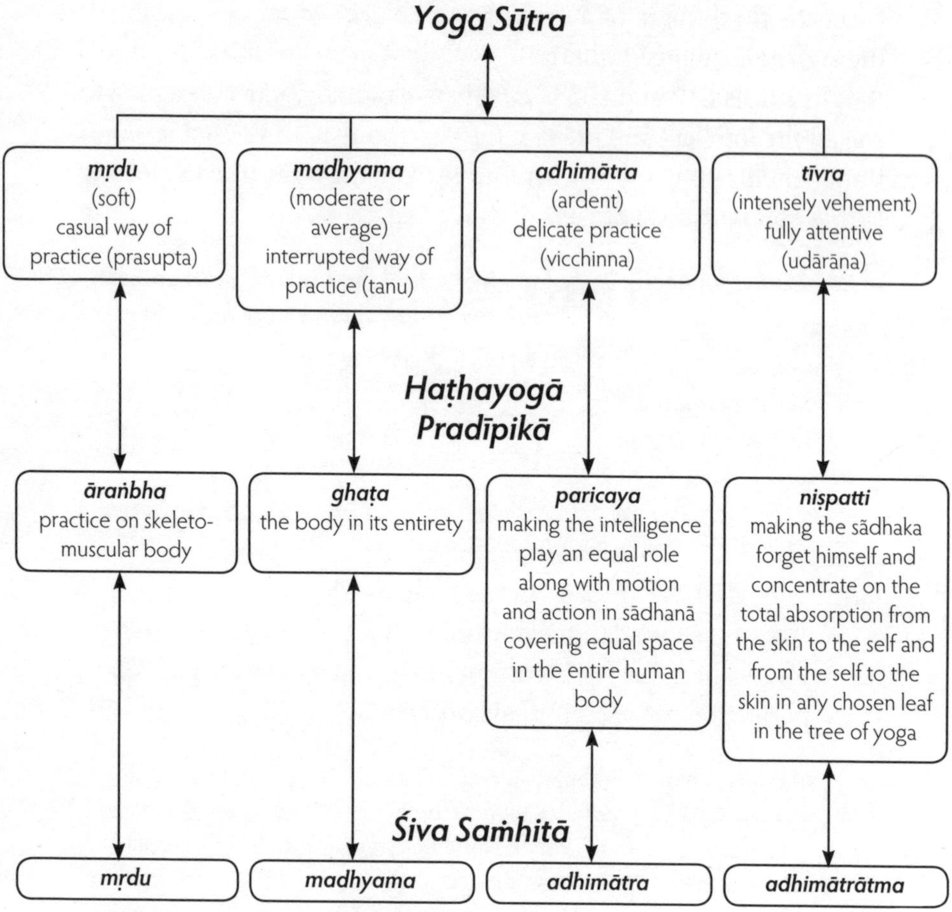

See also: Levels of *sādhaka*s, tables 1 and 3 in *Light on the Yoga Sūtras of Patañjali*.

In order to make full use of energy flow, the *sādhanā* should be supreme, and the *sādhaka* must cultivate and civilise the four psychological functions of the head to co-operate with the four emotional intelligences of the heart and co-ordinate without deviation so that the self is induced to reach not only its own frontier but even to spread throughout the vastness both within and without (*adhyātma prasādana*) (*Y. S.*, I.47).[1]

1 *nirvicāra-vaiśāradye adhyātmaprasādaḥ* (I.47) – From proficiency in *nirvicāra samāpatti* comes purity. *Sattva* or luminosity flows undisturbed, kindling the spiritual light of the self.

I feel that though Patañjali doesn't speak directly about the four lobes of the brain[1] or the four chambers of the heart, one of his main concerns is to bring a harmonious union between the intellect of the head and the intelligence of the heart, creating oneness between the brain and the heart. For me, this is the heart of Patañjali's yoga.

---

1 See *Light on the Yoga Sūtras of Patañjali*, London: Thorsons, 2002, p. 69.

III

Janma Mṛtyu Cakra – The Wheel of Birth and Death

Before proceeding to the subject of yoga itself, it is important to understand the theory of cause and effect and thus the theory of rebirth.

People often attribute both suffering and joy to their past life actions (*prārabdha karma*), requiring them in the present to reflect before acting and thus avoid actions that may boomerang. In this strand of the present, they must improve the quality of their actions so that one day they can be free from the cycle of birth and death.

The concepts of cause/effect and rebirth are closely related to each other. As each cause has an effect, so each effect becomes the cause for creating further effects. This process goes on without interruption and eternally in our lives. These leave an impression, which can be recollected by accomplished yogis (III.18),[1] and they remain until the aspirant becomes pure. When he reaches this state, his actions do not leave any imprints on him.

The concept of rebirth is strongly emphasised in the *Yoga Sūtras* of Patañjali, and I have experienced this in my own life.

---

1 *saṁskāra-sākṣāt-karaṇāt pūrva-jā-ti-jñānam* (III.18) – A yogi will be able to recollect the impressions of past lives when he has reached the state of contemplation (*samāpatti*). We hear often how some at a young age could describe their past birthplace, parents, relatives, friends and surroundings.

I never dreamt in my young days that I would follow the path of yoga, nor did my parents ever think that I would embrace yoga. No members of my family had encountered or had any idea of yoga. As far as I know, no one was interested in *yaugika* or spiritual pursuit. My parents had 13 children. I was the 11th child. Out of 13, only 10 members lived long. No one in my family took an interest in the subject except my immediate elder brother and my younger sister, who dabbled in it for a very short period of time. I stuck to it – which is no less than a reflection of the efforts of my past lives.

Call it God, or the hidden hand of destiny, or the accumulated fruits of my past *karmas*; circumstances in 1934 created the opportunity for my *guru* to initiate me into yoga by teaching me a few *āsanas* to improve my health. Yet he used to tell my colleagues that I was *apātra* (not destined, or unfit, for yoga). But again, the hidden hands of God created the opportunity for me to teach so that I might learn.

Despite all my pains, disappointments and unsuccessful attempts, yoga inspired me to practise enthusiastically. Like a magnet attracting iron filings, yoga attracted me to feel the newness of each day in this God-given body.

With due respect to my *guru* and colleagues, I may have proved them wrong by pursuing yoga despite the odds. I attribute my relentless interest in yoga to the *sādhanā* of my previous lives. I stuck to yoga like the proverbial leech and now, even at the age of 93, I still practise for four to five hours a day. I do so with a lot of inspiration and without any aspirations. As I adore yoga, so it adorns me with fresh developments and thoughts. With this zeal and without hankering for *kaivalya*, I practise watching and capturing new feelings that arise from my *sādhanā* and use them as a platform for further study and investigation.

I am practising with a simple thought – that yoga is embedded and immersed in my head and heart as a base which will enable me to continue my *sādhanā* if I am destined for a human life in my next birth.

Having drawn this small sketch of my practices as a proof that impressions from my previous lives affected me, I must admit that I still do not know how I stuck to my practice without wavering.

The *Bhagavad Gītā* says:

***dehino'smin yathā dehe kaumāraṁ yauvanaṁ jarā / tathā dehāntara-prāptir dhīras tatra na muhyati //* (*B. G.*, II.13)**

A baby undergoes changes from infancy through youth, middle age, old age and death. After death, the soul takes another body. Lord Krishna says that, while living, as we do not feel sorry when physical and psychological changes take place, why should one feel sorry at the time of death?

***jātasya hi dhruvo mṛtyur dhruvaṁ janma mṛtasya ca / tasmād aparihā-rye'rthe na tvaṁ śocitum arhasi //* (*B. G.*, II.27)**

Where there is death, birth is certain, and where there is birth, death is certain. This cycle of rebirth is inevitable. So why lament?

Hence, rebirth continues unceasingly until all impressions are eradicated by the refined *yaugika sādhanā*. For this reason, why grieve on the inevitable truth of rebirth?

How Birth Happens

This present life becomes the storehouse of good or bad actions on account of actions done directly, indirectly or induced due to desire, greed, anger and infatuation with past lives.

***vitarkāḥ hiṁsā--ādayaḥ kṛta-kāritā-anumoditāḥ lobha-krodha-moha--pūrvakaḥ mṛdu--madhya-adhimātrā duḥkha-ajñāna--ananta-phalāḥ iti pratipakṣa--bhāvanam* (II.34)**

The 34th *sūtra* of *Sādhanapāda* explains the root cause of rebirth.

Misunderstanding creates room for greed, anger and delusion to a mild, moderate or intense degree, which in turn brings violence, whether practised directly or indirectly, or abetted. These result in endless pain and ignorance and, on account of it, rebirths take place.

***kleśa-mūlaḥ karmā-āśayo-dṛṣṭa-adṛṣṭa--janma-vedanīyaḥ* (II.12)** As the body is the house of *karma*s, Patañjali explains how these afflictions accumulate the imprints of the merits and demerits of one's past lives, which are made to be experienced in this present life. In the event that they do not come to fruition, these may carry on to future lives.

According to Indian philosophy, actions are of three types: *prārabdha karma*, *sañcita karma* and *kriyamāṇa karma* or *āgāmin karma*.[1]

Prārabdha karma manifests in this life according to the imprints of many past lives. *Sañcita karma*s are the actions of the immediate past life, which have a grip on this life, and *kriyamāṇa karmas* are the actions accumulated in this life, which will act as a springboard to the next life (*āgāmin*).

This relation of cause, action and effect is often compared to water evaporating by the heat of the sun (cause) and becoming clouds; these clouds then come down as rain (action), bringing food and moisture (effect).

***sati mūle tad-vipākaḥ jāty-āyur--bhogāḥ* (II.13)** The present life is fixed with its class of birth, lifespan and experiences on account of the merits and demerits of past lives.

So,

***te hlāda-paritāpa--phalāḥ puṇya--apuṇya-hetutvāt* (II.14)** Accordingly a man's present life is structured on the basis of the assets and liabilities of past lives. If he plans a disciplined way of life to ensure progressive evolution, he will be able to minimise the imprints of actions.

Here it is interesting to note Patañjali's advice: *heyam duḥkham anāgatam* (II.16). He guides us to stick to actions that may not create pains, or pleasures mixed with pains. This *sūtra* is a guide to build up skilful actions that do not inflict pain in this life or the lives to come.

---

1 See *Aṣṭadaḷa Yogamālā*, vol. II, p. 63.

Each action and reaction, as well as understanding, leaves its imprints (*saṁskāra*) in the storehouse of memory. These must be faced in this life and in the coming lives also. Even in the state of *sabīja samādhi*, these imprints remain, though in a state of dormancy. These past imprints should be reduced by reaching a state wherein righteousness and virtuousness pour like rain from a cloud (*dharmamegha samādhi*) as *nirbīja samādhi* (a seedless state of mind). Like a burnt seed that cannot sprout, consciousness in this state is free from cause and effect and hence remains free from the taints or colours of the source itself.

jāti-deśa-kāla- ***-vyavahitānām*** ***apy ānantaryaṁ*** ***smṛti-saṁskārayoḥ*** ***ekarūpatvāt* (IV.9)**	Life is a continuous process, though it may be demarcated by a new form of life, place and time. The subliminal impressions stored in the well of memory remain intact from one life to the other as if there was no separation between births. In most people impressions, memories and desires continue to accumulate and compound one upon the other forever.

Actions are of three types.

karma aśukla- ***-akṛṣṇam yoginaḥ*** ***trividham itareṣām*** **(IV.7)**	The three types of actions (*karma*) are black, white and grey for all of us. But for a real yogi, there is a fourth type of action (*karma*) that is beyond these three types.
tataḥ tad-vipāka- ***-anuguṇānām*** ***eva abhivyaktir*** ***vāsanānām* (IV.8)**	These three types of actions manifest their impressions in one's life. So we have to make use of them to transform them into favourable conditions.

Patañjali says,

hetu-phala-āśraya- ***-ālambanaiḥ*** ***saṅgṛhītatvāt eṣām*** ***abhāve tad abhāvaḥ*** **(IV.11)**	As the impressions and desires of several lives create more desires, these merits and demerits in turn continue the cycle of cause and effect in the form of birth and death. When one reaches the zenith in *yaugika* discipline, then the impressions and memories cease on their own.

***atīta-anāgataṁ sarva-rūpataḥ asti adhva-bhedāt dharmāṇām* (IV.12)**

For a yogi who is in the zenith state of *satcit*, the existence of the past and future is as real as the present.

***tāsām anāditvaṁ ca āśiṣaḥ nityatvāt* (IV.10)**

Just as the universe is without beginning and eternal, impressions and desires are also without beginning and eternal. Besides the ordinary benefits, yoga also offers supernormal powers. However these tempt a yogi, leading him to bondage. Even the seed of these defects has to be eradicated so that the impressions and supernormal powers that arise from *yaugika* practice are used to bring imprints and desires to an end (*see* III.51). Then, birth and death come to an end.

Patañjali speaks of the state of an exalted yogi who has reached *samādhi*, in which he experiences a state of void (*śūnya*) or a state of loneliness. If he assumes this to be the end of *yaugika sādhanā*, then he lives in illusion (*bhrānti-darśana*).

***virāma-pratyaya-abhyāsa-pūrvaḥ saṁskāra-śeṣaḥ anyaḥ* (I.18)**

Patañjali clearly mentions that in the intermittent period between *sabīja* and *nirbīja samādhis*, these impressions remain latent and dormant on account of *svarūpa śūnyāvastha*, or the void of one's essential form. As it is only a seemingly void state, the impressions may arise again. That is why he cautions *sādhakas* to keep aside this felt state of *samādhi* and to continue *sādhanā* with faith, vigour and total absorption.

***bhava-pratyayo videha-prakṛti-layānām* (I.19)**

On account of the void in the *ahaṁkāra*, he may be merged with nature, thinking that this is the end state of yoga. For him, rebirth is certain.

***saṁskāra-sākṣāt-karaṇāt pūrva jā-ti-jñānam* (III.18)**

A person who has mastered yoga gets direct impressions of previous lives and, by pursuing *yaugika sādhanā*, tries to wash them out totally.

Lord Krishna says:

ihai 'va tair jitaḥ sargo yeṣāṁ sāmye sthitaṁ manaḥ / nirdoṣaṁ hi samaṁ brahma tasmād brahmaṇi te sthitāḥ // (B. G., V.19)	Even on the mortal plane, those who have conquered and established impartial minds become established in the existence of the Soul in all creatures, conquering the cycle of birth and death. They get established in God, as He is flawless, appearing the same to one and all.

As a person evolves in spiritual pursuits, he or she cultivates actions without the taints of black, white or grey and moves smoothly on the path of *kaivalya*, or emancipation with intellectual enlightenment.

The paths for enlightenment are said to be *karma*, *jñāna*, *bhakti* and *yoga*. Whatever path is chosen, if one follows it with religious, skilful attention, and without allowing even the smallest interruption in the flow of awareness, one will reach the state where the wheel of birth and death ceases to move. This is illumination or emancipation or liberation.

God has endowed humans with hands and legs for *karma*, intellect in the head for *jñāna* and emotional intelligence in the heart for *bhakti* to do right actions with judicious thinking and to love without attachment. The path of yoga is embedded in all three paths, helping us to remain clean in hand and clear in thought, in order to live in lustless love.

IV

Sṛṣṭikartā – Ādi Puruṣa or Īśvara

It is essential for students of spiritual pursuits as well as yoga *sādhaka*s to have a background of some key concepts such as *Sṛṣṭikartā* (Creator of the universe – God), and the universe with its five elements, their atomic qualities and their organisational and structural interference in creation.

Everything in creation is endowed with inert, vibrant and illuminative qualities (*tamas*, *rajas* and *sattva*). The exception is humanity, which has one difference. As I mentioned before, humans have the power of discernment in the art of speech, thought and the actions or interactions of the body with the mind.

With this special quality of discernment, humans can think and cultivate knowledge and wisdom, to achieve both evolution (going with the current, *pakṣa bhāvanā*), and involution (going against the current, *pratipakṣa bhāvanā*).

With a proper understanding of the reasons and effects of action (*karma phala*), the following chapters explain how to put an end to the perpetuation of life and show ways to experience the state of permanent bliss, or emancipation, through the *yaugika* path of spiritual pursuits.

In order to tread the path of permanent bliss, one must understand the background not only of the *Sṛṣṭikartā*, *Ādi Puruṣa* or *Ādi Daiva* (God) and the creation of the universe, but also of yoga, which is the means to understanding the creator, creation and birth.

As yoga means to associate or to join or to unite, its practice helps the *sādhaka* to understand the connections between God, the universe and himself. So, let us start with an overview of God and creation (*prakṛti*). In subsequent chapters we shall look into the universe, as well as consciousness and its veils.

Despite all scientific discoveries, the enigma of what was before the beginning of the process of evolution remains, and is seldom expressed. What is that hidden force which guides and makes us able to think?

We commonly call the presence of this Special Super Power or Force 'God'. He is the Lord of the universe as this universe (*prakṛti*) is His playground, in which He makes use of and moulds nature.

This God, though one being, has been recognised in different ways by different people, according to their intellectual growth and outlook.

This *Sṛṣṭikartā* has many names, including *Ādi Puruṣa*, *Ādi Daiva*, God, Universal Soul, *Paramātman*, *Parama Puruṣa*, *Puruṣa Viśeṣa*, *Īśvara*, *Viśvacetana Puruṣa*, *Antaryāmin*, and *Śarīrin* (one who possesses a body – *śarīra*).

He is the Supreme Being, eternally free from conflicts and afflictions, unaffected by actions and reactions. He is omnipresent, omnipotent and omniscient. Hence He is within us and outside of us. He is not conditioned by time or space, a matchless seed of all knowledge, the *guru* of all *gurus*, represented by the sacred syllable *āuṁ*, which when repeated with meaning and feeling removes all obstacles and hindrances in the pursuit of spiritual knowledge.

Food that is served on the table may be the same, but each one who eats that food may savour it differently. It is the same with attributes given to God. God is beyond qualities (*guṇātīta*). Yet, He has a *guṇa* that is completely distinct and separate from the common *guṇa*s known as *sattva*, *rajas* and *tamas*. Humanity is full of *kleśa*s (afflictions) and *vipāka* (results). God is beyond these two. This *guṇa* of God is an excellent and auspicious prosperous quality (*kalyāṇa guṇa*). He is *maṅgaḷamaya puruṣa* (God, filled with auspiciousness and prosperity).

kleśa-karma--vipāka-āśayaiḥ aparāmṛṣṭaḥ purṇa--viśeṣaḥ Īśvaraḥ (I.24)

We as human beings are caught in the net of pleasures, pains, sorrows, motivations and results, but *Īśvara* or God is beyond all these.

He, as the Supreme Being, is eternally free from all conflicts and afflictions, unaffected by actions and reactions and untouched by the cycles of cause and effect.

Īśvaraḥ sarva-bhūtānāṁ hṛddeś-e'rjuna tiṣṭhati / bhrāmayan sarva-bhūtāni yantrā-rūḍhāni māyayā // (*B. G.*, XVIII.61)

Lord Krishna says, 'Arjuna, God abides in the hearts of all beings, causing them to revolve according to their *karma* by His elusive power as if they are moving with habitual behaviour, like a machine.'

tam īśvarāṇāṁ paraṁ maheśvaraṁ taṁ devatānām paraṁ ca daivataṁ / patiṁ pātinam paraṁ parastād vidāma devaṁ bhuvaneśam tḍyam // (*Śvetaśvtara Upaniṣad*, 6.7)

He, the Supreme ruler of all rulers, the Supreme Deity of all deities, the Lord of Lords who creates, preserves and destroys, is greater than the greatest ruler of the universe.

vaisayama nairgṛhṇyana sāpikṣtvāt tathā hi darsayati (*Brahma sūtra*, 2.1.34)

No partiality or cruelty can happen from God as He is above all. It is Man according to his *karma phala* who creates conditions and attributes whereas God is above all this. This is what the *Vedas* say.

tatra niratiśayaṁ sarva-jñana-bījam (I.25)

The unrivalled and unexcelled matchless seed of all knowledge abides in this Supreme Being. This is his *prātibha jñāna*, which is no less than divine knowledge.

sa eṣaḥ pūrveṣām api guruḥ kālena anavacchedāt (I.26)

In *sūtra* I.15, Patañjali deals with the qualitative nature (*pratibhā*) of this Supreme Being. Here he suggests this Supreme Being as the first, foremost and absolute preceptor and master (*guru*), who is not bound or conditioned by place, space or time.

***tasya vācakaḥ praṇavaḥ* (I.27)** He is universally represented and received in the sacred syllable *āuṁ* (*pāribhāṣīka prajñā*).

***taj-japaḥ tad-artha--bhāvanam* (I.28)** The *mantra 'āuṁ'* is an incantation for contemplation on its meaning with full significance, through feelings. Actually for me, *japa*, *artha* and *bhāvanā* cover *karma*, *jñāna* and *bhakti* as the threefold *sādhanā*.[1]

***tataḥ pratyak--cetana-adhigamaḥ api antarāya--abhāvaḥ ca* (I.29)** Repetition of *praṇava* with a meditative mind on God removes all hindrances that come in the way of Self-realisation. This shows God's compassion for the practitioner.

As the body is the home as well as the pillar of the soul, so the soul in each of us becomes the home or the pillar of God (*śarīra śarīri bhāva*).

God is a *dharmin*. Though the word may change, He does not change. He is ever virtuous, pious, just and never-changing.

***ajo 'pi sann avyayātmā bhūtānām īśvaro 'pi san / prakṛtiṁ svām adhiṣṭhāya saṁbhavāmy ātmamāyayā //* (*B. G.*, IV.6)** Though birthless and deathless, God manifests himself by his own divine power (*yogamāyā*) for keeping *prakṛti* under control.

***teṣāṁ jñānī nityayuktaḥ ekabhaktir viśiṣyate / priyo hi jñānino 'tyartham ahaṁ sa ca mama priyaḥ //* (*B. G.*, VII.17)** One who is ever established in *me* with absolute devotion, I become extremely dear to him as he is dear to *me*.

1 In order to know the meaning of *āuṁ*, refer to *Light on Yoga*, HarperCollins, 2001.

***śānta udita avyapadeśya dharma anupātī dharmī* (III.14)**

This *sūtra* speaks mainly of the nature (*prakṛti*) of consciousness as we change our thoughts according to the conditions of time and circumstances. I find it applies to God, as it describes the inherent characteristic attributes and principles of virtuosity and righteousness, which remain the same at all times.

God and his powers are beyond our cognition. Yet these descriptions take our understanding of God from *nirguṇa* (without qualities) to *saguṇa* (with auspicious qualities and *sākāra* – form), so that one is drawn towards the feet of God, as the focus for our attention and contemplation. This is the keynote of yoga.

God is attributed as real (*satyam*), eternal (*śivam*) and beautiful (*sundaram*), as well as *satcidānanda* (*sat* = truthfulness, *cit* = the self, and *ānanda* = bliss). If we think about these expressions of God, they represent his auspicious qualities (*sadguṇas*). Most of us pray to God with these attributes of God, and highly advanced souls pray without attributes (*nirguṇas*).

V

Sṛṣṭikrama – The Structure of the Universe

Now, let us try to understand the universe. *Viśva cetana puruṣa* (the Supreme Being) or God creates *puruṣa* (*ātman*). As the soul (*puruṣa*) dwells in the heart of all beings without a form, God endows a power in it with a form of "I-ness" (*ahaṃ-ākāra*). Along with the form in the Self, He creates energy (*prāṇa*), the elements of nature and *guṇas*.

1. Puruṣa (*Ātman*)

According to *Gopatha-Brāhmaṇa* and *Liṅga-Purāṇa*, *pura* means a fortress, a city or a castle, and *īśa* means the Lord of the fortress. Here fortress represents the body, and the Lord of it is the *Puruṣa*.

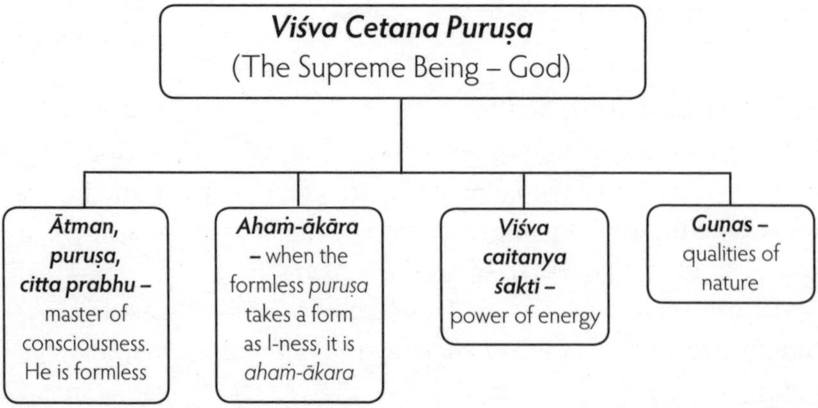

Puruṣa (*Ātman*, Seer, Self or Soul) is the absolute formless, changeless, ever-permanent and brilliant. Though He is above the reality of *prakṛti*, He dwells in the body.

Due to the importance of this concept, I will return to it in Chapter VI.

2. *Ahaṁ-ākāra*

The principle of individuality has a dual presence in human beings. When this individuality originates from *puruṣa*, it is the shape, the form given by God to the immutable *puruṣa* in order to be present at the core of the human beings. But when the principle of individuality originates from *prakṛti*, it is *ahaṁkāra*, the ego or I-maker, with all its qualities and defects.

Based on this, I had to coin the term *ahaṁ-ākāra*. *Ahaṁ* means 'I' and *ākāra* means 'shape'. For me, it means the form of the self. Hence I feel *ahaṁ-ākāra* (*sākāra* or *svarūpa*) as the form of the seer with good nature (*saguṇa*), while the formless *puruṣa* or the soul remains *nirākāra* and *nirguṇa*. The *saguṇa* form of the self interacts with all the particles of nature, as well as with the five organs of action (*karmendiyas*) and five senses of perception (*jñānendriyas*). There are 24 principles of matter, to which I add *ahaṁ-ākāra* as the 25th. *Puruṣa*, or the seer, is the 26th and *Īśvara* the 27th. I have introduced *ahaṁ-ākāra* because the *puruṣa* is *nirākāra* and *nirguṇa*. He remains ever a witness and never an actor. Only when *puruṣa* manifests in form does he come into contact with *prakṛti* and become an actor as well as a witness.

3. *Viśva Caitanya Śakti*

Let us now understand the universal power, or *śakti*, of God. This universal energy (*viśva caitanya śakti*) governs the formation as well as the functioning of nature along with its principles, and this energy in turn is governed by God (*Sṛṣṭikartā*).

The universal energy is structured into five components, to function in five ways. These are *pañca vāyus* – *prāṇa*, *apāna*, *samāna*, *udāna* and *vyāna* – supported by five subsidiary *upavāyus*, pervading the entire creation.

In the human body, *prāṇa* controls the mind, senses, heart, veins, arteries, nerves and motion; *apāna* controls the lower parts, alimentary organs and excretory system, and moves downwards; *udāna* controls the umbilical area, thorax, larynx and also moves upwards to enrich the voice, memory and intellect; *vyāna* controls the entire body and heart, as well as the blood circulation; and *samāna* helps digestion and nourishes the body.

The *upavāyus* and their functions are as follows: *nāga* controls belching; *kūrma* controls the eyelids; *kṛkara* controls hiccups and involuntary coughing; *devadatta* controls yawning and sleep; and *dhanaṁjaya*, which creates phlegm and nourishes the body, remains even after death, inflating the corpse.

Five *Vāyus*, Five Elements and Five *Kośas*

pṛthvī earth	***āp*** water	***tejas*** fire	***vāyu*** air	***ākāśa*** ether
apāna	***prāṇa***	***samāna***	***udāna***	***vyāna***
annamaya kośa	***prāṇamaya kośa***	***manomaya kośa***	***vijñānamaya kośa***	***ānandamaya kośa***

4. *Guṇas*

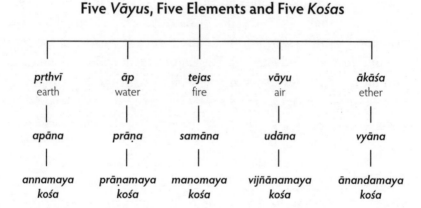

Prakṛti is endowed with three qualities (*triguṇas*) – illumination (*sattva*), vibrancy (*rajas*) and inertia (*tamas*). Though the qualities of the *guṇas* are different, their function is to promote the evolution of the *sādhakas*. The *guṇas* are the base principles of the whole of nature. They are called 'principles' as they cover the evolutionary spectrum in the quality, character and function of things. The *triguṇas* at their root source are in a state of perfect, non-specific, non-distinguishable, signless and traceless nothingness. This is *mūla prakṛti*, or the root of nature. This *mūla prakṛti* is in a state of perfect equilibrium. All things in the beginning are in a noumenal, undifferentiated state, without any sign or mark (*aliṅga*). They become differentiated by conjunction and intermingling activities and by specific transformations (*guṇa parvāṇi*) into phenomenal entities.

Lust (*kāma*), anger (*krodha*), greed (*lobha*), infatuation (*moha*), pride (*mada*) and malice (*mātsarya*) affect those human beings who are influenced by *guṇa*s. God has provided humanity with both possibilities: sensual transient joy and eternal bliss through spiritual pursuits.

The three *guṇa*s either play with their own vibrational movements, creating harmony, balance and concord, or they play in discordant ways with our words, thoughts and deeds. This equilibrium or disequilibrium of the *guṇa*s continues until the individual consciousness evolves to merge in the first principle, the cosmic consciousness, or *mahat*.

As the *triguṇa*s continue the evolutionary change, evolution becomes specified or particular. Yoga is the means for nurturing and culturing these constituents of nature to merge together in bringing rhythm and harmony in life and to make each person a true human being. Though they are not discernable to the senses, they are recognisable to the *citta*, or individualised consciousness.

Ahaṁkāra has three major categories: *bhūtādika ahaṁkāra* of the elements (*bhūta*s) and the infrastructure of the elements (*tanmātra*); *vaikārika ahaṁkāra*, from the organs of action and senses of perception; and *tejas ahaṁkāra*, from the mind. This *tejomaya* mind divides itself between the unbroken chain of stimuli received by the outward-facing senses of perception and the inward reflection of the inner senses (*antar indriya*s). This *tejomaya* mind has the capacity for both. Humanity has evolved with the resources of the outer *indriyas*, the organs of action, the senses of perception and *ekādaśendriya* as the external part of the mind, which together enable us to move towards the inner faculties or the inner parts of the mind (*antara manas*). These are intelligence, the I-maker, consciousness, conscience and, in a way, I-ness.

These external senses or internal faculties plunge us into waves of consciousness. This creates chaotic movements. Restraining the waves of consciousness brings control over the chaos.

The *Yoga Sūtras* explain the role of the *guṇas* and the importance of transcending them.

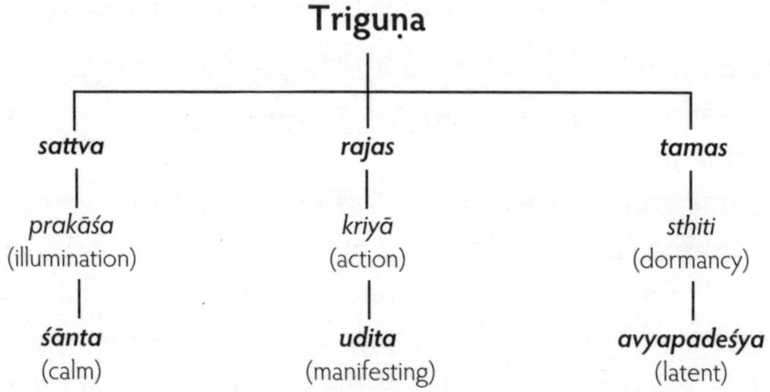

***prakāśa-kriyā--sthiti-śīlaṁ bhūta-indriyā--ātmakaṁ-bhoga--apavarga-arthaṁ dṛśyam* (II.18)**	The five elements with their infrastructure (*tanmātras*) and the *guṇas* activate the *jīvātman*, or individual self, either for sensual pleasures or for spiritual bliss.
***tat paraṁ puruṣa khyāteḥ guṇa vaitṛṣṇyam* (I.16)**	When one transcends the *guṇas*, one reaches the highest state of renunciation, which makes one eligible to perceive the seer or the soul.

In the art of living, the *guṇas* have two roles to play; one is towards *bhoga* and the other is towards *mokṣa*. The former leads to the pleasures of the material world (*bhoga*), whereas the latter invites us to experience the untainted and unalloyed blissful life (*apavarga* or *mokṣa*). *Bhoga* is material joy and *apavarga* is spiritual bliss.

***te vyakta-sūkṣmāḥ guṇā-ātmānaḥ* (IV.13)**

Nature is interconnected with time as past, present and future. The discipline of discernment means that the *guṇa*s wither like dry leaves. Then the gross or subtle components of nature fade, losing the sense of *guṇa* as well as *kāla* (time).

***pariṇāma-ekatvāt vastu-tattvam* (IV.14)**

Changes do occur due to the rhythmic mutation of time and the *guṇas*, but the 'real' abides without mutation. When this 'real' is understood, then the wheel of *guṇas* and time comes to an end. Only stillness in consciousness is felt as the *guṇa*s and time cease to move. When *guṇa*s and time stop moving, then one experiences the seer.

***tataḥ kṛtā-arthānāṁ pariṇāma-krama--samāptiḥ guṇānāṁ* (IV.32)**

Mutations of consciousness are created by the activity of *guṇa*s. 'Thinking' is different from 'thought'. The former is done with conscious intelligence, whereas the latter, being a *saṁskāra-vṛtti*, has its root in 'subconscious intelligence'. Conscious mutations of consciousness can be controlled. Subconscious mutations come to an end only when consciousness is completely refined and the *guṇa*s become quiet and return back to their source: nature. This is the very moment when all mutations automatically fade.

5. *Prakṛti* (Nature)

It is said by the *dārśanika*s that *prakṛti* covers five gross elements (*pañca bhūta*s), five organs of action (*karmendriya*s), five senses of perception (*jñānendriya*s), five subtle elements (*pañca tanmātra*s) and cosmic intelligence (*mahat*), which transforms into consciousness (*citta*) in individuals. *Citta* has three facets (ego, intelligence and mind – *ahaṁkāra, buddhi and manas*).[1]

1 For more details, *see Aṣṭadaḷa Yogamālā*, vol. II, p. 278, table n. 13.

***viśeṣa-aviśeṣa-liṅga--mātra-aliṅgāni--guṇa-parvāṇi* (II.19)** This *sūtra* encompasses the entire structure of nature existing in the body.[1]

Viśeṣa are the five elements, the five organs of action, the five senses of perception and mind.

Aviśeṣa are the five *ahaṁkārika guṇa*s of nature, or the atomic qualities (*tanmātras*) of the five elements of nature. Each one expresses its own egoistic character like the *ahaṁkāra* in an individual, which impersonates and acts as a reflective mirror of the soul. These are not knowable by the *viśeṣa indriyas*.

Liṅga is *mahat* or cosmic intelligence. In an individual it is consciousness encasing the I-maker (*ahaṁkāra*), intelligence as well as the mind.

Aliṅga is the unmanifested state of nature, or *avyakta*. It is the *mūla prakṛti*, the source from which nature sprouts.[2]

When all these are silenced, *guṇa*s (nature's qualities) evaporate and merge in *mūla prakṛti*, and *mūla prakṛti* in *puruṣa*.

Patañjali clearly states that nature is there to serve the seer and that the same nature can also entangle the incarnated seer.

***tad-arthaḥ eva dṛśyasya ātman* (II.21)** *Mūla prakṛti*, the organs and senses, mind, intelligence, *ahaṁkāra*, *citta* and *sākāra* of the self are there for the sake of *puruṣa* as they reveal the seer and his position, and incite him to *see* his true nature.

6. The Conjunction between *Puruṣa* and *Prakṛti*

The relationship between nature (*prakṛti*) and soul (*ātman*) is like the relationship between a righteous husband (*pati*) and his virtuous or faithful wife (*satī*). If there is no husband, then there can be

1 Nature has four divisions. They are differentiable and undifferentiable, phenomenal and noumenal.

2 See table n. 9, in *Light on the Yoga Sūtras of Patañjali*, 'The evolution and involution of prakṛti'.

no question of a virtuous or a faithful wife. Similarly, a wife without a husband has no meaning. It is the same with *prakṛti* and *puruṣa. Prakṛti* has to be made virtuous so that its union with *puruṣa* is divine. Yoga acts as an instrument for this union. This *yaugika* path helps in associating the various sheaths of the body to integrate (*saṁyoga*) with the *ātman.*

If *pati* does not exist, the *satī* also cannot exist. Married life is considered to be the noble *āśrama* out of the four *āśramas* (*brahmacarya, gṛhastha, vānaprastha, sannyāsa*). It is only *gṛhastha* (the householder's life) that offers protection and support and provides health, happiness and prosperity in the material world, as well as in the spiritual world for the other three *āśramas.*

Patañjali makes a sweeping statement about the result of the conjunction between *prakṛti* and *puruṣa:*

***draṣṭṛ-dṛśyayoḥ saṁyogaḥ heya--hetuḥ* (II.17)**	The conjunction between nature, body, consciousness and the soul has to be relinquished so that consciousness blossoms. This removes the obscuring veils of *kleśa* and *avidyā* and frees consciousness from suffering, enabling it to remain aloof from the cluster of worldly thoughts and ambitions.

This *sūtra* is directly connected to those in the fourth *āśrama* – the *sannyāsāśrama.* But, what about common people like us who are caught in the web of the world?

Soon in the same chapter, Patañjali defines the special relationship between nature and the seer. There he explains their ways of connection and what happens to that connection when the purpose of nature is fulfilled:

***kṛtā-arthaṁ prati naṣṭam api anaṣṭaṁ tad-anya--sādhāraṇatvāt* (II.22)**	The vestures for the seer exist so that his position and status are revealed and realised. The moment this happens, the vestures fall off on their own.

Note how he establishes the importance of this conjunction or association of nature with the seer.

***sva-svāmi-śaktyoḥ sva-rūpa-upalabdhi- -hetuḥ saṁyogaḥ* (II.23)**

'*Sva*' stands for the vestures of the seer and *svāmi* stands for the seer as the Lord of the body, mind, intelligence and consciousness. As *puruṣa*, he recognises his own status (*svarūpa upalabdhi*), through this conjunction with elements of the body. By this conjunction, the power of the seer is known.

***draṣṭā dṛśi-mātraḥ śuddhaḥ api pratyayā-anupaśyaḥ* (II.20)**

For us, he speaks about the need of the seer, or *puruṣa*. The *puruṣa* witnesses the functionings of the seen, the body, intelligence and consciousness and, as *ahaṁ-ākāra*, guides us to act with discriminative power so that the thoughts of the *citta* bloom like a flower.

***tad-abhāvāt saṁyoga-abhāvaḥ hānaṁ tad-dṛśeḥ kaivalyam* (II.25)**

However, without this conjunction, it is not possible to eradicate ignorance. As this conjunction matures and blossoms, consciousness breaks its binding contact with its supports and moves towards *puruṣa* with absolute freedom.

Like husband and wife, both *prakṛti śakti* and *puruṣa śakti* or *citi śakti* are needed for the evolution of involution and the involution of evolution.

The involution of evolution in consciousness brings light to the intelligence to free it from pride, and crowns the insight of the soul or *puruṣa*

***sattva-puruṣayoḥ atyantā- -asaṁkīrṇayoḥ pratyaya- -aviśeṣaḥ bhogaḥ para-arthatvāt sva- -artha-saṁyamāt puruṣa-jñānam* (III.36)**

It is possible to distinguish the illuminative consciousness from the insight of the seer.

He further elaborates:

***sattva-puruṣayoḥ śuddhi-sāmye kaivalyam iti* (III.56)**	When the currents of the senses of perception, mind and intelligence involute and move towards the *ātman* (seer), he evolves and moves from his dwelling place and unites with these currents, dissolving the differences between the intellectual position of nature and the blazing luminosity of the seer.

The transformation in the various vestures of the seer happens through *yoga-sādhanā* by merging the elements, the senses, mind and consciousness into the *mahat*, or cosmic intelligence. By this, the mind loses its individuality and the difference between the seer and his vestures disappears.

***etena bhūta--indriyeṣu dharma--lakṣaṇa-avasthā--pariṇāmāḥ vyākhyātāḥ* (III.13)**	As the armour of the seer is polished (like a musical instrument is tuned), the elements, senses, mind, intelligence and consciousness transform from their potential states (*dharma*) to qualitative states of refinement (*lakṣaṇa*). The polishing continues until they reach a state where no further polishing or culture is necessary (*avasthā*).
***bandha-kāraṇa--śaithilyāt pracāra--saṁvedanāt ca citta-sya para--śarīra-āveśaḥ* (III.39)** ***bahiḥ akalpitā vṛttiḥ mahāvideha tataḥ prakāśa-āvaraṇa--kṣayaḥ* (III.44)**	This state is stainless (*vimala*), which is beyond further polishing and cultivation. Otherwise the seer and his armour are wrongly perceived as one. When they are thoroughly and completely polished, the bondage that holds the yogi in the world of illusion is understood. By this the yogi develops the ability to do unimaginable things like entering into a person's body at will. He can also live without a body.

As Patañjali explained in II.19–20, which I have dealt with in detail before, the *ātman* is he who is absolute, distinct from nature, ever aware, real and consistently the same. This is the understanding of the seer or the soul. Read Chapter VI on *Īśvara* and the universe to understand the conjunction of *Īśvara*, *puruṣa* and *prakṛti*.

7. *Citta* (Consciousness)

Muṇḍakopaniṣad (*muṇḍaka* 3, sections 1 & 2) deals with a story of two birds to explain *citta* – or consciousness – having two facets. One is the absolute consciousness (*kūṭastha citta*) and the other is the alternating consciousness (*pariṇāma citta*). *Kūṭastha* means immovable, perpetually and universally remaining the same; *pariṇāma* means to change, alterate or transform, or turning around and about. This *pariṇāma citta* is made to be transformed from the state of evolution towards the state of involution.

If *kūṭastha citta* represents the seer, the *pariṇāma citta* sprouts as *ahaṁkāra*, impersonating the *kūṭastha citta* with clusters of thought waves.

The formless *ātman* is *kūṭastha citta*. Due to ignorance, it becomes *pariṇāma citta*. *Kūṭastha citta* is the cosmic mind. It represents the seer. It is stable, non-oscillating and non-vacillating. When *kūṭastha citta* takes the form of *ahaṁkāra*, it becomes *pariṇāma citta*. Yogis work to transform *pariṇāma citta* to become *kūṭastha citta*.

The story of the *Upaniṣad* describes these two phases of consciousness. There are two birds in a fig tree. One bird hops from twig to twig, pecking at fruits. Not finding the taste it wants, it becomes agitated and flies to far-flung branches, whereas the other bird remains impassive, steady, silent and blissful in its place.

Gradually the wandering bird draws closer and closer towards its quiet companion and eventually stops wavering in further attempts. Losing interest in its wants and desires, it becomes calm, silent and non-attached, filled with blissfulness.

Here the tree represents the body, the two birds the self and consciousness. The different taste of the fruits represents the senses of perception, creating clusters of thought waves in consciousness.

Kūṭastha citta is like the sun, non-wavering and non-waxing; *pariṇāma citta* oscillates, vacillates and wanes and waxes, like the moon. If *kūṭastha citta* represents the pure consciousness (the *puruṣa*, or the seer), *pariṇāma citta* corresponds to the ordinary functioning of consciousness.

I will describe in more detail these two aspects of *citta* in Chapter VII: *Citta Svabhāva*.

VI

Puruṣa – Seer

Viśva puruṣa is God, and *puruṣa* is the Self, or the Seer. *Puruṣa*, the Lord of the body, is called the *ātman*, the Seer, the Self, the Soul, the *citta-prabhu* (Lord of consciousness). Patañjali calls the seer *citi śakti* (*see Y. S.*, IV.34).

In this home of the Lord dwells *ahaṁ-ākāra* (form of the formless *puruṣa*) or the self as *jīvātman*, *antarendriya* (conscientiousness), *citta* (consciousness), intelligence (*buddhi*), *ahaṁkāra* (ego), mind (*manas*), *jñānendriyas* (senses of perception) and *karmendriyas* (organs of action). These constituents in general, and conscientiousness and *ahaṁ-ākāra* or *jīvātma* in particular, act as links with the *puruṣa*.

As the body is the supporter of consciousness (*citta*), consciousness is the foundation or base for the *puruṣa* to realise his position and status. As *citta* has its own disposition (*svabhāva*), *puruṣa* too has his own significant nature.

Puruṣa, or the *Seer*

Puruṣa, *ātman* or the seer, does not rely on nature. It cannot involute. In order to feel the *puruṣa*, one has to reach its final destination – i.e., its evolution and culmination. I have already dealt with nature and its constituents, so here it is essential to remember the role of intelligence in evolution as well as in involution. Intelligence acts as a bridge in connecting the consciousness of nature with the consciousness of the seer. I said before that the alternating individual self or the individual consciousness is the *pariṇāma citta*, and the *kūṭastha citta* is the absolute consciousness or the seer. When the *pariṇāma citta* transforms into *kūṭastha citta*, the seer shines in his own natural state (*svarūpa*).

Pariṇāma citta gets caught in illusory knowledge (*mithyājñānam*). This has to be cleansed with the glowing intelligence, so that the seer shines in his own self-luminous light. This clears the way for the personalised individual to transform into a luminous and impersonal auspicious *asmitā*.

In this state, the roving *citta* or *pariṇāma citta* ceases to function. As the mutation of time ceases, *guṇa*s return to their source for the absolute consciousness or *kūṭastha citta* to shine as *puruṣa*.

***tadā draṣṭuḥ svarūpe avasthānam* (I.3)**

The seer, or the *ātman*, dwells in his home. When the coverings of the *ātman* – namely, the five elements and their counterparts (the body, organs of action, senses of perception, mind, intelligence and consciousness) – are quietened, the core *puruṣa* (*bindu*) reveals himself. Then he moves to surrender himself to God (*Īśvara praṇidhāna*).

***draṣṭā dṛśi-mātraḥ śuddhaḥ api pratyaya-ānupaśyaḥ* (II.20)**

The *ātman* is pure and absolute. Without knowing the characteristic quality of the *puruṣa*, we cannot experience the *puruṣa* dwelling in his home. So Patañjali first explains the pure characteristic (*dharmin*) quality of the *puruṣa* for us to experience his restful states of *nirākāra* and *nirguṇa*.

Here, he explains how, depending on the enthusiasm of the practitioner in his *yaugika sādhanā*, nature begins to involute towards the seer, enabling him to witness nature without depending upon it.

***tad-arthaḥ eva dṛśyasya ātmā* (II.21)**

Nature with its *guṇa*s exists solely in the service of the seer for him to realise his position. Though these vehicles of nature lead one towards the pleasures of the senses or towards emancipation, Patañjali clearly mentions that the vehicles of nature (*prakṛti*) are there to serve the *ātman*, motivating him to discover himself (II.23).[1]

Consciousness (individualisation of *mahat*) exists in close proximity to the seer and is able to serve the seer (IV.24).[2]

Through *yaugika sādhanā*, the yogi untangles and disassembles all the constituents of *prakṛti* to their respective states (*dharma lakṣaṇa avasthā pariṇāma*), dismantling the illusion that the Self is connected to the modifying *vṛttis* and revealing its true splendour, never seen before or realised.

It takes *prakṛti* to its pristine state, bringing an end to the appearance of the seer as a distorted or sullied entity. At this state the *prakṛti* adores the *puruṣa*, and *puruṣa* adorns the *prakṛti* with its purity.

***bhuvana-jñānaṁ sūrye saṁyamāt* (III.27)** Like the sun that gives light to the world, the soul lights the individual self fully with the flame of knowledge.

As the sun never fades in the universe, the *ātman* as sun (*sūrya*) never fades in the body. By *saṁyama* on the *puruṣa* (sun), the *sādhaka* obtains knowledge of the contents of the nature's constituents.

Due to a lack of the right knowledge and understanding on the part of *citta*, the *ātman* appears to be enamoured by the pleasures of the world. Hence, Patañjali suggests two wings of *yaugika* discipline: *abhyāsa* (practice), which covers *tapas*, *svādhyāya* and *Īśvara praṇidhāna* (II.1);[3] and *vairāgya* (renunciation of desires), which

---

1 *sva-svāmi-śaktyoḥ sva-rūpa-upalabdhi-hetuḥ saṁyogaḥ* (II.23) – The conjunction of the seer with the seen is for the seer to discover his own true nature.

2 *tat-asaṇkhyeya-vāsanābhiḥ citram api para-arthaṁ saṁhatya kāritvāt* (IV.24) – Though the fabric of consciousness is interwoven with innumerable desires and subconscious impressions, it exists for the seer on account of its proximity to the seer as well as to the objective world.

3 *tapaḥ-svādhyāya-īśvara-praṇidhānāni kriyā-yogaḥ* (II.1) – Burning zeal in practice, self-study and study of scriptures, and surrender to God are the acts of yoga.

lead the *sādhaka* to dwell in his own splendour of purity. These two wings of *yaugika* discipline will be explained in the chapter on *aṣṭāṅga yoga* (Chapter XIV).

I must mention here that though *sūtras* III.27–30[1] speak of the universe, which we identify as the cosmos with its stellar and planetary bodies, they can also be thought of as representing the human body.

***sattva-puruṣa--anyatā-khyāti--mātrasya sarva-bhāva--adhiṣṭhātṛtvaṁ sarva-jñātṛtvaṁ ca* (III.50)**

When the *sādhaka* is illuminated, he recognises the difference between *citta* and *puruṣa*, as well as the difference between material or worldly knowledge (*laukika jñāna*) and spiritual knowledge (*vaidika jñāna*). This is spiritual enlightenment. The *sādhaka* realises that the seer is immovable, immutable and changeless, while nature is transient and changing with the intermingling of the *guṇas*.

***sadā-jñātāḥ citta--vṛttayaḥ tat-prabhoḥ puruṣasya apariṇāmitvāt* (IV.18)**

Īśvara is the Lord of all *puruṣas*. *Puruṣa* or *ātman* being ever alert, ever illuminative and brilliant, knows the movements, moods and modes of the senses of perception, mind, intelligence, I-maker and consciousness. So He is the master of consciousness (*citta-prabhu*). He is pure *prajñā* (awareness), whereas *jīvātman*, the formful *puruṣa* is a blend of *prāṇa* (energy) and *prajñā* (awareness). *Jīvātman* is the individual soul; it departs when *prāṇa* leaves.

---

1 *bhuvana-jñānam sūrye saṁyamāt* (III.27) – The yogi will gain knowledge of the seven worlds by studying the sun. (These seven universal astronomical bodies may also be read as seven cosmic centres in the body).

candre tārā-vyūha-jñānam (III.28) – By *saṁyama* on the moon the yogi will know the orderly disposition of the planets or the galaxy of stars (as *sūrya* does not wane or wax, and is ever bright, so the *puruṣa* never wanes or waxes). But the moon wanes and waxes, so it is consciousness waning and waxing, creating clusters of thoughts.

dhruve tad-gati-jñānam (III.29) – As the pole star is the guide for navigation, so too the intelligence is a pole star that navigates the cluster of thought waves in the right direction to gain correct understanding and steadiness, and move towards the seer.

nābhi-cakre kāya-vyūha-jñānam (III.30) – By full control on the navel region, the yogi acquires perfect knowledge of the body, which means control on *prakṛti*.

citeḥ apratisaṁkra-māyāḥ tad-ākāra--āpattau sva-buddhi--saṁvedanam (IV.22)	The *ātman*, being changeless, has the power to distinguish acquired knowledge from the knowledge of experience while abiding within his own intelligence, wearing the crown of wisdom.
sattva-puruṣayoḥ atyantā--asaṁkīrṇayoḥ pratyaya-aviśeṣaḥ bhogaḥ para--arthatvāt sva-artha--saṁyamāt puruṣa--jñānam (III.36)	[1]Intelligence being the pinnacle of nature, its instinctive quality is transformed through *yaugika* discipline to stand equal to the intuitive intelligence, knowledge and wisdom of the seer. On account of this oneness between the two, the real seer becomes experienced.

Patañjali ends the *sūtra* by referring to *puruṣa* as *citi śakti:*

puruṣa-artha--śūnyānāṁ guṇānāṁ pratiprasavaḥ kaivalyaṁ sva-rūpa--pratiṣṭhā vā citi--śaktir iti (IV.34)	Given the *ātman's* visage or natural condition (*puruṣa svarūpa*), Patañjali states that when the vehicles of nature become separated and are no longer obscuring, *puruṣa* shines in his own glory.

Thus, *citi śakti* is nothing less than *puruṣa*, who is beyond the four aims of life (*dharma*, sense of duty; *artha*, means and pursuits; *kāma*, love and gratifications; *mokṣa*, emancipation), and who transcends the qualities of nature (*guṇa*), breaking the bondage of the material world to live in bliss. Later on, I will explain this concept in detail.

Īśvara praṇidhāna is the total surrender of both consciousness (*citta*) and soul (*citi*) to finally rest in the lap of God.

The inner layer of the skin radiates with instinctive intelligence and the seer is resplendent with intuitive intelligence. By *yaugika* practices, the instinctive potencies of nature are subdued

---

1 By *saṁyama*, the yogi easily differentiates between the intelligence and the soul, which is real and true.

by continuous involvement and the filtering of intuitive wisdom. By this, the filtered intuitive intelligence flows evenly and without interruption from the skin towards the Self and from the Self towards the skin, breaking through all divisions in the intelligence.

VII

Citta Svabhāva – The Natural State of Consciousness

After explaining *puruṣa* and the link between *puruṣa* and *citta*, I will now consider the natural state of *citta*. By traditional notions, *citta* or consciousness is constituted of *ahaṁkāra* (I-maker), *buddhi* (intelligence) and *manas* (mind).

The *annamaya* (anatomical) body and *prāṇamaya* (physiological) body include the senses of perception and organs of action. The psychological aspect of the external mind in conjunction and interaction with the senses is called *ekādaśendriya* (the 11th sense) or *bāhyendriya* (external mind). When the same external mind is made to involute towards the body of *vijñānamaya* (intelligence), *ahaṁkāra* (I-maker) and *ahaṁ-ākāra* (I-ness), it becomes the inner mind (*antara manas*). This involution of mind leads to a state of emancipation and unalloyed bliss with a consciousness that is both passive and pensive.

The seer (soul) is *nirākāra* (formless). When the formless soul transforms into a form (*sākāra*), it becomes I-ness (*ahaṁ-ākāra*). Due to ignorance (*avidyā*), this I-ness is identified with the I-maker or *ahaṁkāra*.

1. *Ahaṁkāra* (I-maker), a Mirror of the Seer and the Seen

As I explained already, the word *ahaṁkāra* conveys two meanings:

When *ahaṁkāra* is taken as a single word, it conveys the ego or the I-maker.

If the same word *ahaṁkāra* is divided and separated, it becomes *ahaṁ* and *ākāra*. *Ahaṁ-ākāra* is nothing less than the formless *puruṣa* transformed into a personified self (*sākāra*). This personified form of the self is still a pure state of the Self.

If *ahaṁ-ākāra* (I-ness) is a personified form of the formless Self, *ahaṁkāra* acts as an impersonator of the Self (I-maker).

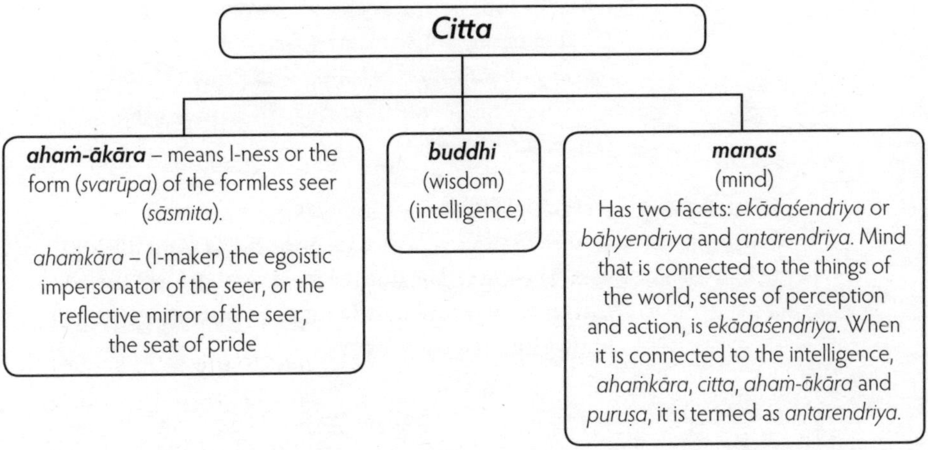

It is exceedingly rare to see the relationship evenly placed as depicted in this chart (I.3).[1] Each one supersedes the other. If pride overrules, then the intelligence (*buddhi*) is hidden. If mind overrules, the intelligence and pride subside. Mind without the contact of intelligence is like a horse that has bolted. This is how they function for us, whereas in the case of saints and yogis they all balance evenly.

---

1 *tadā draṣṭuḥ svarūpe avasthānam* (I.3) – Then, the seer dwells in his own true splendour.

Patañjali explains the nine *antarāyas*, or obstacles, which get in the way of spiritual pursuit (see *sūtra* I.30)[1]. If one assesses *antarāyas* carefully, one will find an intrinsic order in them. *Vyadhi* and *ālasya* are physical; *avirati* is somatopsychic (affecting the mind through the body); *saṁśaya* and *pramāda* are mental; *bhrāntidarśana* is intellectual; and *alabdhabhūmikatva* and *anavasthitatvāni* are spiritual distractions.

dṛg-darśana-śaktyoḥ eka-ātmatā iva asmitā **(II.6)**	Due to ignorance or want of spiritual knowledge, the I-ness (*ahaṁ-ākāra*) thinks as if it is a part of consciousness and changes into ego, projecting itself as if it is the real seer. This want of understanding (*avidyā*) makes the I-ness (*sākāra puruṣa*) become a part of consciousness and get involved with the fluctuating consciousness (*see Y. S.*, I.4, *vṛtti--sārūpyam itaratra)*,[2] bristling with pride. This is the *tāmasika* or *rājasika* state of I-ness (*ahaṁkārika asmitā*).
nirmāṇa-cittāni asmitā-mātrāt **(IV.4)**	Anything that springs from consciousness with a sense of pride or ego is taken as if it is from the seer. This *sūtra* explains the need to transform the ego or the arrogant I-maker into an instrument of knowledge and wisdom.[3]

Ahaṁkāra, as the impostor of the Self, acts like a mirror (*biṁba*), reflecting the seer. This mirror re-reflects (*pratibiṁba*) on the mind in multiple ways. *Ahaṁkāra*, in fact, has a double role:

❊ it is the impostor of the Self;

---

1 *vyādhi-styāna-saṁśaya-pramāda-ālasya-avirati-bhrānti-darśana-alabdha-bhūmikatva-anavasthitatvāni citta-vikṣepāḥ te antarāyāḥ* (I.30) – These obstacles are disease, inertia, doubt, heedlessness, laziness, indiscipline of the senses, erroneous views, lack of perseverance, and backsliding.

2 At other times, the seer as individual self gets involved with the fluctuating consciousness.

3 *Sūtras* II.6 and IV.4. Please refer to the explanation under the heading '*Pariṇāma citta*' in section 5, below.

❊ it can be transformed into a recipient of *jñāna* by using the power of disccerning intellect (*vicāra jñāna*). Then the *ahaṁkāra*, being a part of intellectual consciousness of the head, is made to descend and merge with the intelligence of the heart, enabling it to become sublime. When *ahaṁkāra* reaches this state of sublimity, *citta* becomes quiet and pure. Wisdom is established, true *jñāna* dawns and that *jñāna* is transformed into *bhakti* (devotion).

2. Buddhi (Wisdom, Intelligence)

Buddhi is another component of *citta*. It is an instrument that acts as the true assessor. It helps to acquire the reliable and untainted knowledge that comes from experience. Its power of discernment is the lustre of wisdom.

See what Lord Krishna says on *buddhi:*

***vyavasāyā-atmikā buddhir eke'ha kuru-nandana / bahu-śākhā hy anantāś ca buddhayo 'vyavasāyinām //* (*B. G.*, II.41)**

The refined knowledge of experience, earned through strenuous determined effort, is steady, singular and complete. It does not create oscillations in the mind but keeps it completely stable. Knowledge that does not come from experience, being on the verbal level, or at an unripe state of experience, branches into innumerable permutations and combinations. Therefore the true lustre of knowledge (*rasātmaka jñāna*) gained by experience (*ānubhavika jñāna*) is *vyavasāyātmikā buddhi*.

Owing to our past impressions, the qualities of our thinking and action become adulterated.

***pariṇāma-tāpa--saṁskāra-duḥkaiḥ guṇa-vṛtti-virodhāt ca duḥkham eva sarvaṁ vivekinaḥ* (II.15)**

A man of wisdom realises that all things that appear pleasant are coated with sorrow. Hence he, as a wise man, keeps aloof from them. This is *buddhi*.

Buddhi is the axial constituent of *citta*. It acts as a gravitational force to draw the *citta* towards the seer. It is the mediator. It is the judging faculty that orientates the other instruments on the inner path. This intelligence serves the *sādhaka* in orientating the inevitable sorrows that are coated in pleasant experiences.

It positions itself as the pole star, guiding the journey of the *citta* towards the source. Like consciousness, intelligence too is tied on the threshold between worldly pleasures and liberation from them. This is why it is essential to study and reflect to discern the differences between intelligence and consciousness.

If one does not take note of the distinction between immature intelligence (1) and mature intelligence (2), then the gate leading to the supreme intelligence (3) is closed. Only on the basis of extreme refinement, indicated by Patañjali, does this lustrous intelligence, or *buddhi*, attain the level of purity of the seer. Then the intelligence turns inwards and becomes attracted by the gravitational pull of the seer, causing the *citta* to know directly the true light of *puruṣa*.

viveka-khyātiḥ aviplavā hāna- -upāyaḥ **(II.26)**

In *sādhanā*, discriminating wisdom should flow ceaselessly without interruption.

When the judged, uninterrupted and unfailing flow of discriminating knowledge dawns, then ignorance, disharmony and imbalance in body, mind and intellect vanish and right word, work and wisdom, or right thought, word and deed (*trikaraṇa śuddhi*) occur.

---

(1) Immature intelligence – crude, conceited, competitive, constantly making comparisons in worldly affairs.

(2) Mature intelligence – knows from experience, inference and deduction the outcome of actions, knows that pleasent experiences will eventually have a trace of pain in them, and chooses to act skilfully. Knows the adjustment required in *āsana* to bring stability and lightness, and maintains an even flow of single-focused attention.

(3) Supreme intelligence – can tell the difference between the true luminosity of the seer and the reflected luminosity of *citta*.

This *sūtra* conveys the end of wisdom when it reaches from the core to its frontier – the body, as a single unit of awareness.

***dhruve tad-gati--jñānam* (III.29)**	Just as the pole star (*Dhruva*) is the guide for navigation, intellectual wisdom is the constant unmoving pole star in the individual, which navigates us to move on towards the continual process of evolution – i.e., the one goal, eternal freedom from bondage.[1]
***sattva-puruṣa-anyatā-khyāti--mātrasya sarva-bhāva--adhiṣṭhātṛtvaṁ sarva-jñātṛtvaṁ ca* (III.50)**	When the yogi knows the difference between the mind (*manas*), knowledge (*jñāna*), acquired knowledge (*vidyā*), the intelligence of experience (*buddhi*), the ego (*ahaṁkāra*), consciousness (*citta*) and the seer, he reaches the pinnacle of knowledge and wears the crown of wisdom, which remains constant at all times.
***kṣaṇa-tat-kramayoḥ saṁyamāt viveka--jaṁ jñānam* (III.53)**	For example, if we maintain a single, focused awareness of the moment, without getting caught in the sequential movement of moments, then our consciousness not only experiences freedom from the constraints of time and space but is radiant in wisdom.
***tārakaṁ sarva--viṣayaṁ sarvathā viṣayaṁ akramaṁ ca iti viveka-jaṁ jñānam* (III.55)**	The yogi with this radiant wisdom does not become involved in the movement of moments, but stays in the moment. He then transcends nature and gains clear knowledge of the light of the seer or the *ātman*.

1 Dhruva, etymologically fixed, firm and immovable. According to a beautiful legend (*Mahābhārata* and especially *Viṣṇu Purāṇa*), Dhruva was humiliated as a child and made a vow to reach a high and unattainable position. He became a child-hermit and performed a very severe penance till Lord Viṣṇu appeared to him and granted him a place higher than the planets and stars: Dhruva, or the pole star.

***sattva-puruṣayoḥ śuddhi-sāmye kaivalyam iti* (III.56)**	When the instinctive intelligence is cultured, it reaches the mature state that is on a par with the intuitive intelligence of the seer. It means that he has reached the state of emancipation, illumination and freedom from bondage.
***tadā viveka--nimnaṁ kaivalya--prāgbhāraṁ cittam* (IV.26)**	When this crown of wisdom is ablaze, consciousness is luminescent and reaches the state of purity equal to the seer. Perfectly radiant in the light of the seer, it becomes divine and absolute. As intelligence and consciousness are the first principles of a man, they are drawn like a magnet by the seer to become one with him, extinguishing the seed of division or separateness.

3. *Manas* (Mind)

The mind connects and co-ordinates the five senses of perception and five organs of action. At the same time it acts as the innermost sense (*antarendriya*), the agent connecting the *buddhi* and *ahaṁkāra* with the *puruṣa*. The mind plays a double (*dvandva*) role. Its role is to connect the 10 organs (*indriyas*) on the one hand, and, on the other, to connect the intelligence, consciousness and the core. This dual role of the mind affects the *citta* so that it plays a double game. The mind being the gross part of consciousness needs to distinguish between subject and object.

Let me give you an idea of how the mind plays multiple roles. The different facets of mind are:

caitanya-śila manas	(biological mind)
svabhāva-śila manas	(physical mind)
grahaṇa-kṣama manas	(sensory mind)
laukika manas	(temporal mind)
sendriya manas	(organic mind)
prāṇika manas	(energy mind)
naitika manas	(ethical mind)
nṛvaṁśiya manas	(ethnic mind)

mānasika manas	(emotional mind)
ahaṁkārika manas	(egoistic mind)
cittaja manas	(dominant mind)
vyāvahārika manas	(habitual mind)
preraṇa manas	(impulsive mind)
saṁskārika manas	(instinctive mind)
śaṇkara manas	(confused mind)
vyutthāna manas	(wandering mind)
chidra manas	(perforated mind)
atiprasaṇga manas	(impressionable mind, deriving thoughts from elsewhere)
janukīya manas	(genetic mind)
karmaja manas	(predestined mind)
pañca prāṇika manas	(five energies of mind)
guṇaja manas	(qualitative mind)
viparyaya manas	(misperceiving mind)
vikalpa manas	(misconceiving mind)
smṛti manas	(mind working with memory)
nidrā manas	(inert mind)
vitarka manas	(analytical mind)
vicāra manas	(synthesising mind)
nirodha manas	(restraining mind)
śanta manas	(tranquil mind)
ekāgra manas	(attentive mind)
prabhāva-śila or *tejas manas*	(enlightening mind)
ānanda manas	(joyful mind)
vedāntika manas	(selfless mind)
divya yaugika manas	(divine mind)

I must add here that the *buddhi manas* and *vijñāna manas* are a subtle way to evolve through analysis, used by *sādhaka* throughout his *tapas* to progress, to gauge his progression and to avoid pits and downfalls in life and precipices on the path.

sattva-śuddhi- *-saumanasya-* *-eka-agrya-indriya--* *jaya-ātma-darśana-* *-yogyatvāni ca* (II.41)	When the senses of perception and mind are controlled, cleansed and made to involute towards the internal senses through *yaugika* practices, then the very same mind develops a benevolent, cheerful and divine state, enabling it to become a fit instrument that leads towards the sight of the seer or *puruṣa* (*ātmadarśana*). *See also* II.28, wherein Patañjali identifies *yaugika* practices as the means.[1]
grahaṇa-svarūpa- *-asmitā-anvaya-* *-arthavattva-* *-saṁyamāt* *indriya-jayaḥ* (III.48)	Being uniquely positioned on the threshold between the inner and the outer senses, the mind, after understanding the power of the senses and the seer, connects (*saṁyoga*) and integrates (*saṁyama*) the external senses with the internal senses, and enables the seer to feel his excellence.

For this, one has to cultivate the outer layer of the *citta* – i.e., the senses and mind – and move closer to the intelligence and consciousness, to remain wholeheartedly in a single focus on the seer. See, *viṣayavatī vā pravṛttiḥ utpannā manasaḥ sthiti-nibandhanī* (I.35).[2] As an example, in my early days of *sādhanā* I was totally engrossed in the external aspects of yoga. When I began penetrating the interior aspects of the body with careful practice, I began to surrender to the finest aspect of yoga — i.e., towards an awareness of the seer. For a *sādhaka* like me, this is the way to develop constancy.

Patañjali emphasises how *prāṇāyāma* also helps its practitioner to gain that state of attention:

tataḥ kṣīyate *prakāśa-āvaraṇam* (II.52)	The obscuring veils are the afflicted states of mind orbiting around ignorance, covering the light of knowledge. It is uncovered by *prāṇāyāma*.

---

1 *yogā-aṅgā-anuṣṭhānād aśuddhi-kṣaye jñāna-dīptiḥ ā vivekakhyāteḥ* (II.28) – By dedicated practice of the various aspects of yoga, impurities are destroyed: the crown of wisdom radiates in glory.

2 Or, by contemplating on an object that helps to maintain steadiness of mind and consciousness.

***dhāraṇāsu ca yogyatā manasaḥ* (II.53)**	Then both mind and consciousness become fit instruments to concentrate with a single, focused attention.
***pracchardana--vidhāraṇābhyāṁ vā prāṇasya* (I.34)**	Patañjali advises us to get acquainted with this sort of *prāṇāyāma*, wherein he explains the passive retention after the out-breath for consciousness to remain quiet, passive and pensive.
***tato mano-javitvaṁ vikaraṇa-bhāvaḥ pradhāna-jayaḥ ca* (III.49)**	From this conquest of mind (*manojaya*), alertness sets in to embrace the cosmic intelligence (*mahat*), the first principle of nature.

This *sūtra* brings to our understanding that the mind which plays multiple roles in thought and action (II.48) is transformed to become a single, universal, cosmic mind.

Consciousness is an enigma. In order to move towards restraining its waves or clusters of thoughts, it is better to know its character as well as its characteristics.

In Chapter V, I explained *kūṭastha* and *pariṇāma cittas*. I feel that I must develop these notions further before explaining the characteristics of *citta*.

4. *Kūṭastha Citta* (Big 'I')

Absolute pure consciousness is nothing less than the seer, which remains ever impassive, steady, silent and blissful. This pure facet of consciousness remains unchanged from birth to death. This *kūṭastha*, or absolute consciousness, appears as self-abiding (*svastha*) in the form of the Big 'I' (*ahaṁ-ākāra*), whereas the alternating consciousness impersonates the real consciousness and becomes the ego (*ahaṁkāra*).

5. *Pariṇāma Citta* (Small 'i')

The other face of consciousness is *pariṇāma citta*. It is the fluctuating state of consciousness, which moves in different directions with alternating views, agitating and jumping from one thought to another and becoming enamoured by various clusters of thoughts. I call this state of ever-changing *citta* ego, *ahaṁkāra* or the small 'i'. I am using small 'i' in order to differentiate it from the non-changing consciousness. This alternating *citta* is a transformation from the non-oscillating *citta*. *Kūṭastha citta* is pure consciousness, whereas *pariṇāma citta* is the tainted consciousness.

vṛtti-sārūpyam itaratra **(I.4)**	The mirror cannot reflect the image clearly when it is covered with dust. In the same way, when the seer is veiled by the taints of senses of perception, he is influenced by them and becomes a fabricated consciousness.
nirmāṇa-cittāni asmitā-mātrāt **(IV.4)**	When the mirror is cleaned, it reflects clearly. In the same way, if the seer is made to move away from his identifications with the cluster of thought waves, he shines alone in his own glory, reflecting his purity without refraction. Often the fabricating consciousness masquerades as the real *asmitā-citta*. Hence one has to train this consciousness and cultivate it so that it transforms itself into its real state.

We can see from these two *sūtras* that the understanding of *asmitā* may vary depending on context. From the perspective of Chapter IV of the *Yoga Sūtras*, *asmitā* is the individuality that is sprouted from the seer. It identifies with its source as pure consciousness. But from the perspective of Chapter II, it is the individuality of the immature consciousness which claims itself as the pure consciousness, causing *kleśas*.

In order to understand the difference between *kūṭastha* and *pariṇāma citta* from a practical point of view, let me explain how you can realise the presence of the big 'I', or pure consciousness of the seer in *prāṇāyāma*, *āsana* and *dhyāna*.

In *prāṇāyāma*, the in-breath begins from the seat of the *kūṭastha citta* and transforms into *pariṇāma citta*. In retention after the in-breath (*antara kuṁbhaka*), the *kūṭastha citta* mingles with *pariṇāma citta* and unites with it as one. In exhalation, as the out-breath is made to move out, *pariṇāma citta* recedes towards *kūṭastha citta*, and in retention after exhalation (*bāhya kuṁbhaka*) the *pariṇāma citta* merges and unites with the seer (*kūṭastha citta*).

While performing the *āsanas*, the *kūṭastha citta* transforms into *pariṇāma citta*, forgetting its true, steady nature. This can be seen in people doing the *āsanas* (like the second bird with the wandering and fluctuating mind in the story from *Muṇḍakopaniṣad*). Some limbs of the body are over-stretched, some are under-stretched, some parts hold the *āsanas* with fear, some suffer pain (*bādhanā*), whereas some parts feel a pleasant sweet sensation (*bhāvanā*). In the same way some muscles act positively and attentively, some parts remain negative or inattentive, and some remain indifferent, making no response or challenge.

As the *āsanas* are done mainly with the help of the *pariṇāma citta*, the practitioner has to take the centre part of the body from the crown of the head to the perineum as the site of *kūṭastha citta*. Now he has to perform *āsanas* in such a way that the *pariṇāma citta* (here, the sides of the body) are made to balance with the line of *kūṭastha citta*. Or the intelligence (*buddhi*) must be made to flow and spread singularly, like oil that flows steadily when it is poured from one vessel to another.

As an experienced *sādhaka*, I feel that when the deviated flow of intelligence is made to become one single flow of intelligence from one end to the other end of the body, such a presentation of the *āsana* is *sthiram sukham āsanam*. When *pariṇāma citta* transforms into *kūṭastha citta*, the wandering *cittan* transforms into a single *cittan*. This is *vedānta*. *Veda* means knowledge and *anta* means the culmination (of knowledge and wisdom). When performing the *āsanas*, the rays of the intelligence of the seer are made to extend, expand and engulf without interruption, spreading themselves evenly over the body. This is the perfection of the *āsanas*. When the light of the seer reaches from the source towards its periphery and from the periphery towards the source, it is the finality of each *āsana* – or the *vedānta* of each *āsana*. This is *sthira sukham āsanam* (II.46).

This oneness of intelligence flowing from the core to its frontier is well explained in *Y. S.*, II.26.

Only when one reaches the state of *vivekakyāti* (*see Y. S.*, II.26) can one realise the true meaning of II.48:

tatah dvaṇdva--anabhighātaḥ **(II.48)**	In a perfect presentation of the *āsanas*, one has to break the dualities of consciousness and experience an undisturbed state of unicity.

In *dhyāna*, the *pariṇāma citta* is constituted by the senses, mind, intelligence, *ahaṁkāra* (ego) and consciousness. In the state of contemplation (*dhyāna*) these parts of *pariṇāma citta* are made to involute towards the *kūṭastha citta*. They are then made to move towards the seer, so that both *citta*s merge into one, single entity.

In *dhyāna*, *pariṇāma citta* is made to unite with the *kūṭastha citta* so that the *kūṭastha citta* stays constant and without interruption, with focused awareness. This is *ekātānatā dhyānam* (III.2).

If each *sādhaka* practises *āsana*, *prāṇāyāma* or *dhyāna* in this way, he will experience directly the untainted state of the *citta* without mutations of the *guṇa*s of nature.

kṣaṇa-pratiyogī pariṇāma-aparānta--nirgrāhyaḥ kramaḥ **(IV.33)**	As the mutations of *guṇa*s cease in their functions, the movement in the moment also stops. Hence, the feeling of time fades. The experience of this state is *kūṭastha citta*, and this state is experienced in that noblest practice of *āsanas* and *prāṇāyāma*. From here on, the seer moves towards God.

This is how a yoga *sādhaka* quietens the fluctuations of the *guṇa*s of nature (*prakṛti laya*) and moves to work towards the conquest of nature (*prakṛti jaya*), which is nothing less than *kaivalya*.

In Chapter IV of the *Yoga Sūtra*s, Patañjali offers an exhaustive study of the character and characteristics of consciousness and its possibilities for transformation. Through this understanding, it is possible to eradicate the adverse (*pratikūla*) thought waves and retain the favourable (*anukūla*) thoughts towards evolution in involution, through *yaugika* discipline.

In some people, the imprints of the *sādhanā* of their previous lives may mean that their consciousness is in a ripe state. Keeping this in mind, Patañjali speaks in the opening *sūtra* of the *Kaivalya Pāda* about five types of accomplished yogis with powers (*siddhis*). These are: a) a yogi by birth, whom we call a genius (*janma*), b) a yogi who has experienced divinity through herbs or elixirs (*auṣadha*), c) a yogi who has gained experience through the charms of *mantras*, d) a yogi who has gained experience by ascetic practice (*tapas*), and e) a yogi who has gained experienced by profound observation and absorption (*samādhi*). As the last two yogis have gained experience via yoga, see what Patañjali says in the succeeding *sūtra*:

***jāti-antara- -pariṇāmaḥ prakṛti-āpūrāt* (IV.2)**	Through devoted *yaugika sādhanā*, the abundant flow of divine energy transforms them towards favourable thoughts (*anukūla vṛtti*). Whereas in others the anti-currents of thought waves (*pratikūla vṛtti*) put a break in the involution.

In these five classes of yogis, it is nature that has the potential to lift them up if they are caught in the mesh of physical or mental disturbance.

To be free from the mesh of psychosomatic or somatopsychic disturbances requires will-power. This is true even for those who are highly evolved and refined yogis. Patañjali says that they should have a strong balanced state of discerning intelligence, *nirmāṇa- -cittāni asmitā-mātrāt* (IV.4),[1] so that even when celestial beings seduce such yogis with temptations (III.52), the chances of the yogi getting involved with those attachments are avoided.

1 Fabricating mind (*citta*) springs from the sense of individuality (*asmitā*).

6. *Citta Nirūpaṇa* (Representation or Definition of *Citta*)

The main characteristic of *citta* is to be the bridge connecting the seer with the principles of nature that exist in his body. The seer is inherently illuminative but *citta*, which is a part of nature, is not.

***eka-samaye ca ubhaya-anava-dhāraṇam* (IV.20)**

Citta cannot comprehend the seer and itself at the same time.

Citta, not being civilised, claims itself as the seer because it is in close proximity to the seer. The essential need of the *sādhaka* is to purify itself from all obstacles that impede its acceptance of the supremacy of the seer.

***pravṛtti-bhede prayojakaṁ cittaṁ ekam anekeṣām* (IV.5)**

Though consciousness is one, it appears to act as many due to our capacity and power of understanding. As mind is part of conciousness, the various facets of mind given on pages 56–7 stand also for the multiple tendencies of consciousness.

***vastu-sāmye citta-bhedāt tayoḥ vibhaktaḥ panthāḥ* (IV.15)**

The substance of an object may be the same. On account of qualitative variations in the development of our intelligence, the way we perceive an object may vary, but its essence or substance remains the same. There is a famous allegory describing six blind men touching an elephant. Their different perceptions, or their lack of understanding, makes each conceive the same elephant differently. In the same way, we may view the same object differently according to the quality of development in our intelligence and consciousness (*mūḍha*, *kṣipta*, *vikṣipta*, *ekāgra*, *niruddha*).

***na ca eka-citta--tantraṁ ced vastu tat-apramāṇakaṁ tadā kiṁ syāt* (IV.16)**

The existence of an object or its essence cannot be denied because consciousness does not conceive it. When an object is not perceived by the mind and consciousness, this does not mean that the object does not exist. Even when an object is perceived, each person conceives it differently.

***tad-uparāga--apekṣitvāt cittasya vastu jñāta-ajñātam* (IV.17)**	Due to the conditioning of consciousness, it may misinterpret the object it sees because it cannot perceive it correctly.
***sadā jñātāḥ citta-vṛttayaḥ tatprabhoḥ puruṣasya apariṇāmitvāt* (IV.18)**	The seer, or the *puruṣa*, is changeless, eternal and self-illuminative. He is the Lord or master of consciousness (*citta*).
***na tat-svābhāsaṁ dṛśyatvāt* (IV.19)**	*Ātman* is inherently illuminative. It can act at the same time as a subject or as an object, as an actor or a witness. *Citta*, being a knowable object to the seer, has no light of its own. Hence it is perceivable and knowable to the seer.
***citta-antara-dṛśye buddhi-buddheḥ atiprasaṅgaḥ smṛti-saṅkaraḥ ca* (IV.21)**	Consciousness is one. Due to ignorance, heedlessness and immaturity, it appears in plurality, leading towards confusion. Like the facets of a diamond, it creates the illusion that the faculties of intelligence and the mind are many. This creates a situation of perpetual confusion.

Reflecting on these *sūtras* (*see also sūtras* IV.22–24 and IV.32 in the next chapter), we can understand the complex ways of the functioning of consciousness and the treacherous and difficult ground that the yogi has to walk through. It is only through judicious handling of the latent impressions (IV.28),[1] with supreme focused awareness, that the yogi can come within sight of achieving his quest.

1 *hānam eṣāṁ kleśavat uktam* (IV.28) – In the same way as the *sādhaka* strives to be free from afflictions, the yogi must handle these latent impressions judiciously to extinguish them.

VIII

Citta Lakṣaṇa – Characteristics of Consciousness

The body and consciousness are part of nature (*prakṛti*). This means that *mūla prakṛti* is the support of consciousness. Since consciousness is a part of *prakṛti*, we should examine its nature and its principles before trying to understand its *lakṣaṇa*, or characteristic changes. (*See table opposite.*)

Before considering the central role of *citta* in this table, I would like to recall your attention to the correspondence between the senses of perception and the infrastructure of the elements:

Ears	represent	ether's quality	sound (*śabda*)
Skin	represents	air's quality	touch (*sparśa*)
Eyes	represent	fire's quality	form (*rūpa*)
Tongue	represents	water's quality	taste (*rasa*)
Nose	represents	earth's quality	smell (*gandha*)

As it is described in the table, *citta* or the individual consciousness springs from the first principle of nature, the cosmic or the universal consciousness (*mahat*). Before distinguishing the components of *citta*, let us understand its function. This in turn may help us understand why the path of yoga exists.

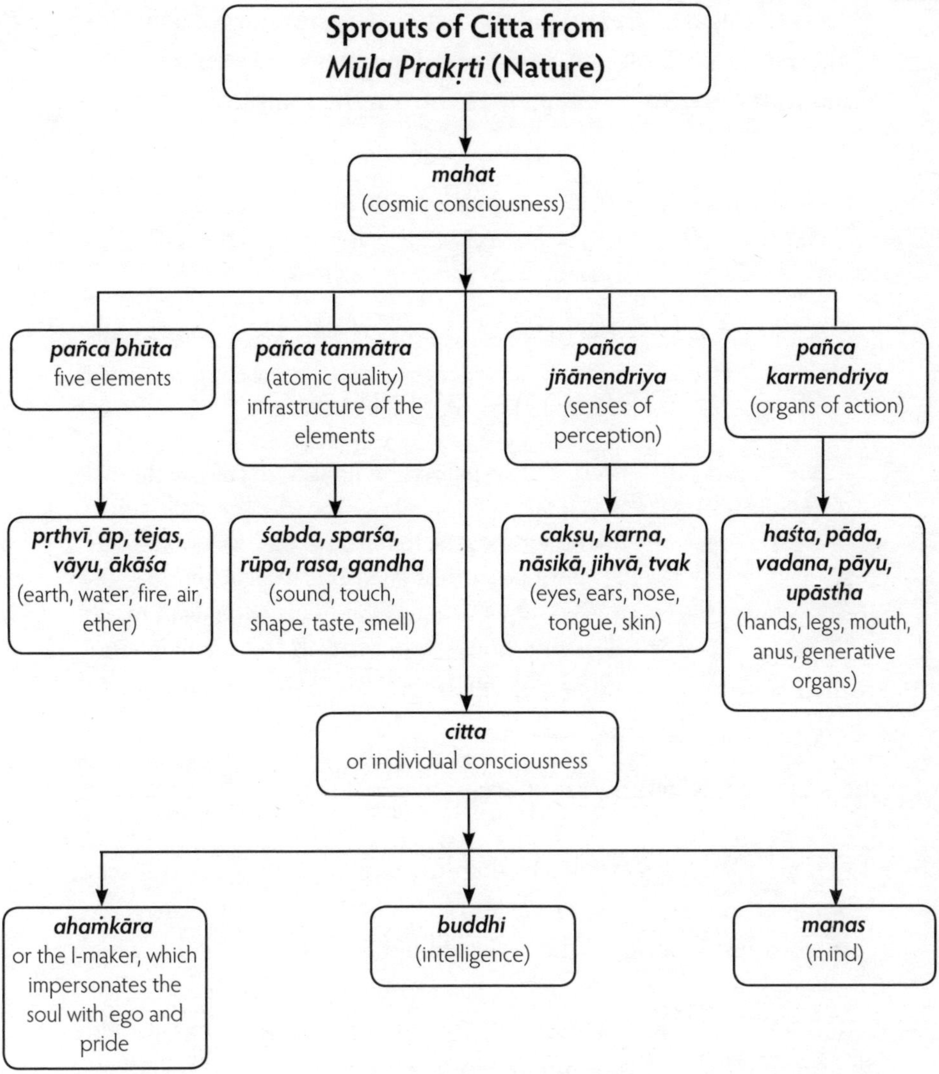

Citta is not a fixed reality; it changes. Its real seat is in the heart, which is where our highest intelligence and spiritual aspirations abide. Awareness of the changeable nature of *citta* brings to light its own limitations and reveals the supremacy of the seer, which is ever-constant.

Describing the properties or qualities of *citta*, Patañjali explains its weaknesses and its inclination and attraction towards objects of desires. He proclaims that *citta* is simultaneously close to the seer and to objects of nature. Hence it is crucial to understand it in order to be emancipated from the temptations of seen objects.

candre tārā-vyūha--jñānam (III.28)	As the moon waxes and wanes, so *citta* waxes and wanes according to variations in thought permutations and combinations.
hṛdaye citta-saṁvit (III.35)	The seat of consciousness is the spiritual heart (seer or soul). Knowledge of consciousness arises through the inner light of the spiritual heart.
dhruve tad-gati--jñānam (III.29)	*Dhruve* is the pole star. It has a fixed place in the sky. If the moon stands for consciousness, the sun stands for the soul. In the same way, *dhruve* stands for intelligence (*buddhi*). Mind gathers imprints and conveys them to the intelligence (*buddhi*) to discriminate and judge correctly and communicate back to the mind how it has to react to these imprints.

Dhruva, the son of King Uttānapāda in *Purāṇa*s, acts as a guiding star for navigation, and here he navigates the right course for the mind.

Though the stars are there when the sun rises, they are not seen. Moonlight allows the stars to be clearly visible. In the same way, consciousness (moon) is the reflected light of the soul (sun), which allows the starlight of intelligence to orientate our wayward thoughts.

All objects illuminated by the *puruṣa* are knowable, examinable and seeable through the *yaugika* journey. Hence *puruṣa*, being ever illuminative and changeless, witnesses consciousness, intelligence, the mind and their *vṛtti*s, and helps in the evolution of man to move closer to the *puruṣa*.

1. *Citta Bhūmi*

Before proceeding to know the qualities (*lakṣaṇa*) of consciousness (*citta*), one should have an idea of its *bhūmi* (its soil or ground).

Citta's evolution has five divisions or states. These states are epitomised by the five elements. Inevitably intelligence and mind also depend on these five states, arranging themselves according to the principle they embody.

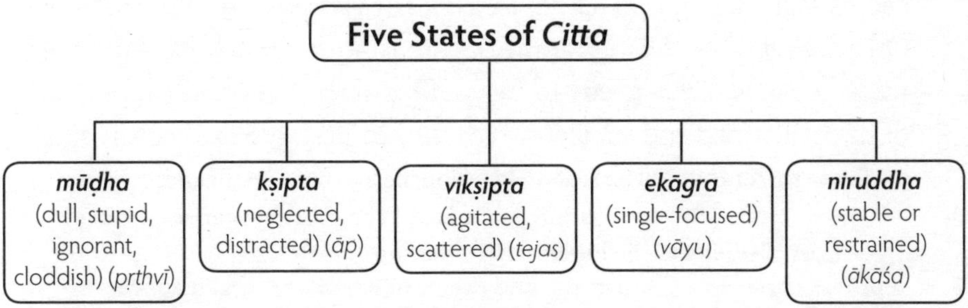

Citta has to be refined and polished to move towards illumination and emancipation. Sage Vyāsa defines these states, starting from a dull *citta*, *buddhi* or *manas*, and progressively moving by refining the mind and intelligence to cross the bridges of *kṣipta* and *vikṣipta* and reach *ekāgra* and *niruddha*. These five states correspond to the growth and evolution of the intelligence. They imply that the evolution of mind and intelligence is harmony with the five elements – *pṛthvī*, *āp*, *tejas*, *vāyu* and *ākāśa*. These have their own characteristics:

Pṛthvī (earth element)	strength, hardness and odour.
Āp (water element)	softness and smoothness or rhythmic flow, taste.
Tejas (fire element)	heat, glow, sight.
Vāyu (air element)	dryness, transparency and touch.
Ākāśa (ether element)	porosity, hearing, sensitivity to vibration.

2. *Citta Lakṣaṇa*

Let us now look at the qualities of *citta lakṣaṇa*.

We already saw that the main characteristic of *citta* is to act as a bridge to connect the seer with the principles of nature through the body. Its function is dependent upon the seer, who is self-illuminative. *Citta* is not self-illuminative. It is dependent upon the light of the seer. As we saw before, consciousness cannot comprehend the seer and itself at the same time (IV.20). Consciousness, being close to the seer, claims that when it is in a *mūḍha, kṣipta* or *vikṣipta* state, it is the seer. On account of *avidyā* (ignorance), *citta* is prone to *mūḍha, kṣipta* or *vikṣipta* states. *Citta* needs to be purified from the *mala* (impurity) of its oscillations and vacillations as they impede it from recognising and accepting the supremacy of the seer.

***pravṛtti-bhede prayojakaṁ cittaṁ ekam anekeṣām* (IV.5)**	Consciousness is one, but according to one's capacity and power of understanding, it appears to act in innumerable spheres.
***sadā jñātāḥ citta-vṛttayaḥ tat-prabhoḥ puruṣasya apariṇā-mitvāt* (IV.18)**	The seer or the *puruṣa* is changeless, eternal and self-illuminative. He is the Lord, the master, the knower of consciousness, which is composed of *ahaṁkāra, buddhi* and *manas*.

It may be easy for readers to understand the state of *kūṭastha cittan* and *pariṇāma citta* by the following example. The *mūla vigraha* is installed permanently as a subject of prayer in temples with *prāṇapratiṣṭhā* (the rites of bringing life into the idol). The replica of the original in the form of *utsava vigraha* is taken out in procession on festival days as a representation of the *mūla vigraha*.

The *mūla vigraha* represents *kūṭastha citta*; and its replica, the *utsava vigraha*, represents *pariṇāma citta*.

***na tat-svābhāsaṁ dṛśyatvāt* (IV.19)**	*Ātman* is self-illuminative but *citta* is not. *Citta* is a perceivable and knowable object to the seer. Its principal characteristic in its relationship with the seer is its knowability or perceptibility.
***eka-samaye ca ubhaya--anava-dhāraṇam* (IV.20)**	*Citta* is unable to comprehend the *ātman* as well as itself or another object at the same time.

***citeḥ apratisaṁkramāyāḥ tad-ākāra-āpattau sva-buddhi--saṁvedanam* (IV.22)**

Consciousness has the power to distinguish its limitations as well as to identify its Master, the Lord.

***draṣṭṛ-dṛśya--uparaktaṁ cittaṁ sarva-arthaṁ* (IV.23)**

The *citta* is the connecting link between the body (*prakṛti*) and the seer (*puruṣa*), and it realises that its light is borrowed from the seer. Then it no longer prides itself as all-pervading and all-knowing.

***tat-asaṅkhyeya--vāsanābhiḥ citram api para-arthaṁ saṁhatya-kāritvāt* (IV.24)**

Consciousness is part of *prakṛti*, with its desires (*vāsanā*) of the world and subliminal impressions (*saṁskāra*) of the past, and is also in close proximity to the seer. Its function is to evolve the senses and mind so that these connect to the seer. Unfortunately, most of the time it is drawn towards the net of desires, ambitions, motivations and pleasures. On account of this close connection with the objects of the world, consciousness with its components must be restrained, civilised and cultivated through *yaugika* practices so that it is drawn closer towards the seer.

***tataḥ kṛtā-arthānāṁ pariṇāma-krama--samāptiḥ guṇānāṁ* (IV.32)**

The *citta* has to weigh and balance the value of knowledge of the world (*laukika jñāna*) for it to be cleansed, eradicating the taints that arise from the objects of the world. *Citta*, along with the organs of action, senses of perception, mind and intelligence, must be immersed in the Self and reach its destination, merging in the *ātman*.

So far, I have explained the significance of consciousness, which can be cultivated, uplifted and nurtured from a state of dullness to reach a dispassionate state.

IX

Citta Śreṇi –
Stages of Consciousness

In the previous chapter, I explained about the various characteristics of consciousness having distinctive marks and functions. I also explained about the various facets of the mind. Here I shall deal with the various stages of the *citta* as explained by Patañjali in order to understand the successive progressions and transformations that take place to realise the ultimate goal of reaching the heart of Pātañjala yoga and experience the divine state of consciousness.

Let me begin with the various states of awareness in the individual consciousness that springs from the first principle of nature, termed the *mahat* or the cosmic consciousness.

Yoga Sūtra II.27 says:

tasya saptadhā prānta-bhūmiḥ prajñā (II.27)	The human consciousness has seven fundamental states or stages or spheres of awareness (*prajñā*). This sūtra speaks of seven states, stages or spheres of consciousness in the form of awareness (*prajñā*). Patañjali explains these seven states as provinces

(*śreṇi*) of consciousness in the following sūtras. *Y. S.* III.9, 10, 12; IV.27 and 29.[1]

Seven Provinces of the *Citta*

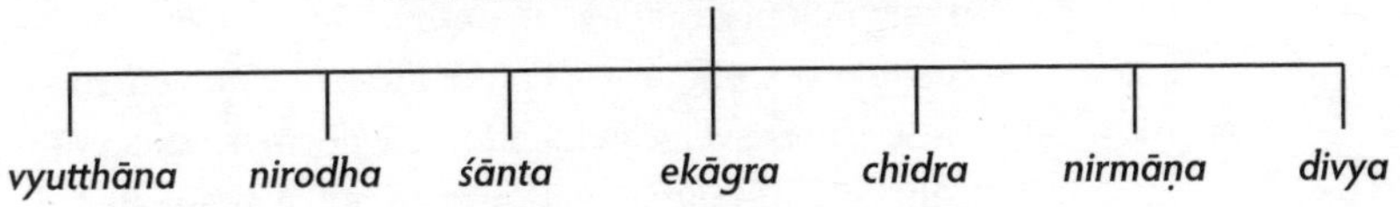

1. *Vyutthāna Citta* and *Nirodha Citta*

***vyutthāna-nirodha--saṁskārayoḥ abhihava--prādurbhāvau nirodha-kṣaṇa--citta-anvayaḥ nirodha-pariṇāmaḥ* (III.9)**

Vyutthāna citta is the wandering consciousness and *nirodha citta* is the restraining consciousness.

Normally we oscillate between the wandering mind and the restraining mind. Between these two states, there is a non-deliberate pause, which we do not think about at all. Patañjali wants us to observe this pause or space that occurs in between these two states of consciousness.

During this pause, consciousness experiences a state of silent quietness. This is the third stage of consciousness, a state of silence and quietude. If we capture this quiet state, it helps us to realise the higher and nobler states of consciousness.

---

1 *vyutthāna-nirodha-saṁskāryoḥ abhibhava-prādurbhāvau nirodha-kṣana-citta--anvayaḥ nirodha-pariṇāmaḥ* (III.9) – *vyutthāna citta* is the rising or wandering state of consciousness. Studying the silent moments between rising and restraining subliminal impressions is the transformation of consciousness towards the restraint (*nirodha pariṇāmaḥ*).

tasya praśānta-vāhitā saṁskārāt (III.10) – The restraint of rising impressions brings about an undisturbed flow of tranquillity.

tataḥ punaḥ śānta-uditau tulya-pratyayau cittasya ekāgratā-pariṇāmaḥ (III.12) – When rising and falling thought processes are brought under control, single-focused consciousness emerges. Maintenance of this state of awareness with keen intensity is *ekāgratā pariṇāma*.

tat-chidreṣu pratyaya-antarāni saṁskārebhyaḥ (IV.27) – If one is careless in this state of attention, then past hidden impressions arise, creating fissures that express the divisions between consciousness and the seer.

prasaṁkhyāne api akusīdasya sarvathā viveka-khyāteḥ dharma-meghaḥ samādhiḥ (IV.29) – The yogi who has no interest even in this highest state of evolution, and maintains supreme attentive, discerning awareness, attains *dharmamegha samādhi*: he contemplates the fragrance of virtue and justice.

***pramāṇa-viparyaya-vikalpa-nidrā-smṛtayaḥ* (I.6)**

The provinces for the thought waves of wandering consciousness are of five types: direct perception or proper understanding; perverse perception or wrong judgement and/or contrary thoughts; fanciful imagination; sleep; and memory. This analysis furthers our enquiries. Out of these five movements, sleep and perverse perception are dormant states of consciousness, imagination is a state of attenuated consciousness and memory interrupts the flow of consciousness. Direct perception is a fully active state of *citta*. Regarding *nirodha citta*, Patañjali begins the text by describing the restraint of consciousness before dealing with its wandering state.

***yogaḥ cittavṛtti-nirodhaḥ* (I.2)**

Patañjali defines the cessation (*nirodha*) of the movements or fluctuations of consciousness (*vyutthāna citta*) as yoga. He explains that *pramāṇa*, *viparyaya*, *vikalpa*, *nidrā* and *smṛti* cause *vyutthāna citta*, or wandering thoughts. As these thoughts run deliberately or non-deliberately helter-skelter, Patañjali advises us to discipline consciousness by restraint.

In *sūtra* III.9, he elaborates upon *sūtras* I.2 and I.6.[1] He respects both the wandering and the restraining states of consciousness, and tries to find the middle line between these in order to tame the wandering *citta*.

At this point I would like to draw your attention to *prāṇāyāma*, where *prāṇa staṁba vṛtti* or *kuṁbhaka vṛtti* (the retention of breath after the in-breath or out-breath) are discussed. I can relate this *prāṇa stambhana vṛtti* to consciousness where a pause takes place between *vyutthāna* and *nirodha citta* and between *nirodha* and *vyutthāna citta* as *citta staṃbha vṛtti*.

***bāhya-abhyantara-staṃbha-vṛttiḥ deśa-kāla-saṁkhyābhiḥ paridṛṣṭaḥ dīrgha-sūkṣmaḥ* (II.50).**

In I.34 (see the chapter on *manas*) Patañjali suggests that the restraint of the breath after exhalation helps to restrain the fluctuations of consciousness.

The *prāṇa staṃbha vṛtti* (restraint of breath) is

1 *pramāṇa-viparyaya-vikalpa-nidrā-smṛtayaḥ* (I.6) – They are caused by correct knowledge, illusion, delusion, sleep and memory.

like the silent moment or peaceful state that happens in between the wandering state and the restraining state of consciousness.

With this connection, we can infer a close relationship of the breath, or *prāṇa*, with the *citta prajñā*.

2. *Śānta Citta*

tasya praśānta-
-vāhitā saṁskārāt
(III.10)

The pause (*nirodha kṣaṇa*) between the wandering and the restraining thought waves of consciousness makes us experience the moment of silence and the perennial flow of tranquillity.

Patañjali wants us to observe this perennial silent state of consciousness and then to expand these moments to experience equipoise (*samāhita citta*).

3. *Ekāgra Citta*

tataḥ punaḥ śānta-
-uditau tulya-
-pratyayau cittasya
ekāgratā-pariṇāmaḥ
(III.12)

As we build up this silent tranquil state of consciousness, the wandering consciousness transforms itself to develop stability to hold on to single-focused attention (*ekāgra citta*).

4. *Chidra Citta*

tat-chidreṣu
pratyaya-antarāṇi
saṁskārebhyaḥ
(IV.27)

After acquiring *ekāgra citta*, if one becomes proud of success and careless or inattentive, the force of the past latent impressions is able to overrule, creating fissures that breach the closeness of the *citta* with the seer.

citta-antara-dṛśye
buddhi-buddheḥ
atiprasaṅgaḥ
smṛti-saṅkaraḥ ca
(IV.21)

Such self-inflicted fault lines may fissure consciousness. Likewise, the power of concentration may intoxicate the practitioner. These seismic shifts rupture one's intellectual stability as well as that of one's consciousness.

Through this breach unwelcome fluctuations and afflictions enter.

Patañjali says, about the effect of *chidra citta:*

hānam eṣāṁ kleśavat uktam **(IV.28)**	[1]If this happens, then it is the downfall of practitioners in their *yaugika* achievements and they have to begin yoga again from the start to return to their illuminated state.

Besides the explanations mentioned above, *chidra citta* can occur through *saṅkara citta* or *saṁskāra citta* (see Chapter X, *saṅkara citta* in *pratikūla vṛtti* and *saṁskāra citta* in *anukūla vṛtti*).

5. *Nirmāṇa Citta*

This state of *citta* is nothing less than a distinguished pure state of consciousness of being one within itself.

vitarka-vicāra- -ānanda-asmitārūpa- -anugamāt saṁpra-jñātaḥ **(I.17)**	Analysis and conjecture, reasoning and synthesising, elation of an inexplicable bliss, and knowing actually the true form of the determined consciousness lead one to feel and experience the illuminative state of the seer. This is *asmitārūpa citta* or *nirmāṇa citta*.
nirmāṇa-cittāni asmitā-mātrāt **(IV.4)**	This established, constant state of consciousness is the sign of an illuminated state of consciousness, which is achieved through practice (*abhyāsa*).

Patañjali explains the states of the wandering consciousness (*citta vṛtti*) in *sūtra*s I.6 to 11. These *vṛtti*s can either taint and distort or construct and guide one to know the true nature of consciousness.

One should consciously channel the thought waves so that one develops, refines and builds up intellectual sensitivity to achieve *nirmāṇa citta* – cultured consciousness or *saṁprajñāta citta* (*sāsmitā-citta*) (I.17).

---

1 The yogi has to relinquish all powers. Otherwise, he will be caught in the web of afflictions at once.

6. *Divya Citta (Paripakva Citta)*

Divya citta is pure *citta*, or divine consciousness.

When supreme intellectual attentiveness and absolute awareness appear, then pure virtues pour from the heart, as rain pours from clouds. In this state the yogi experiences the divine state of evolution. This is the heart of the *yaugika sādhanā*.

When this illuminated wisdom fades, one experiences the *nirbīja samādhi*, which has no seed or ground. This is *ātman sākṣātkāra*, or the heart of the Self.

***tadā sarva-āvaraṇa-mala-apetasya jñānasya ānantyāt-jñeyam alpam* (IV.31)**

When the veils of all impurities are extinguished, the infinite subjective wisdom of experience is sighted, and thereafter all finite things appear trivial.

***puruṣa-artha-śūnyānāṁ guṇānāṁ pratiprasavaḥ kaivalyaṁ sva-rūpa-pratiṣṭhā vā citi-śaktiḥ iti* (IV.34)**

In the final state of involutory evolution, all the principles of nature return to their unmanifested (*avyakta*) state for the seer (*citi*) to manifest (*vyakta*) in the final state of the *sādhanā*. With this manifested state, the seer moves towards surrendering totally to God, culminating in *Īśvara praṇidhāna*.

Thus the *Yoga Sūtra* begins from a state of disarranged, wandering consciousness to reach the stabilised state of consciousness via the path of *yaugika* discipline, according to the zeal with which one practises it.

Though I have dealt with the higher and nobler aspects of consciousness, I would like to remind readers that it is not easy to experience the highest divine state of consciousness, as we find ourselves in a snake-pit of undisciplined thought waves and afflictions, which disturb and impede consciousness. These disturbances and impediments may be hidden, and only surface when one begins to take to *sādhanā*.

In order to overcome these drawbacks, Patañjali explains that one should not only face these hurdles but also cross over them through correct *yaugika* methodology. Hence the next chapter discusses *kleśa*s, *vṛtti*s and *antarāya*s.

X

Kleśa, Vṛtti and *Antarāya* – Afflictions, Fluctuations and Impediments

In the *Yoga Sūtras*, Patañjali speaks of *citta vṛtti*s and *antarāya*s first (Chapter I) and then of *kleśa*s (Chapter II). Here I have taken them in reverse order since today's lifestyle means it is easy to have a better understanding of the states of disturbances. Both *kleśa* and *antarāya* are conscious feelings, which motivate one to find means to get rid of them, whereas it may take time for anyone to realise how *citta vṛtti* functions and affects the body, mind and self. *Kleśa*s and *antarāya*s are exclusively subjective, whereas *citta-vṛtti*s are objective as well as subjective.

*Kleśa*s and *antarāya*s affect the body first and then the mind. They can be thought of as somato-psychic disorders. *Vṛtti*s knowingly or unknowingly may create confusion and doubt, leading to psycho-somatic disorders.

We have already seen that each one of us is reborn according to the imprints of merits and demerits from past lives. These create mental fluctuations in the form of thought waves (*vṛtti*s), psycho-physiological afflictions (*kleśa*s) and emotional upheavals or intense feelings of joy tinted with pain, anger or sadness. These disturb the equilibrium between the body, mind and self, creating obstacles or impediments (*antarāyas*) in our ways of living.

Like the sparks from a fire, which are scattered, vary in size and spread out unpredictably in different directions, thought waves and afflictions sprout from the disc of consciousness and move in various directions with or without reason.

Patañjali enumerates five afflictions (*kleśas*), nine obstacles (*antarāyas*) and five thought waves (*vṛttis*). Though these afflictions, obstacles and fluctuations appear as if they function independently, they are definitely interrelated and interwoven.

Patañjali states that the five movements of the mind may be *kliṣṭa* (painful, perceptible or knowable) or *akliṣṭa* (non-painful, imperceptible or unknowable). Sooner or later, these *vṛttis* create imbalances in one's psychological and mental faculties, causing disturbances. Yet, they can also be used to bring about a positive mental balance and stability in the mind and consciousness.

Afflictions (*kleśas*) may be somatic or somato-psychic, psychic or psycho-somatic, creating imbalances at physical, physiological, ethical, psychological, emotional or intellectual levels.

Most of us can recognise the root problems caused by afflictions, as they corrode not only the body but the mind, disturbing one's intellectual calibre and consciousness.

Therefore, irrespective of one's intellectual calibre, one must give equal attention not only to the thought waves but also to bodily afflictions. Otherwise one ends up with grief, distress and sorrow. These in turn lead to an increase in nervous energy and laboured breathing, adding further distractions to consciousness (I.31).

Patañjali speaks of nine impediments in I.30 and four in I.31, which run concurrently. The last four impediments of I.31 seem more like symptoms of disease rather than impediments. They are like the symptoms used to diagnose disease today and can be investigated according to modern scientific approaches.

Patañjali, being a man of medicine, speaks in clear terms of the ill-effects that affect the body and mind due to fluctuating thought waves and afflictions. Even contrary thought waves (*pratikūla vṛtti*) lead one towards sorrow, distress, pain and physical suffering. It is also possible that sorrow and distress affect the mind in generating contrary thoughts.

*Vṛtti*s and *kleśa*s are closely related and interdependent. They intensify contrary thoughts, fuelling further fears, worries and anxieties.

If one develops favourable *vṛtti*s by accepting the conditions of the body and mind, and works through *yaugika* discipline, these *kleśa*s and *antarāya*s are eradicated or minimised, and one acquires the power to proceed in spiritual pursuits.

There is an old story of a farmer who was proud of the fruits produced in his orchard. There was one diseased tree that never produced anything of value but merely took up space in the orchard. He tried everything, but couldn't get rid of that tree. He tried cutting it down, but it would grow again from a shoot. He tried poisoning it, but it never quite died. Then one day, following someone's advice, he planted many healthy trees around it. They were vigorous and healthy trees that suited the environment well. Soon it was difficult to see where that diseased tree was amongst them. Gradually those beneficial healthy trees took over the entire space and when the farmer looked for his old adversary, that diseased tree couldn't be found; it had become healthy and on its branches were growing splendid crops of beautiful fruits.

This is *sahavāsa guṇa*, or the qualities one develops through good companionship.

Kleśas are five in number:

avidyā-asmitā-rāga--dveṣa-abhiniveśāḥ kleśāḥ **(II.3)**

These are ignorance (*avidyā*), ego or pride, which acts as an imposter of the seer (*ahaṁkāra-asmitā*), attachment (*rārga*), aversion (*dveṣa*), and anxiety or fear of death (*abhiniveśa*), as if life were eternal.

anitya-aśuci-duḥkha--anātmasu-nitya-śuci--sukha-ātma-khyātiḥ avidyā **(II.5)**

Thinking of what is not permanent as permanent, impure as pure and clean, pain as pleasure and non-eternal as eternal is ignorance (*avidyā*).

What is *asmitā?*

***dṛg-darśana-śaktyoḥ eka-ātmatā iva asmitā* (II.6)**	False identification of the seen for the seer or the conception of the ego as the seer is *asmitā*.
***draṣṭṛ-dṛśya--uparaktaṁ cittaṁ sarva-arthaṁ* (IV.23)**	Mistaking the knowable consciousness as the seer and considering it to be all-comprehending is an illusive knowledge. This *sūtra* explains how egoist *asmitā* creates deep afflictions, which disturb the healthy functioning of consciousness.

The feeling of *asmitā* is the result of the conjunction of the seen with the seer. But this conjunction is definitely essential in order to know the reality of the seer: if one develops a mature intelligence and makes use of this conjunction to study, reflect and understand, the false *asmitā* is dispersed and transformed into a true state of *asmitā*.

***sukha-anuśayī rāgaḥ* (II.7)**	Pleasure leads to attachment, which triggers desire after desire as if enjoyments were eternal bliss.
***duḥkha-anuśayī dveṣaḥ* (II.8)**	Want of satisfaction from pleasures and joys brings irritation, frustration, hatred and malice. This is why a wise man identifies attachments as being eternally tinged with sorrow and pain and tries to keep aloof from attachment and aversion (*see* II.15).
***svarasa-vahī viduṣaḥ api tathā rūḍhaḥ abhiniveśaḥ* (II.9)**	The subtlest of all afflictions is attachment to life and fear of death. The more we identify with the seen – *avidyā* and *asmitā* – the more we fear death and struggle to project the life of the ego even beyond death. This type of attachment does not leave even the wisest of the wise men.

If *avidyā* and *asmitā* have their source in the weaknesses of the intellect, *rāga* and *dveṣa* develop from the weak intelligence of the mind (mental heart), and *abhiniveśa* is the latent impression of past experiences (*pūrva saṁskāra vṛtti*). Let us consider *abhiniveśa*. Here it is the fear of death. This fear of death comes from the egoistic self and, paradoxically, it is the desire for the continuation of the *citta*. At least this fear of death makes us do good in this life, fearing that something bad may affect the next life.

***te pratiprasava- -heyāḥ sūkṣmāḥ* (II.10)**	If these afflictions penetrate deep inside consciousness, they corrode the mind, creating psycho-somatic problems. *Avidyā* could be eradicated through the process of de-coding old thoughts and re-coding the thinking process in order to make the senses of perception run in the right direction. This right way of thinking is possible if one either dissociates from the seen permanently or understands the purpose of the seen and works out ways to use it to discover one's own true nature.

This *sūtra* conveys two ways of thinking:

- If one goes on thinking over and over about afflictions, it becomes a foothold for psycho-somatic or somato-psychic illnesses and makes one succumb to the nine *antarāyas*.
- Or, if the *sādhaka* meditates on what is eternal, involuting his senses of perception, mind and intelligence towards the seer, he will be able to eradicate totally these afflictions or minimise their impact on the body and mind. (See I.24 and 29.)[1]

By now, the reader must have obtained a clear picture of how fluctuating thought waves, sorrows, pain and anxieties cause obstacles and how these can be minimised or totally eradicated by the pursuit of *yaugika sādhanā*.

---

1 *kleśa-karma-vipāka-āśayaiḥ aparāmṛṣṭaḥ puruṣa-viśeṣaḥ Īśvaraḥ* (I.24) – God is the supreme being, totally free from conflicts, unaffected by actions and untouched by cause and effect.

tataḥ pratyak-cetanā-adhigamaḥ api antarāya abhāvaḥ ca (I.29) – Meditation on God with the repetition of *āuṁ* removes obstacles and leads towards mastery of the inner self.

1. *Vṛttis*

The sun's rays do not affect us just before rising and after setting. Similarly, consciousness is without thought when asleep or when awakening from sleep. When it becomes fully active, thoughts flash and flicker out from the seat of consciousness like sparks from a fire.

As the sun rises and reaches the zenith, it emits millions of light-rays, making it impossible for anyone to stare directly at it. Similarly, consciousness, in its normal day-to-day functioning, fluctuates with many thought waves. At any moment, it may connect to the self within or to the objects of the world. At different times it reacts with right knowledge and perception of facts, with wrong notions, or with fanciful ideas, and at other times it reverts to a particular state of mind, such as sleep, or acts according to memory.

Following the definition of *sūtra* I.2, '*yogaḥ citta-vṛtti-nirodhaḥ*'[1] this fluctuating consciousness has to be restrained for the seer to reveal himself in his true form. Until consciousness is trained and re-conditioned enough to restrain its own functioning (*vṛtti*), we remain affected by confused thought fluctuations, modulations and modifications.

*Citta vṛtti*s are classified into five categories:

vṛttayaḥ pañcatayyaḥ kliṣṭa--akliṣṭāḥ **(I.5)**

These five thought waves can be either painful (*kliṣṭa*) or non-painful (*akliṣṭa*), perceptible or imperceptible, active or non-active, dormant or non-dormant, and helpful or non-helpful. If thought waves move in line with spiritual pursuits, then they are termed favourable (*anukūla*) *vṛtti*s. If the power of thought waves moves against the true aims of life, these are termed non-favourable thought waves (*pratikūla vṛtti*s).

These painful (*kliṣṭa*) or non-painful (*akliṣṭa*) thought waves are like the rim of a bicycle wheel where the inflated tyre is trapped between the two edges of the wheel rim.

1 Yoga is the cessation of movements in consciousness.

These five types of *vṛtti*s (which are explained later) can:

help the practitioner make a dynamic progress towards acquiring spiritual knowledge;

or

bind him to perpetual cycles of lives, pointlessly searching for fulfilment that brings only pain.

If the *sādhaka* resists any active response between the two rims of thought waves, his path will then be vibrant and luminous. If he is caught and gets entangled in the net of thoughts without reflection or consideration, then the same thought waves trap his progress, creating not only a state of constant restlessness but also hindering him from knowing the self.

We have already seen that the movements of these five types of thought waves define and decide the course of lives to come. Their restraint is the decisive and defining act in their return to the true state of the Self. We shall take a deeper look into the significance of these five through the following *sūtra*s.

pratyakṣa-anumāna- -āgamāḥ pramāṇāni **(I.7)**	Valid knowledge may come through the proper and direct understanding of experience; through investigation, inference or reasoning; or through study of the authoritative scriptures or masters.

Hidden in this *sūtra* is a description of the threefold path undertaken by followers of yoga. We begin by studying and taking guidance from experienced masters, or their recorded testimony. We practise, learn and experience what was condensed in those teachings through our own investigation and experience to arrive at the state whereby we see, understand and experience directly, gaining insight into the true status of our relationship with the seer.

viparyayaḥ mithyā- -jñānam atad-rūpa pratiṣṭham **(I.8)**	Misperception or contrary thoughts, twisting the basic facts or reversing the facts arises due to the erroneous understanding or perception of an object.

***śabda-jñāna-anupātī vastu-śūnyaḥ vikalpaḥ* (I.9)**	Misconception, hearsay, conjecture, surmise, assumption and imagination are just verbal knowledge, which lacks substance and ends in fancy.
***abhāva-pratyaya--ālambanā vṛttiḥ nidrā* (I.10)**	In sleep there is an absence of knowledge and understanding as well as a state of absent-mindedness; the senses are in inertia, without awareness, stunned, numb and thoughtless. At the same time, sleep is refreshing, due to the quietening of the senses. A good, deep sleep may be described as a sound sleep. Here the awareness of the seer witnesses the sleep and expresses its effect. This is the twofold characteristic of the seer.
***anubhūta-viṣaya--asaṁpramoṣaḥ smṛtiḥ* (I.11)**	Memory is nothing but an unmodified collection of words and experiences.

The function of memory is to remember, recollect and recognise. These points of memory can be used for progression or regression. If it is used as a base towards refinement, it enables progress. If a person lives in memory and does not make constructive use of it, then his acts become repetitive and stale.

These *vṛtti*s may help to obtain right knowledge and understanding – or they may put a brake on acquiring right knowledge. Making use of right knowledge and understanding may restrain the *vṛtti*s, leading towards evolution; the difference between right and wrong judgements is immediately obvious.

Being negligent and heedless may introduce agitation, dullness and a wrong interpretation of memory or facts.

The effects of *vṛtti*s depend on the way one interprets and uses their form and content. As such, even *āgama* (authoritative scriptures or testimony of realised masters) can be *kliṣṭa* or *akliṣṭa*, depending on the intellectual capacity of the reader and his interpretation. In the case of someone who gets confused after reading books, for example, the *āgama* becomes *kliṣṭa* as it creates *saṅkara citta vṛtti*s.

This is why I classify favourable thoughts (*anukūla vṛttis*) and unfavourable or adverse thoughts (*pratikūla vṛttis*) in terms of the support or lack of support they offer for the pursuit of the self.

2. *Saṁskāra Vṛtti*

Before dealing with the very important subject of favourable and unfavourable *vṛttis* and their interactions, I will discuss some *sūtras* that are of interest for intensifying the *sādhanā*. These are *sūtras* on latent impressions of actions in word, thought and deed (*saṁskāras*), which are earned and stored. Some of these *saṁskāras* are conducive to *yaugika* practices and may help the *sādhaka* to practise with further intensity and keenness.

Though it is said that *saṁskāras* or imprints have to be discarded at the time of reaching seedless *samādhi* or *nirbīja samādhi*, they do play an important role because the merited (*puṇya*) or unmerited (*pāpa*) *saṁskāras* have a close relationship with memory.

For example, Patañjali says that in between *sabīja samādhi* and *nirbīja samādhi* there is an intermission or pause.

virāma-pratyaya-abhyāsa-pūrvaḥ saṁskāra-śeṣaḥ anyaḥ **(I.18)**

In this state, *citta* is kept free from pleasures and sorrows or wants and desires. Similarly, *citta* is a non-oscillating state between thoughts. Hence, one has to increase or enhance this state of pause in between thoughts.

As one progresses in *sādhanā*, new developments take place, creating further *puṇya saṁskāras*.

taj-jaḥ saṁskāraḥ anya-saṁskāra-pratibandhī **(I.50)**

Though latent impressions remain quiet, the knowledge and wisdom gained in the *virāma pratyaya* state must be made use of so that previous impressions are left behind and new ones are presented.

saṁskāra-sākṣāt-karaṇāt pūrva-jā-ti-jñānam **(III.18)**

With this new direct perception, knowledge and wisdom, subliminal impressions may arise. These must also be kept away.

It is interesting to know that though many think that all imprints begin and end in each life, and each life is independent of residual imprints, Patañjali says that life is a continuous process that bears residual imprints until one reaches the state of emancipation.

tāsām anāditvaṁ ca āśiṣaḥ nityatvāt **(IV.10)**	Though these latent impressions, memories and desires co-exist eternally, they can be extinguished, like dry leaves dropping off a tree, through *yaugika sādhanā.*

The next *sūtra* clearly mentions that it is possible to get rid of all past and present impressions.

hetu phala āśraya ālambanaiḥ saṅgṛhītatvāt eṣām abhāve tad abhāvaḥ **(IV.11)**	Impressions and desires are dependent upon the principles of cause and effect. If one ceases to function, the other also ceases to function.

All these *saṁskāras* can be utilised to maintain *sādhanā* and achieve further refinement.

3. *Anukūla* and *Pratikūla Vṛtti*

Vṛttis are such that some may help the *sādhaka* in the goal of spiritual pursuits or they may regress a *sādhaka* by putting a brake on his spiritual path.

Here, I am presenting both aspects of the *vṛttis* so that the *sādhaka* can plan to move in the right direction on the chosen path to Self-realisation (*see table overleaf*).

4. *Anukūla Vṛtti*

I already mentioned that *anukūla vṛttis* are helpful, friendly and favourable. Carelessness, heedlessness and arrogance may play against *anukūla vṛttis* and mar one's progress on the chosen path.

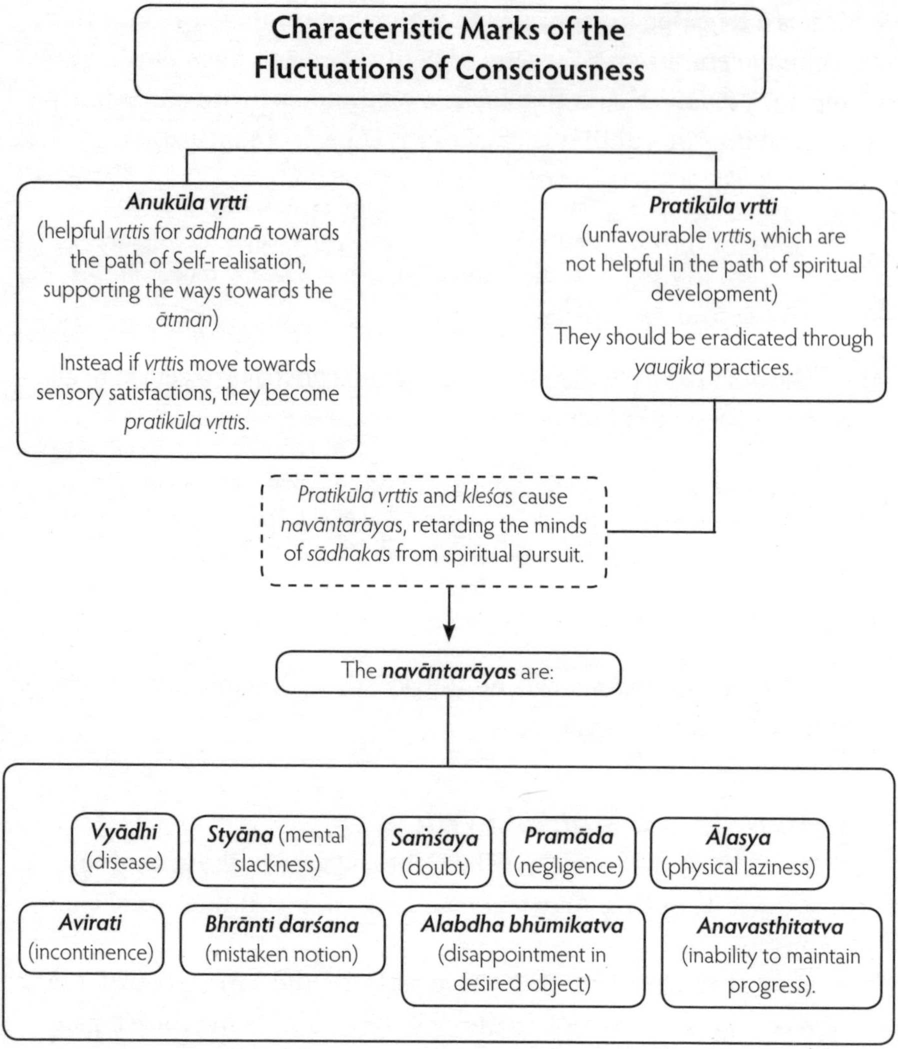

The following *sūtras* help the *sādhakas* directly to build up the qualities needed to stop unfavourable thoughts and help in removing wants, desires and impressions. From *sūtra* I.33, Patañjali explains indirectly the eight petals of yoga, explaining their functions without going into detail. These are explained in detail in the *Sādhana Pāda*.

maitrī-karuṇā- ***-muditā-upēkṣāṇāṁ*** ***sukha-duḥkha-*** ***-puṇya-apuṇya-*** ***-viṣayāṇāṁ*** ***bhāva-nātaḥ-citta-*** ***-prasādanam*** **(I.33)**	Patañjali suggests that one should cultivate friendliness towards one and all, show compassion particularly towards the needy, develop joyousness to those who are better placed than oneself or to be grateful to God (for one's positive life condition) when looking at those placed beneath you, build indifference to pleasure and pain, virtue and vice, and then create conditions that help one's consciousness to maintain itself evenly in all circumstances. By cultivating this state of consciousness, all deviations and differences in thought waves are favourably disposed, enabling one to move towards the spiritual path.
maitrī-ādiṣu balāni **(III.24)** ***baleṣu hasti-*** ***-bala-ādīni*** **(III.25)**	The effects of *maitrī* in the form of moral and physical strength are mental stability, grace, endurance and a memory like that of an elephant.

On the face of it, *sūtra* I.33 appears to convey a message of social health and well-being. Yet, if the message of this *sūtra* is objective, there is also an underlying subjective message where friendliness and compassion stand for *yama* and *niyama*, while joy and indifference correspond more to the practice of *āsana*s and *prāṇāyāma*s in order to eradicate the nine obstacles or impediments.

Now, when in I.31–32 he enumerates the *antarāya*s, I feel that some defects like *vyadhi* and *styāna* are objective since they are defects in the body, whereas some other defects like lack of alignment and symmetry (*see* verse 13 in chapter VI of the *Bhagavad Gītā*) are subjective, having causes outside the body, like habits of life or acquired defects. *Sūtra* I.33 stipulates that these *antarāya*s must be eradicated with the means of *āsana-abhyāsa* (I.32) and, once cured, fixed, stabilised or under control, one must treat them with *muditā* and *upekṣa*. The latter means, in this sense, *vairāgya*.

Then from the next *sūtra* (I.34)[1] Patañjali introduces gradually and systematically the different aspects of *aṣṭāṅga yoga* from *prāṇāyāma* onwards until *dhyāna* (I.39).[2]

The body has its own constitution and systems with the mind as well as numerous muscles, joints, organs and so forth. When the functions of the body are disturbed, the harmony of the mind too is disturbed. Hence, I feel that this *sūtra* implies a message as well as an approach to treat the body with friendliness and compassion and to be glad when it can look after itself. Then, when it can do so on its own, to be indifferent to it. Without this thoughtful attention to all the various layers of our inner and outer lives, there is no way to encourage consciousness towards evolution.

In today's conditions, I would like to apply this *sūtra* to the body since true health covers physical, moral, mental and intellectual provinces. People have lost their sensitivity to be able to work intelligently with the body, which is the soul's support. Through application of *maitrī*, *karuṇā*, *muditā* and *upekṣā*, we can attain harmony within ourselves. Sensual enjoyment and pleasures have become the fashion of the day in place of the true culture of physical, moral, mental and emotional harmony.

Therefore I am particularly referring to the body's ethics: morality begins by looking after the soul's prop or the envelope – the body – in order to make life noble and worth living.

Patañjali suggests an alternative way to make the body – the envelope of the soul – divinely healthy so that it opens the gate of the soul that is hidden deep inside it.

***pracchardana- -vidhāraṇābhyāṁ vā prāṇasya* (I.34)**	Patañjali says that with retention (*bāhya kuṁbhaka*) after complete exhalation, the mind automatically gains quietness by which consciousness becomes quiet, passive and pensive.

---

1 *pracchardana-vidhāraṇābhyāṁ vā prāṇasya* – Or, by maintaining the pensive state felt at the time of soft and steady exhalation and during passive retention after exhalation.

2 *yathā abhimata-dhyānāt vā* – Or, by meditating on any desired object conducive to steadiness of consciousness.

As he speaks of *prāṇāyāma* here, and *pratyāhāra*, *dhāraṇā* and *dhyāna* later, I feel that *maitrī*, *karuṇā* and *muditā-upekṣā* together stand for *yama*, *niyama* and *āsana*. Being friendly to the body, needing compassion when it is affected by obstacles and needs, being clad when it is healthy, and showing non-attachment (*upekṣā*) when it can take care of itself on its own.

***viṣayavatī vā pravṛttiḥ utpannā manasaḥ sthiti--nibandhanī* (I.35)** Focusing on a subject or an object that helps the *citta* to remain steady (*kūṭastha* state) is yet another method suggested to achieve mind control (*pratyāhāra*).

This *sūtra* guides the *sādhaka*'s mind to get away from external means and move towards the internal means to acquire maturity and steadiness in consciousness.

The internal disturbances that occur in the forms of sorrow, mental disturbances, unsteadiness of the body and laboured or heavy breathing (I.31) have to be understood, realised and acted upon with faith and will, using memory as a springboard to encourage profound awareness and supreme devotion in the *sādhaka*. (I.20)[1]

A similar emphasis is again laid on awareness:

***deśa-bandhaḥ cittasya dhāraṇā* (III.1)** *Dhāraṇā* is the focusing of attention inside or outside the body, which helps in stilling the oscillations and vacillations of the intelligence and consciousness.

From consciousness, the *sūtra*s take us towards the seer.

***viśokā vā jyotiṣmatī* (I.36)** As the *antaryāmin* (*puruṣa*) is luminous, sorrowless and radiant, focusing on that *antaryāmin* can be correlated to *anukūla vṛtti*, which brings stability in consciousness and serenity in the self. The focus on

1 *śraddhā-vīrya-smṛti-samādhi-prajñā-pūrvakaḥ itareṣām* (I.20) – Practice must be pursued with trust, confidence, vigour, keen memory and power of absorption to break this spiritual complacency.

luminosity works to raise and bring lightness to the texture of consciousness itself.

***vīta-rāga-viṣayaṁ vā cittam* (I.37)**

Thinking of the lives of fearless, enlightened saints, sages and philosophers like Vyāsa, Bhartṛhari, great *ācārya*s, Saint Jñāneśvara, Tukārāma, or prophets like Mohamed, Moses, Christ or Zarathustra, who were free from desires, affections and attachments, practitioners following their ways of living can make the wandering, restless or anxious mind calm, steady and stable. Their lives provide a refuge for the heart that is inspirationally uplifting.

This and the next *sūtra* speak about gaining total absorption.

***svapna-nidrā-jñāna--ālambanaṁ vā* (I.38)**

Maintaining a steady state of awareness during transition periods between dreamy, sleepy and wakeful states, and recollecting those dreamy and sleepy mental states while awake, helps us to gain a single state of stable *citta*. It is one aspect of *dhyāna*.

We must keep in mind that *dhyāna* in its relationship with *vṛtti*s can be either constructive or destructive. For example, a positive approach to conquer *vṛtti*s with the motto of 'I face it' may be considered a constructive *dhyāna*, whereas the idea of 'I lose' when facing somato-psychic *vṛtti*s is a destructive approach.

***yathā-abhimata--dhyānāt vā* (I.39)**

The seeker on the path of spiritual pursuit can choose whatever object is conducive to achieve a steady consciousness. He should be totally engrossed in it. Knowing about the 'I' or the individual self (*jīvātman*) that is freed from the possessiveness of clinging and aversion is the most conducive object, as 'I' is the closest to the seer.

Reaching this state of stable consciousness, once develops direct perception and conceives with comfort, and without depending on *anumāna* or *āgama*. Having reached this un-altering *jñāna* and wisdom, one has no more need of scriptures for furthering *sādhanā* (*see* I.7 and I.49).

In I.7 Patañjali says *pratyakṣa anumāna āgamaḥ pramāṇāni* – i.e., the requirements for spiritual *sādhanā* are direct experienced knowledge, reasoning or reference to sacred books.

He clarifies later that:

***śruta-anumāna--prajñābhyām anya--viṣayā viśeṣa--arthatvāt* (I.49)** When one has reached the un-oscillating state of knowledge (*paripakva asmitā* state) through direct perception, the first-hand knowledge and shining wisdom (*vivekaja jñāna*) dawns, enabling one to proceed in pursuit of the genuine and authentic light of the soul. Then one no longer depends on knowledge gleaned through books, the precepts of others or testimony (I.7).

5. *Pratikūla Vṛtti*

***tasya hetuḥ avidyā* (II.24)** The cause for adverse currents of thought waves is ignorance or want of understanding as well as the demerits of past lives.

In *citta vṛttis*, I already discussed *pramāṇa, viparyaya, vikalpa, nidrā* and *smṛti*. However, these five *vṛttis* are referred to here under this epigraph of *pratikūla vṛtti*. In fact, when any of the five kinds of movements or fluctuations of consciousness is not conducive towards the stillness or restraining of *citta*, it is to be considered as adverse (*pratikūla*) *vṛttis*. Hence Patañjali classified the *pañca vṛtti* as *kliṣṭa* or *akliṣṭa* (tormenting and non-tormenting).

In this chapter I want to add one more *vṛtti: saṅkara citta vṛtti* (admixture of thoughts), which impedes evolution. *Saṅkara citta* is the admixture and confusion of thoughts, or the mixing of different types of thoughts (see *Y.S.*, IV.21). *Bhagavad Gītā* also explores the concept of the admixture of thoughts, or *saṅkara citta*, in I.41–43.

Pramāṇa as valid knowledge is earned through direct perception, inference and authoritative scriptures. These may misguide those who see it in a wrong way or who draw inferences, as a person with jaundice sees everything tinged with yellow. Just as clear sight is restored as soon as the jaundice is cured, the same is true of *vikalpa*. Take as an example a person who mistakes a rope for a serpent; the moment he sees with a right perspective that it is a rope and not a serpent, his imagination is silenced. Similarly, too much sleep or an induced sleep creates a dull state of mind, whereas good healthy sleep makes one active and fresh. Even memory, when coloured, influences one with imaginative or mixed thoughts, creating disturbances that bring unfavourable thoughts.

This mixture of ideas and thoughts occurs to all of us in varying degrees as our words, along with their sounds and meanings, superimpose and lose their connections. For a yogi with mature wisdom, the word, and its meaning and feeling, are very clear without any change or division between them.

***śabda-artha- -pratyayānām itara-itara adhyāsāt saṅkaraḥ tat-pravibhāga- -saṁyamāt sarva- -bhūta-rūta-jñānam* (III.17)**

Mixed words, objects, ideas and purposes may get superimposed, creating confusion.

If all superimposed thoughts are transformed towards favourable thoughts, the journey towards *ātma-darśana* becomes easy.

Good *saṁskāras* act favourably while bad *saṁskāras* act unfavourably on our path of evolution, creating fissures in our consciousness and resulting in confused states. Only a master yogi can transform such *vṛttis* into favourable *vṛttis* (through *sādhanā*).

6. *Nava Antarāya* (Nine Types of Impediments)

In order to experience the sight of the Self (*ātma-darśana*), one has to undertake a journey, and for that journey four paths are given. These are: the path of action (*karma mārga*), the path of knowledge (*jñāna mārga*), the path of spiritual love (*bhakti mārga*) and the path of yoga (*yoga mārga*). Each path can be seen and followed distinctly. But the paths of *karma*, *jñāna* and *bhakti* are wholly encompassed in *yoga mārga*. So, these three paths can be collectively seen as facets of the one path.

As I said before, in spiritual pursuits, adversaries present themselves in the form of *pratikūla vṛtti*, *kleśa* and *antarāya*. When adversaries come, one should not lose hope, but accept them and continue on the path already chosen (the path of *śraddhā*). We have to accept that our present circumstances are the result of our actions in previous lives (for both good and bad). With right thoughts let us stick to right actions in this present life (*kriyamāṇa karma*) so that we build a good foundation to reach the end of the *sādhanā* in the form of experiencing the *ātma-prasādana*.

All these paths have two goals – one is enjoyment of pleasures (*bhoga*) and the other is sight of the self (*ātma-darśana*) as well as the sight of God (*Paramātma-darśana* or *viśva cetana śakti*). *Kleśas* and *antarāyas* issue from cluttered *vṛttis*, which form the basic material for spiritual evolution. Rejecting these means rejecting the path as well. All these impediments are a blessing in disguise on the journey towards the realisation of the *puruṣa* (seer) and *Parama puruṣa* (God).

karma aśukla-
-akṛṣṇam yoginaḥ
trividham itareṣām
(IV.7)

Everyone is caught in performing *kṛṣṇa* (black), *śukla* (white) or grey (the mixture of white and black) actions. We accumulate these obstructions in our vocational pursuits, but the yogi cultivates actions that are beyond these three and carries out a fourth kind of action, which is non-black, non-white and non-mixed.

It is easy to guess what the black and white actions might be, but there are a thousand tints and tones of grey in between. Often our actions may not necessarily be wholly evil (black), or completely pure (white), but in between. If we are free from desire or aversion, our actions are mostly white. If our actions are filled with selfish motives, then our actions are more grey. The yogi's action goes beyond the axis of good and evil (*puṇya* and *apuṇya*). A yogi does all actions just for the sake of refining the actions skilfully, without any other motivation, and remains as a witness to action. He is free from the influence of the *tri-guṇa*, which leave no trace in his actions. This is the fourth type of action.

Hence in this life we have to reconstruct our thoughts, words and deeds (*kriyamāṇa karma*) and act to continuously lessen the black, white or grey actions, so that we may reach the goal – the sight of the soul – in this life or in the lives that follow.

Patañjali explains nine major impediments or obstacles that get in the way of our *sādhanā* and spiritual pursuits, along with four further impediments that act together.

***vyādhi-styāna-*
-saṁśaya-pramāda-
-ālasya-avirati-
-bhrānti-darśana-
-alabdha-
-bhūmikatva-
-anavasthitatvāni
citta-vikṣepāḥ te
antarāyāḥ (I.30)**

These are disease, mental laziness, indecision, carelessness, heedlessness, laziness, self-gratification or a lack of moderation, living under illusion, and the inability to maintain practice due to doubt that the final result will be achieved. These are the obstacles. They can be gross or subtle.

Besides these main nine impediments, four more impediments run concurrently:

***duḥkha-*
daurmanasya-
-aṅgam-ejayatva-
-śvāsa-praśvāsāḥ
vikṣepa-sahabhuvaḥ
(I.31)**

I think these four can be observed when we are faced with major obstacles, and present as symptoms recognised by modern medical science that can be observed when we are faced with major obstacles. These are grief or sorrow; mental pain, dejection or despair; shakiness or tremors in the body; and laboured breathing. Like oil to fire, these four factors act as fuel for the main nine obstacles in distracting the practitioner. Some interrupt and disturb the *sādhaka* on a physical level; others impede on mental and intellectual levels; and the last two, on the spiritual level. They create a blaze of mental fluctuations and physical afflictions.

Charge the intelligence with the battery of analysis and synthesis. Co-ordination between these two aspects of intellect in action will gradually eradicate ignorance and heedlessness.

***avidyā kṣetram uttareṣāṁ prasupta--tanu-vicchinna--udārāṇām* (II.4)**	Adverse thoughts (*pratikūla vṛttis*), afflictions (*kleśas*), impediments (*antarāyas*) and symptoms of obstacles occur on account of ignorance (*avidyā*), which may be dormant, attenuated, interrupted or fully active.

These distinctions may be further categorised as feeble (*mṛdu*), moderate (*madhyama*), intense (*adhimātra*) and supremely intense (*tīvra*).

From this, one can understand the importance of yoga and why it must be practised.

***tataḥ tad-vipāka--anuguṇānām eva abhivyaktiḥ vāsanānām* (IV.8)**	All types of *karma* or actions, whether *manovṛtti karma*, *kleśa karma* or *antarāya karma*, leave their impressions, if not attended to, and manifest firmly in the body and mind. By attending to these adverse conditions, they can soon be converted and transformed into favourable conditions for reaching the desired goal – the *ātma-darśana*.

Thus, this chain of cause and effect can be gradually minimised and phased out by following actions and thoughts with righteousness and virtuousness.

When absolute and experienced knowledge and wisdom are acquired, this chain of cause and effect culminates. With this acquisition of wisdom, consciousness does not waver but remains the same (*samatvam*) in all circumstances. Pure devotion (*parā bhakti*) now passes through the gates of the seer in order to bring adverse thoughts under control, hence the importance of yoga and the reason why it must be practised.

XI

Citta Parivartana through Yoga – Transformation of *Citta* through Yoga

In the previous chapter, I discussed *kleśas*, *vṛttis*, *antarāyas* and the transformation of unfavourable thought waves into favourable thought waves. Now let me explain how the eight aspects (*aṅgas*) of yoga help consciousness (*citta*) to reach a prosperous state of absoluteness, free from tinges of thought waves, afflictions and obstacles, and leading the *sādhaka* towards the establishment of the seer or *citi* (*puruṣa*).

Yoga is a discipline meant to bring cohesion between body, mind, intelligence, consciousness and the seer. It draws those who are interested, holds their interest and shows them why it needs to be practised.

The main reason to practise yoga is to unify the traditional 24 principles (*tattvas*) of nature (*prakṛti*) with the ever-brilliant *puruṣa* – the seer.

When I do my *sādhanā*, my practice makes my senses, mind and consciousness involute towards the seer, and at the same time I feel the seer embracing the involuting *citta* and its accessories, namely mind, intelligence and ego. My *sādhanā* enables me to access the seer who constricts and hides himself, whereas many *sādhakas* may find it hard to do so. I am fortunate that in my practice I can make this infinitesimal atom (*paramāṇu*), the self, become great within this *bhūmi* – the body – to cover every inner layer from the source (*cidākāśa*), just like the universal sky (*mahat ākāśa*).

This way one has to subdue first the five elements along with the five layers of the Self (*kośas*) and their constituents to move towards the sight of the *ātman*.

Through the conquest of the elements and their subtle qualities, supernatural powers (*siddhis*) accrue. I will deal with them later after explaining the mechanism of *saṁyamas*. At present, I like to describe them as indications of transformations within consciousness.

The gross body takes its shape according to the pervasiveness of the four layers of the inner body, namely: physiological (*prāṇamaya*), mental (*manomaya*), intellectual (*vijñānamaya*) and self (*ātmamaya*). Watching the formation of the gross body and reshaping it enables one to reflect on the inner body, which reacts, creating harmony and balance between these two bodies.

***sthūla-svarūpa--sūkṣma-anvaya--arthavattva--saṁyamāt bhūta-jayaḥ* (III.45)**

The five elements (*mahābhūtas*) are earth (*pṛthvī*), water (*āp*), fire (*tejas*), wind or air (*vāyu*) and space (*ākāśa*). Each element has five forms. These are mass (*sthūla*), subtle or fine (*sūkṣma*), form or shape (*svarūpa*), conjunction or interpenetration (*anvaya*) and means and purposes (*arthavatva*).

***tato' ṇima-ādi--prādur-bhāvaḥ kāya-saṁpat tad-dharma--anabhighātaḥ ca* (III.46)**

The five forms of elements, namely gross, subtle or fine, form, conjunction and means have their own characteristics. I feel that there is an intrinsic correspondence between the five elements (*pañcamahābhūtas*), their infrastructural qualities (*pañcatanmātra*) and the five sheaths (*pañcakośas*): the solidity and smell of the earth element corresponds to *annamaya kośa*; the fluidity and taste of the water element corresponds to *prāṇamāya kośa*; the warmth and sight of the fire element corresponds to *manomaya kośa*; the mobility and touch of the air element corresponds to *vijñānamaya kośa*; and the

> volume and sound of the space element corresponds to *ānandamaya kośa*.
>
> The *ātman* is free from the contents of the elements and their sub-atomic structures. Studying their purposes and ways of utilising them to achieve integration brings unity. Focused, concentrated examination of their structural relationships and function reveals their true character – being changeable, mutable and made up of the insubstantial matrix of nature. Close examination of their structural relationships and function reveals their true character. They being changeable and mutable, and the Self being non-changeable and non-mutable, the *sādhaka* understands the characteristic relationship between the matrix and the Self.

Patañjali clearly explains in a sequential order the gradual effects that result from the mastery of these constituent contents of nature, which are covered in the five layers of the Self.

If III.45 describes *bhūtajaya* (conquest of the five elements), III.46 describes *tanmātrajaya* (conquest of the subtle qualities of the elements), from where the wealth of the body or *kāya saṁpat* accrues.

Commentators have referred to the *aṣṭa siddhi*s or the eight super-normal or supernatural powers in connection with this 46th *sūtra*. These are:

1) *aṇiman*, the power of making oneself infinitely small;
2) *mahiman*, the power of increasing size at will;
3) *gariman*, the power to become heavier and heavier;
4) *laghiman*, the power of becoming as light as cotton;
5) *prāpti*, the power of obtaining anything;
6) *prākāmya*, power to attain anything by will or freedom of will;
7) *vaśitva*, power of subjugation;
8) *īśatva*, power of supremacy over all.

As Patañjali deals with the supernatural or super-normal powers in Chapter III (*sūtra*s 17, 18, 19, 21, 26, 34, 37, 42, 43 and 44), I feel that this *sūtra* has nothing to do with *aṣṭa siddhis*. Here the word *aṇimādi* stands only for the atomic structure of the elements.

In the subsequent *sūtras*, he speaks of the conquest of the body (*śarīra jaya*), conquest of the senses (*indriya jaya*), conquest of the mind (*manojaya*), and the true nature of the seer. As such, the *aṣṭa siddhis* are irrelevant here.

rūpa-lāvaṇya- -bala-vajra- -saṁhananatvāni kāya-saṁpat **(III.47)**	As the elements and their qualities are brought under control through *yaugika sādhanā*, the body (*pañca bhautika śarīra*) gains its wealth in the form of beauty, grace, strength and compactness, and shines like the brilliance of a diamond. In short it is *śarīra jaya*, or loveliness and liveliness of the body.

When Arjuna beheld Lord Krishna's true form, he could not withstand the luminous light of God. He requested the Lord bless him with eyes to see that light clearly (*B. G.*, XI.4–9). If that was so in Arjuna's case, what about weaklings like us? How are we to bear the sight of the seer when it occurs?

Patañjali says that the body is made as hard and as compact as a diamond, so that when the *puruṣa* is sighted, it can withstand and withhold the brilliance of the luminous light of *puruṣa*.

grahaṇa-svarūpa- -asmitā-anvaya- -arthavattva- -saṁyamāt indriya-jayaḥ **(III.48)**	The practice of yoga keeps the senses of perception (*jñānendriyas*) under control (*indriya jaya*), so that their contact with the objects of the world is put aside and made to move towards the direction of the Self. Engaged on this inward path, the external mind (*bāhyendriya manas*) changes into inner mind (*antarendriya*). This *antarendriya manas*, *buddhi*, *ahaṁkāra*, *citta* and conscience realise their distinguished aspect, which is nothing less than movement towards the sight of the seer.
tataḥ mano-javitvaṁ vikaraṇa-bhāvaḥ pradhāna-jayaḥ ca **(III.49)**	As the senses of perception are brought under control, the mind is also controlled and subdued (*manojaya*). Being free from the senses of perception, the mind understands its position and merges with the first principle of nature, cosmic consciousness (*mahat*).

In this state, consciousness, which till now appeared as an individual entity, is transformed into a Universal or Cosmic consciousness.

***sattva-puruṣa--anyatā-khyāt-imātrasya sarva--bhāva--adhiṣṭhātṛtvaṁ sarva-jñātṛtvaṁ ca* (III.50)**

As the discursive *citta* dissolves in the singular universal cosmic consciousness (*mahat*), the *guṇas* cease stirring the elements of nature. Then the intelligence realises its significance and surrenders to the seer, enabling him to dwell in his true splendour: *tadā draṣṭuḥ svarūpe avasthānam* (I.3).

Patañjali warns the *sādhaka* at this particular moment to be careful that the infinitesimal seed of blemishes (*doṣa bīja*)is burnt out fully and totally (*see* III.51 below), otherwise it may sprout. Then, he will be caught again by delusion and infatuation (*moha*).

***sthāni-upanimantraṇe saṅga-smayā--akaraṇaṁ punar-aniṣṭa-prasaṅgāt* (III.52)**

If the *doṣa bīja* (the seed of blemishes) is not totally eliminated, celestial beings try to seduce him and pull him down from the grace of yoga.

As the invisible seeds in a mountain sprout forth when the rains arrive, so too defects can manifest later in our lives. These hidden seeds must be totally eradicated so that we may gain maturity and wisdom in *sādhanā* as defined in III.51. That is why Patañjali uses the word *kaivalya* here – nothing that can disturb progress can grow in this state, due to the absence of destructive seeds.

***tad-vairāgyāt api doṣa-bīja-kṣaye kaivalyam* (III.51)**

Destroying the seeds of bondage and renouncing all super-normal powers brings eternal emancipation. Therefore, this *sūtra* guides us to conquer infatuation (*moha*) to experience freedom from attachment (*mokṣa*).

Patañjali explains the high level of achievement that the matured consciousness reaches after giving us glimpses of the wonderful effects of yoga: conquering the five elements, the body and the senses. At the same time, he warns the *sādhaka* that fissures may arise even in this state, due to past impressions that have yet to fruit. After overcoming this last difficulty, the yogi will attain the zenith of yoga.

When the seeds of bondage are destroyed, the power or the *śakti* of *prakṛti* (*prakṛty-āpūrāt* – *Y. S.*, IV.2)[1] flows in abundance (commonly attributed by yogis to *kuṇḍalinī śakti*). From here on, one is free from nature's influences:

***tatra dhyāna-jam anāśayam* (IV.6)**	When one is free from nature's influences and merged in the seer, only then one can gain freedom from influences of latent impressions.
***draṣṭṛ-dṛśya--uparaktaṁ cittaṁ sarvā-arthaṁ* (IV.23) (study it with II.20)** ***citeḥ apratisaṁkramāyāḥ tad-ākāra-apattau sva-buddhi--saṁvedanam* (IV.22)**	Nature's intelligence (*svabuddhi*) changes and assumes an intelligence that is equal to the seer (*svāmibuddhi*), and both intelligences now remain undifferentiated. As the river upon joining the sea transforms into the sea, so the river of consciousness joins the ocean of the seer and transforms into the seer. With this pure consciousness, the seer no longer is the witness, but rather is the beheld. The knower and the knowable unite with each other and are no longer distinguishable.
***tat-asaṅkhyeya--vāsanābhiḥ citram api para-arthaṁ saṁhatya-kāritvāt* (IV.24)**	The innumerable fabrics of thoughts of consciousness, which are close to *prakṛti*, take a U-turn to be near to the *puruṣa*.
***viśeṣa-darśinaḥ ātma-bhāva--bhāvanā-nivṛttiḥ* (IV.25)**	When the relationship between *prakṛti* and *puruṣa*, i.e. *citta* and *ātman*, is known and understood, *prakṛti* and *puruṣa* lose their identities. Only *prajñā* (the intellectual attention and awareness) remains, and nothing else.

---

1 *jāti-antara-pariṇāmaḥ prakṛti-āpūrāt* (IV.2) – The abundant flow of nature's energy brings about a transformation in one's birth, aiding the process of evolution. I feel that the power of *prakṛti* is nothing less than *kuṇḍalinī śakti*.

***tadā viveka-nimnaṁ kaivalya--prāgbhāraṁ cittan* (IV.26)**

Patañjali establishes that consciousness is drawn closely towards the *puruṣa* due to the gravitational pull of the seer. But if pride in the form of a destructive seed (*doṣa bīja*) raises its hood like the cobra, then this merging of *citta* in the seer is disturbed. At this stage there is no choice but to start again from the beginning.

The *sādhaka* must strive again judiciously to extinguish the disturbances and disharmonies and regain that exalted state of illumination: *hānam eṣāṁ kleśavat uktam* (IV.28).[1]

***tataḥ kleśa-karma--nivṛttiḥ* (IV.30)**

After reaching this exalted state of absoluteness through *yaugika* discipline, the *sādhaka* will not commit any action that brings afflictions, but perform only actions which are non-painful (*akliṣṭa*). One has to reach this state of intelligence through yoga.

***tadā sarva-āvaraṇa--malā-apetasya jñānasya ānantyāt--jñeyam alpam* (IV.31)**

He (the *sādhaka*) carries out non-inflicting deeds because he realises that all the knowledge so far acquired is trivial compared with the present state of purity in intelligence:

***tataḥ kṛtā-arthānāṁ pariṇāma-krama--samāptiḥ guṇānām* (IV.32)**

[2]By the result of *dharmamegha samādhi* or *nirbīja samādhi*, one gains knowledge and understanding of how far yoga is essential in this God-given life to attain the four aims of life (*puruṣārthas*), thus making life useful, worthwhile and noble.

When all the dust of ignorance (*avidyā*) is eradicated by *yaugika sādhanā*, all knowledge so far earned appears trivial before this new knowledge of wisdom.

---

1 As a *sādhaka* strives to be free from afflictions, the yogi must again handle these latent impressions judiciously to extinguish them by sticking to the *Sādhanā*.

2 By this the *guṇa* involute and disolve in nature, having fulfilled their duties.

By study, the *sādhaka* must maintain this exalted state of knowledge that never wanes or waxes, nor oscillates or vacillates. He must practise for practice's sake, to reach the zenith of all knowledge – the sight of the seer.

XII

Sādhanā Krama – Method of Practice

Sādhanā is an attempt to investigate and accomplish at the earliest moment possible the union of the individual self with the Universal Self.

Sādhaka must be a skilled and accomplished practitioner of *sādhanā*.

Before going on to the practical aspect of yoga, we should discuss *sādhanā krama*, or various methods of sequences in practice.

First of all, *sādhanā* is a very difficult concept to explain, as it is completely subjective. In 1934 at the age of 15, I was introduced to yoga by my *guru*, but this was purely on the physical level. As I was tremendously stiff, it may be possible that my *guru* taught me with the fixed assumption that the practice of *āsana*s was enough for me. Whatever form he taught, it was certainly yoga, even at my tender age.

With little background on the practical aspect and with none on the theoretical aspect, I was sent to Pune for six months to teach students in schools and colleges, mainly for their physical well-being. At the *yogaśālā* of Mysore, yoga was taught purely on the physical level. I began teaching yoga in the same spirit.

Destiny was responsible for making me learn on my own. I started to think of the behavioural patterns of my own body, brain, mind and intelligence as well as of those who came to me to learn. Many times it happened that my body and mind were not co-operating; my practice was often without direction. When other sheaths of my being were not obliging, I used to scrutinise my mind at the time of practice. Often the body was willing but the intellect of the head and heart seemed non-existent. This was exhausting my physical strength and will-power. Often I was led towards negative thinking. In order to overcome these negative thoughts, I intensified my practices, hoping for the light to dawn.

To investigate, I sometimes practised with my body without involving the mind, and at other times I practised only from the mind, studying and observing the reactions on the body. This way I used to shift my thoughts to the body when the mind was not willing, and used the mind when the body had no strength to continue. Many times I treated the body and mind as separate from myself, and practised involving the Self directly. At other times I maintained myself separately from body and mind, and used these tools in practice.

This method built my confidence and brought me clarity. It showed me a homogenous approach that involved moving the body, mind and self together to find an even balance of attention, extension and expansion in the body, mind and Self. This way of practicing the *āsana*s enabled me to connect the gross physical body with the subtle body – the mind – and then enabled them to integrate with the Self, which is nothing but the causal body. The gross body or the outer body (*sthūla śarīra*) is the musculoskeletal body. The physiological body, the organs of action, senses of perception and the external mind often remain close to this outer layer. When the external mind makes a U-turn, it becomes the inner mind. This inner mind is called *antarendriya*. This *antarendriya manas*, *buddhi*, *ahaṁkāra* and *citta* are the components of the subtle layer (*sūkṣma śarīra*) of the inner mind. *Dharmendriya* (conscience) and *sākāra puruṣa*, or the form of the seer (*ahaṁ-ākāra* or *jīvātmān* or the *ātman* with life), constitute the causal body (*kāraṇa śarīra*). All these are the vehicles of the *puruṣa* for enlightenment, but the very same vehicles may cause the *sākāra puruṣa* to be attached to the thought waves of consciousness (see *Y. S.*, I.4).

After so many years of practice, I am now in such a state that the body (the field – *kṣetra*) immediately sends messages to the seer (the fielder – *kṣetrajña*) if any part of my body is neglected.

With these various efforts, some right and some wrong, I began to discern when and how congenial feelings from the skin to the seer and from the seer to the skin can be brought together. Today, my practice is effortless and I feel no difference between my body and the seer. I practise in such a way that I make the elements and the infrastructural qualities of the five elements (*tanmātras*) flow evenly without deviations and variations, keeping the mind, intelligence and consciousness perennially in touch with the movements of the body. In this way, I practise and surrender myself with *sādhanā* to that invisible force – God – who resides within all of us. I am now in this state of the *sādhanā*.

The educational institutes extended my services in Pune every six months for the next three years, and people also began to attend the classes. Their physical and emotional problems opened my eyes, brain and mind and showed me how I could solve their problems with *āsanas*. The rubbing and brushing of my brain with the body began to work together. I began to practise making my brain penetrate the interior body, and I felt the changes and adjustments that were taking place. This trained my mind to experience inner reactions.

In this process of inner search I had to act, reflect, re-reflect and react to find the range of actions and vibrations on each muscle that provoked a feeling of contentment. If dissatisfaction, untoward and unrhythmic feelings came up, I would find ways to remove them.

This inward exploration led me to judge my actions on each and every part of the joints, capillaries, fibres, tendons, ligaments and muscles. This experimental approach gradually led me, through trial and error, to understand the functions of the body and what type of changes have to occur in the mind. I began introducing these adjustments to those who came to me with their somatic or somato-psychic or psycho-somatic problems. Watching what changes these brought in their minds and bodies made me penetrate deeper and deeper into the subject.

In the early stages, failures, disappointments and anxieties hampered me in my quest and I was in two minds whether to continue or not in my quest. But years of forceful and uninterrupted practice had prepared my mind to accept the challenges of pains, failures and disappointments. With my determined will-power to endure, I began investigating and inspecting my own practice until my mind gained confidence. With this confidence I continued my practices until the comeliness in the body and lustre of elegance in the mind settled in myself.

I reflected on the defective movements of the muscles and joints affected by pain, comparing them to the correct sense of comfortable movements on the same parts of the other side. This made me un-do and re-do the *āsana* with proper adjustments to improve the afflicted side and to judge the actions of each muscle, tendon, fibre and flow of energy and intelligence in them, like the balancing scale of justice.

tat-pratiṣedha--artham eka-tattva--abhyāsaḥ **(I.32)** Correct adjustments in the unrhythmic musculoskeletal structure of the body, and the feeling of the non-movement or movement of intelligence in the various sheaths of the body through *āsanas*, which I practised with single-minded effort, became the key-note in my *sādhanā*.

1. *Sādhanā Krama*

Sādhanā is a key concept. It implies the idea of effort, but actually the sense of effort goes beyond it. *Sādhanā* demands an investigating and examining mind if the action is to purify (*śodhana*). Desiccation and absorption (*śoṣaṇa*) are needed to remove the body's defects and for an auspicious presentation (*śobhana*). When the effortful efforts transform into an effortlessness state then one experiences the calm and soothing state of *śamana*. If all these four aspects (*śodhana*, *śoṣaṇa*, *śobhana* and *śamana*) are followed from the beginning with the precise performance of each *āsana*, *prāṇāyāma* or *dhyāna*, then one can experience the stages that are explained on *saṁprajñāta samādhi* in I.17: *vitarka-vicāra-ānanda--asmitā-rūpa-anugamāt saṁprajñātaḥ*. In this *sūtra* I relate *śodhana* to the *vitarka* level of logical study; *śoṣaṇa* to *vicāra* or investigation and synthesis; *śobhana* to *ānanda* or comeliness in the body; and *śamana* or lustre of elegance to *asmitā-rūpa prajñā* (awareness of the Self). Thus these four stages of *sādhanā* become the ground (*kṣetra*) for the *sādhaka*.

The next step, *śoṣaṇa*, is related to the *vicāra* stage where all the parts have been analysed and carefully rectified. This is the stage of absorption. The period of absorption becomes *ānanda* or *śobhana* (auspicious presentation). With this absorption, efforts and expressions subside; the *sādhaka* exists in the simple and pure state of *asmitā prajñā*, where there is neither loss nor gain, neither excess nor deficiency.

In the true *sādhanā*, one soaks the flesh in the stream of blood, rubs the mind with each cell and brushes the intelligence to burn the defective seeds so that *prāṇa* flows smoothly, invigorating the very core of the being.

To achieve this level, *āsana*s play a perfect role in positioning the joints, tissues, fibres and bones without any distraction, contraction or refraction.

Lastly, *āsana*s are meant to spread the Flame of the Self all over the body as if the Self is performing the *āsana*s using the body, mind, intelligence and consciousness as its agents.

This experience is the nectar of the *sādhanā* and should be savoured by all *sādhaka*s.

Patañjali describes this profound *yaugika sādhanā* as having two facets. One is total surrender of oneself to the Supreme Being (*Īśvara praṇidhāna*), and the other is *aṣṭāṅga yoga*. If the former is the path of renunciation (*vairāgya*), or freedom from worldly joys and attachment to *Īśvara*, the latter is a method (*abhyāsa krama*) of practice.

Please remember that these two facets are complementary and supplementary to each other. They are interwoven as parts of the same *yaugika* process. If the eight limbs of *aṣṭāṅga yoga* are the indirect petals towards Self-realisation, *Īśvara praṇidhāna* (I.23) is a direct route for it.

***Īśvara-praṇidhānāt vā* (I.23)**	*Īśvara praṇidhāna* is total surrender of oneself to God, who is the first and foremost *guru*, untouched by afflictions and actions as well as by the fruits of actions.

As total surrender is difficult for all *sādhaka*s, the other facet of *sādhanā* is *aṣṭāṅga yoga*, which is also considered by Patañjali as *kriyā yoga*, where practice (*abhyāsa*) and renunciation (*vairāgya*) are involved through *tapas*, *svādhyāya* and *Īśvarapraṇidhāna* (II.1) as *sādhanā traya* or three facets of *sādhanā*.

2. *Sādhanā Kriyā*

I consider *sādhanā kriyā* from three angles. These are *sādhanā traya*, *sādhanā krama* and *sādhanā stambha*.

1. *Sādhanā traya*: The three tiers of *sādhanā* are *bahiraṅga*, *antaraṅga* and *antarātman*. When *bahiraṅga* and *antaraṅga sādhanās* become one, they culminate in *antarātman sādhanā*, as all functions and actions originate from the *antarātman* and culminate there.
2. *Sādhanā krama*: This is the progressive classification of *tapas*, *svādhyāya* and *Īśvara praṇidhāna*.

***tapaḥ-svādhyāya-Īśvara-praṇidhānāni kriyā-yogaḥ* (II.1)**	Action in yoga is *tapas*. This term stands also for zeal or passion for the subject. Extending and expanding the intellect of the head with the intelligence of the mind in the practice of *āsana*, *prāṇāyama* and *dhyāna* is *svādhyāya*. Making the core of the being (*puruṣa*) to come in contact with, intermingle and make his presence felt in the cells of the body is *Īśvara praṇidhāna*.

3. *Sādhanā stambha*, or the pillars of practice: These are the essential qualities that the *sādhaka*s must develop in order to reach the goal of yoga, which is no less than the sight of the seer. Here surrender to God and the petals of *aṣṭāṅga yoga* come close together, leading us to savour the *sādhanā*.

To acquire self-knowledge through scriptures and then to practically transmit this studied knowledge (*svādhyāya*) is *sādhanā*. Lastly, surrendering oneself to God is *Īśvara praṇidhāna*. All these acts are *yaugika sādhanā*. Actually these three actions of yoga represent the seed *mantra āuṁ*. *Āuṁ* as *japa* or prayer covers *artha*, the purpose and means, and *bhāvanā*, the felt feelings of the *mantra*. If *akāra* stands for *tapas*, *ukāra* stands for *svādhyāya*, and *makāra* represents *Īśvara praṇidhāna*.

I am not going to refer in this chapter to *sūtras* II.43 to II.45, where Patañjali explains *tapas*, *svādhyāya* and *Īśvara praṇidhāna* as parts of *niyama*. But, I consider here that these three concepts lead one to the higher and nobler stages of the *sādhanā*, according to the contents detailed in the table below:

Tapas is *bahiraṅga sādhanā*, *svādhyāya* is *antaraṅga sādhanā* and *Īśvara praṇidhāna* is *antarātman sādhanā*. *Annamaya* and *prāṇamaya kośa*s, or the musculoskeletal body and organic body, represent the external sheaths (*bahiraṅga*) of the self; *manomaya* and *vijñānamaya kośa*s, or mental and intellectual bodies, represent the internal sheaths (*antaraṅga*); and *ānandamaya kośa* represents the innermost sheath (*antarātman*).

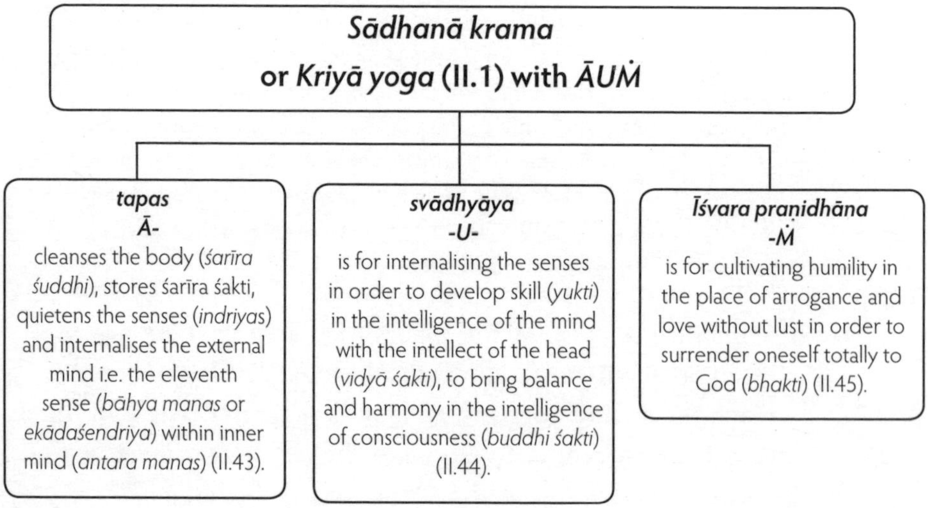
Sādhanā krama
or Kriyā yoga (II.1) with ĀUṀ
tapas
Ā-
cleanses the body (śarīra śuddhi), stores śarīra śakti, quietens the senses (indriyas) and internalises the external mind i.e. the eleventh sense (bāhya manas or ekādaśendriya) within inner mind (antara manas) (II.43).
svādhyāya
-U-
is for internalising the senses in order to develop skill (yukti) in the intelligence of the mind with the intellect of the head (vidyā śakti), to bring balance and harmony in the intelligence of consciousness (buddhi śakti) (II.44).
Īśvara praṇidhāna
-Ṁ
is for cultivating humility in the place of arrogance and love without lust in order to surrender oneself totally to God (bhakti) (II.45).

The Self is essentially the seed that helps the *sādhaka* control the external sheaths (*bahiraṅga*) and cleanse the internal sheaths (*antaraṅga*), so that he penetrates further to trace and realise the Self. Hence the four stages of *sādhanā karma* have to be followed as these outer-related aspects comprise both the means and the end.

3. *Tapas*

Tapas covers *yama*, *niyama*, *āsana* and *prāṇāyāma*. *Tapas* is nothing less than a determined effort in *sādhanā*:

***tatra sthitau yatnaḥ abhyāsaḥ* (I.13)**	It begins with steadfast, effortful practice to eradicate the impurities (*malas*) of the body and then to constrain and still the movements of consciousness (*cittavṛtti*) in order to reach a single-focused attention (*ekāgrata citta*).
***sa tu dīrgha- -kāla-nairantarya- -satkāra-āsevitaḥ dṛḍha-bhūmiḥ* (I.14)**	To establish a firm ground to further the effort, this practice has to be continued assiduously for a long time, with intensity and profundity.
***krama-anyatvaṁ pariṇāma-anyatve hetuḥ* (III.15)**	This requires constant study of the changes and transformations that occur in mind, intelligence and consciousness while adopting and adapting the sequential stages in practices that are explained in *sādhanā krama*.

Maturity in stilling consciousness is reached through steadfast effort defined from III.9 onwards.

***vyutthāna-nirodha- -saṁskārayoḥ abhibhava- -prādurbhāvau nirodha-kṣaṇa-citta- anvayaḥ nirodha- -pariṇāmaḥ* (III.9)**	Experiencing through observation these profound tranquil impressions that happen between the waxing and waning thought waves, one has not only to increase these silent moments but also make these moments steady, continuous, effortless and natural.

tasya praśānta- *-vāhitā saṁskārāt* (III.10)	This steady, effortless and natural tranquil state helps consciousness move towards spiritual absorption or *samādhi pariṇāma*.
sarvā-arthatā- *-ekāgratayoḥ kṣaya-* *-udayau cittasya* *samādhi-pariṇāmaḥ* (III.11)	In spite of steadfast effort, it is natural for the mind to wane and wax without one's knowledge. Hence it is essential to maintain a single-focused attention (I.13) with long, uninterrupted and alert practice (I.14).
tataḥ punaḥ śānta- *-uditau tulya-* *-pratyayau cittasya* *ekāgratā-pariṇāmaḥ* (III.12)	Even with the experience of single-focused attention (*ekāgrata*) or the feel of *samādhi*, one must not stop the *sādhanā* but pursue it (*see also* I.20).

Tapas is the *śodhana kriyā* of the *sādhanā*.

4. *Svādhyāya*

Giving attention to and reflecting and re-reflecting in practice is essential to develop skilfulness in *sādhanā* so that the hidden impurities clouding the intelligence are eradicated.

tat-pratiṣedha- *-artham eka-tattva-* *-abhyāsaḥ* (I.32)	Unpleasant sensations, or wrong actions and feelings (qualities of *viparyaya*, *vikalpa*, *rāga* and *dveṣa*) as well as the defects in one's own practices have to be removed and corrected not only with a single-minded attention, but also with careful detection, distinctive observation and reflection. Throughout the *sādhanā*, one has to feel the flow of energy (*prāṇa*) and awareness (*prajñā*) running together smoothly and without interruption, filling each cell of the body.

Sādhanā is where balance and receptivity combine with reflection and help one to develop intellectual skill (*tejas*), enabling the *sādhaka* to connect the gross (*pṛthvī* and *āp*) and the subtle (*vāyu* and *ākāśa*) elements within the seer.

As the macrocosm is in the microcosm and vice versa, the five elements are the five sheaths (*kośa*) of the Self. *Annamaya* or the muscular-skeletal body represents *pṛthvī*; *prāṇamaya* or the organic body, the *āp* element; mind, the *tejas* element, air, *vijñāna* or intellectual sheath; and the vãyu element and *ānanda* or Self, the *ākāśa* element.

All these five sheaths, with the co-operation and co-ordination of the elements, help to realise the seer.

This covers the *śoṣaṇa kriyā* of the *sādhanā* with self-study (*svādhyāya*).

Svādhyāya covers all the petals of yoga from *yama* to *dhyāna* in general, and in particular from *pratyāhāra* to *dhyāna*. Without the background of *tapas*, it is impossible to follow the *sādhanā* with *svādhyāya* alone.

5. *Īśvara Praṇidhāna*

It is interesting to study how Patañjali connects yoga with *bhakti mārga* in the first chapter, teaching how to quieten the movements of consciousness through total surrender to God. Probably realising that it might not be possible for everyone to reach directly that state of total surrender, he introduced a progressive and augmented approach in the form of *aṣṭāṅga yoga*.

***samādhi-siddhiḥ Īśvara-praṇidhānāt* (II.45)**	It is possible for the *sādhaka* to experience *samādhi* and to reach perfection in it through full surrender and resignation to God (*Īśvara*).

Progression in sequential rhythmic adjustments in *sādhanā* transforms the qualities of *pañca bhūta*s of the body, senses, mind and intelligence and purify each sheath to reach the zenith of refinement. The body, mind, intelligence and consciousness are refined to the state of a pure, transparent jewel. I have no doubt that there is a close connection between the three gradations described in Chapter II (*tapas*, *svādhyāya* and *Īśvara praṇidhāna*) and the transformations (*pariṇāma*) that take place in *sādhanā*.

***etena-bhūta- -indriyeṣu dharma-lakṣaṇa- avasthā- -pariṇāmāḥ vyākhyātāḥ* (III.13)**

Let me explain this more fully. The state of Being remains in the *tāmasika* nature (*dharma*). This *tāmasika* state of Being has to be nudged towards the *rājasika* state in order to change the *tāmasika* Being into Becoming (*lakṣaṇa*). This requires cultivating and refining all the vestments of the Self. Then this Becoming is transformed into the illuminative *sāttvika* state of Being, which is the ultimate zenith (*avasthā*) of the *sādhanā*. If this zenith state is maintained, then surrendering to God is easy to follow (III.56).

This is the *śobhana kriyā* of *sādhanā krama*.

Uninterrupted and zealous practice of *sādhanā* allows transformation to take place. The *sādhanā* (*tapas*) becomes his *dharma*; the transformation that leads towards refinement becomes his *lakṣaṇa* in the form of self-knowledge (*svādhyāya*); and then he reaches the exalted state of the union of consciousness with the Self, the real state or *avasthā*. Here, the inner voice of the self suggests union with *Īśvara*, culminating in *bhakti*. This is the final goal of *sādhanā*.

***sattva-puruṣayoḥ śuddhi-sāmye kaivalyam iti* (III.56)**

When the elements in the body, mind and intelligence are transformed to the level of the illuminative intelligence of the seer, the difference between the *kṣetra* and *kṣetrajña* fades and only awareness (*prajñā*) shines. This is perfection of the *sādhanā*.

This is *śamana kriyā* of the *sādhanā krama*.

Aṣṭāṅga yoga is considered an art (*kalā*), a science (*vijñāna*) and a philosophy (*vedānta* or *prajñāna*).

Patañjali covers *kalā* or the art of living with the principles of *yama* and *niyama*. On the one hand, *āsanas* may to an extent be considered an art; on the other, and along with *prāṇāyāma* and *pratyāhāra*, they act as an experimental science (*vijñāna*). *Dhāraṇā*, *dhyāna* and *samādhi*, being close to the Self, are purely experiential (*prajñāna*).

***trayam ekatra saṁyamaḥ* (III.4)**

Patañjali names *dhāraṇā*, *dhyāna* and *samādhi* together as an integrated whole (*saṁyama*).

trayam-antar- -aṅgaṁ pūrvebhyaḥ (III.7)

He says that the later three aspects of yoga are *antaraṅga* compared with the previous five aspects or petals of yoga. I feel strongly that *āsana*, *prāṇāyāma* and *pratyāhāra* must be *bahiraṅga saṁyama* since Patañjali speaks of *antaraṅga saṁyama* and brackets *dhāraṇā*, *dhyāna* and *samādhi* as three in one. As *yama and niyama* are universal principles for life, this part becomes the *kalā*, or the art of leading a life.

These three divisions of *aṣṭāṅga yoga* bring a transformation in the *sādhaka*, helping him to realise the level of *yaugika* he has reached in his *sādhanā*. Besides this, it helps him to recollect the finer and nobler states of consciousness.

nirmāṇa-cittāni asmitā-mātrāt (IV.4)

The constructed consciousness (*pariṇāma citta* or *nirmita citta*) springs from the sense of the I-maker, the *ahaṁkāra*. When this constructed or built-up consciousness is transformed into the purest state of absolute I-ness (*ahaṁ-ākāra*), this cultivated consciousness is distinguished as *asmitā* or *sāsmitā* (*sa*, auspicious; *asmitā*, self – *see also* I.17). This is *kūṭastha citta* or *nirmāṇa citta* becoming *divya citta*.

śruta-anumāna- -prajñābhyām anya- -viṣayā viśeṣa- -arthatvāt (I.49)

On reaching this state comes first-hand knowledge and wisdom, which are distinct and superior to knowledge gleaned through books, inference or testimony (I.7).

tasyā-api nirodhe sarva-nirodhāt nirbījaḥ samādhiḥ (I.51)

He eliminates all experiences and feelings that have been felt so far, just as a flame is extinguished the moment that the wood (its fuel) is taken from the fire. Here he experiences the seedless state (*nirbīja samādhi*) as the purified *citta* transforms itself into a seer.

This is the *antarātman* aspect of yoga, or the ultimate state in *sādhanā* as all residues of imprints and impressions evaporate from consciousness.

Let us consider *Bhagavad Gītā*, IX.26 below:

***pattraṁ puṣpaṁ phalaṁ toyaṁ yo me bhaktyā prayacchati / tad ahaṁ bhakty--upahṛtam aśnāmi prayata-atmanaḥ //* (*B. G.*, IX.26)**

This *śloka* on the surface appears very simple. It says: 'Whosoever offers a leaf, a flower, fruit or even water to me with devotional love and pure heart, I accept.'

This *śloka* has relevance to all of us as *sādhakas* are the *bhaktas* of their chosen art.

For me, as a *bhakta* of yoga, *patra* or leaves stand for mind (*manas*), *puṣpa* or flower for intelligence (*buddhi*), *phala* or fruit for consciousness (*citta*) and *toya* or water for taste or flavour (*rasa*), which is *ahaṁkāra*.

The latter part of the verse is very important to *sādhakas* like us, as it speaks of a person who has dropped *ahaṁkāra* totally from his *citta* and become sinless, stainless and selfless with a pure heart.

The *dharma* of *citta* is *cintana. Cintana* means reflecting upon objective thoughts. These thoughts may be sorrowful or joyful.

Offering a leaf, a flower, a fruit or water with an auspicious state of *citta* represents surrender to God, and God accepts it with love.

In the context of this verse, I feel the leaves represent the mind that is swayed (like a leaf in the wind) either by thought waves that are sensual or spiritual. If sensual thoughts lead one towards negative thoughts, spiritual thoughts lead towards positive thoughts. The leaves move according to the wind. At the same time, when the leaves move, they help the tree to absorb energy for it to grow healthily.

Most human beings do not think of turning the cluttered mind towards constructive single-focused attention. So cultivating the mind is necessary to develop a sinless and disinterested mind. If consciousness dwells on sensual joys (*bhogārtha*), life ends in grief. If thoughts are diverted towards eternal bliss (*apavargārtha*) through *yaugika* practice, consciousness transforms itself into a ripe state of wisdom. Then that consciousness is a sinless consciousness.

When this is achieved, intelligence blooms like a flower that bears delicious fruits. I call it *paripakva citta* (fully ripened consciousness).

In order to develop this ripe consciousness as the fruit of *jñāna* and *karma*, the mind, *buddhi* and *citta* must be nourished by *ahaṁkāra*, which represents *toyam* or water. As the water flows downstream, *ahaṁkāra* (I-maker), which has its seat in the brain, must spread and flow downwards to nourish the consciousness that is seated in the heart region, so that the *rasa*, or flavour, flows, moistening the *citta* with thoughts of spiritual wisdom.

If the *āsana* or a breath is offered to God with this clean mind, mature intelligence, diffused *ahaṁkāra* and ripened consciousness, the Lord accepts and partakes in the joy of the *sādhaka* with love. Here the *sādhaka* needs not even offer a leaf, a flower, a fruit or water, but simply offer the *āsana* or a breath with a pure sinless head and heart.

This may happen soon for someone like the great *ācārya*s of the past, or saints like Śrī Rāmakrishna, Śrī Ramaṇa of Aruṇācala. But we may not achieve it in this life, and we may need further lives to reach that state (*see sūtra* III.23).[1]

nābhi-cakre kāya--vyūha-jñānam **(III.30)**	Contemplation on *nābhi cakra* or *maṇipūraka cakra* is the *bahiraṅga saṁyama* (*āsana*, *prāṇāyāma* and *pratyāhāra*). This brings clear and complete knowledge and understanding of the entire body.

In the same way, studying the mind, intelligence, the I-maker and consciousness through *dhāraṇā*, *dhyāna* and *samādhi* brings:

prātibhāt vā sarvam **(III.34)**	Clarity in the intellect of the head,
hṛdaye citta-saṁvit **(III.35)**	and cleanliness in the intelligence of the heart,

1 *sa-upakramaṁ-nirupakramaṁ ca karma tat-saṁyamāt aparānta-jñānam ariṣṭebhyaḥ vā* (III.23) – By *saṁyama* on his actions, a yogi sooner or later gains foreknowledge of the final fruits of his actions and learns the exact time of his death.

mūrdha-jyotiṣi siddha-darśanam (III.33)	and guidance in the spiritual field from great masters or *gurus*.
sattva-puruṣayoḥ atyantā-asaṁkīrṇayoḥ pratyaya-aviśeṣaḥ bhogaḥ para-arthatvāt sva-artha-saṁyamāt puruṣa-jñānam (III.36)	When the intelligence is clean and consciousness is pure, not only does the sādhaka realise the difference between the self-interested material world, he also experiences a selfless state of the spiritual world.

6. *Sādhanā Stambha* (Pillars for *Sādhaka* and *Sādhanā*)

In order to reach this state, one must forget the four pillars that act as a springboard, enabling the leap to the finest level of *sādhanā*.

śraddhā-vīrya-smṛti-samādhi-prajñā-pūrvakaḥ itareṣām (I.20)	As there are four types of *sādhakas* (*mṛdu*, *madhyama*, *adhimātra*, *tīvra*), there are four pillars for *sādhanā*. These are: a) trust (*śraddhā*); b) physical, moral, mental, intellectual will-power (*vīrya*); c) recollection and permanent imprints that accrue from practice as memory (*smṛti*); and d) profound contemplative awareness in reaching the soul (*samādhi prajñā*). These are the four essential pillars of the *sādhanā*.

Thus *sādhanā krama* builds a firm foundation, preventing and removing the disharmonies that appear in body as well as in *sādhanā*. It also protects and supports the *sādhaka* through the first four petals, *yama*, *niyama*, *āsana* and *prāṇāyāma*, which are achieved by a mentality of friendliness, compassion, gladness and indifference towards failure and success. When all these disharmonies are removed, it is possible to reach the inner gates of the mind, in the quest for a holistic life.

NOTE

Please read and re-read the following *sūtras* concerning *sādhanā* – I.12, 14, 32, 33; II.15, 16, 30, 32, 33, 35, 36, 37, 38 and IV.3.

XIII

Adhaḥpatana Rekhā in *Sādhanā* – The Razor Edge of Yoga

Patañjali cautions the *sādhaka* at several places to be watchful so that he does not fall from the grace of yoga due to the pride of success.

Almost all commentators and masters on yoga comment on the upaniṣadic saying that practising yoga is like walking on a precipice or on a razor's edge. This description appears very apt. Here are some *sūtra*s describing a fall, as expressed by Patañjali.

For example, the nine *antarāya*s – disease, sluggishness, idleness, indecisive behaviour, inadvertence, lack of judgement, illusion, the inability to pursue the undertaken task, and the inability to maintain progress (I.30) – cause sorrows and grief (II.3). Fluctuating states of consciousness, with painful and non-painful or perceptible and imperceptible thoughts (I.5) – bring distress, dejection and laboured breathing (I.31), whether knowingly or unknowingly. These in turn draw the seer towards involvement (I.4) due to ignorance. It is also possible that the power of the impostor (*ahaṁkāra*) may mean these interruptions obscure the seer.

For this reason the *vṛtti*s must be restrained. When *citta vṛtti*s are not restrained, the small self gets trapped by *citta* and *citta vṛtti*s. In fact, this small self comes so close to the functioning of *citta* that it identifies itself as part of the *citta*.

Both the small self and the Big Self dwell in one home. It is possible that the small self is ensnared by the waves and movements of consciousness (*citta vṛttis*), which disturb the harmony in the conscience, I-maker, intelligence and mind (*antarendriyas*), displacing the splendour in the seer.

vṛtti-sārūpyam itaratra **(I.4)**	Ignoring his own nature, the *puruṣa*, by his *sākāra rūpa* (form), is enticed by the objects of the senses, which make him forget that He is in His home.

As a flame is covered by smoke, mirrors by dirt, and the embryo by the amnion, so is the *puruṣa* covered with the above impediments as the *buddhi* is coated with the psycho-somatic or somato-psychic disturbances. This affects both the lower self and the higher self (*B. G.*, III.38).

Even if the *sādhaka* reaches the state of *samādhi*, he must maintain his practice so that he does not develop pride in his success. The second description from Patañjali is *virāma pratyaya*, which is a *siddhi* or an accomplishment. This *virāma pratyaya* is like a plateau between *sabīja* and *nirbīja samādhis*. If the *sādhaka* thinks that he has reached the state of *manolaya* (which is certainly a great success in yoga) and neglects his practice, he will not reach the state of *manojaya*, which may also lead to his downfall.

virāma-pratyaya--abhyāsa-pūrvaḥ saṁskāra-śeṣaḥ anyaḥ **(I.18)**	Though it is said that in this state of *manolaya*, the seer experiences the states of pause and repose, it appears that this state is not *manojaya*. This stopgap between *sabīja* and *nirbīja samādhi* is a state of void (*śūnya*), from which one moves towards *manojaya*, or a non-void (*aśūnya*) state. Otherwise, one experiences the state of *anavasthitatva* (inability to maintain progress).
bhava-pratyayaḥ videha-prakṛti--layānām **(I.19)**	It is possible that this state of void may make the *sādhaka* believe that he has reached the final state, as he experiences a state of bodilessness. He may be merged in the first principle of *mūla prakṛti*, the *mahat* or cosmic consciousness. Patañjali reconfirms

that this merging of individual mind in *mahat* is not the final goal.

***sūkṣma-viṣayatvaṁ ca aliṅga--paryavasānam* (I.45)** Having merged with the first principle of nature (*mahat*), the *sādhaka* may remain in this stage, thinking that it is the end of the *sādhanā*.

***tataḥ mano-javitvaṁ vikaraṇa-bhāvaḥ pradhāna-jayaḥ ca* (III.49)** The individual mind moves towards its master, the cosmic mind. In this transformation, the individual mind (*manas*) is freed from the clutches of the senses and merges with the cosmic consciousness (*mahat*).

***sthāni-upanimantraṇe saṅga-smayā--akaraṇaṁ punar--aniṣṭa-prasaṅgāt* (III.52)** Celestial beings or enchanting humans may entice *sādhakas* at this stage and make them their prey, causing them to fall from the grace of yoga. But if these *sādhakas* stick to *yaugika* practices and remain indifferent to these temptations as well as to the super-normal powers that accrue, the seeds of temptation are destroyed and they dwell in the house of the seer (*kaivalya*).

***te samādhau upasargāḥ vyutthāne siddhayaḥ* (III.38)** Patañjali further cautions that the attainments of even *samādhi* may impede the *sādhaka* if he becomes enamoured by success. He emphasises that though this is an accomplishment greatly admired by any onlooker and considered to be *siddhi*, a true *sādhaka* should not be trapped by those successes.

***dṛg-darśana-śaktyoḥ eka-ātmatā iva asmitā* (II.6)** Non-cultivated intelligence may pretend to be the seer, creating a sense of perplexity or confusion.

***nirmāṇa-cittāni asmitā-mātrāt* (IV.4)** This perplexity can be washed out by the right judgement that comes with study. This can change that intelligence into a cultivated state of *sāsmita* or *nirmāṇa citta*. When this mature state is reached, the impostor (ego) fades out from the *sādhaka*'s heart and he feels the real 'thou art that'.

The problem for humans in general and *sādhakas* in particular is that nature plays multiple roles. It may engage with the seer or with the objects of desire. The danger of these multiple roles is beautifully expressed in Chapter II and throughout the *Bhagavad Gītā*.

For example, Lord Krishna says to Arjuna, 'You grieve for those who should not be grieved for' (*B. G.*, II.11); 'The contact between the senses and their objects give rise to transitory and fleeting pleasures tainted with pains' (*B. G.*, II.14); and 'When one thoroughly dismisses all cravings of the senses and mind and dwells in the real Self, one is considered to have a stable mind' (*B. G.*, II.55). As the tortoise draws its limbs in from all directions, so if one withdraws the senses from the sense objects is it possible to remain stable in mind (*B. G.*, II.58).

prakāśa-kriyā-sthiti--śīlaṁ bhūta-indriya-ātmakaṁ bhoga-apavargā-arthaṁ dṛśyam **(II.18)**	By walking on both the edges of the razor, the *sādhaka* faces the good and bad sides of nature and learns to be unattached to both. *Prakṛti*, with the elements of nature, may lead one to get caught in a worldly life of sensual pleasures (*bhogārtha*). But, by withdrawing thoughts from the attractions and pleasures of the senses, p*rakṛti* may lead towards freedom and bliss (*apavarga*).

The effect of yoga depends upon one's motivations. The motivation for practice may be to float in sensual pleasures or to achieve illumination and liberation from the sensual pleasures. If maturity in intelligence and clarity in motivation are generated, a good foundation is built, from which it is possible to reach bliss in this very life.

On account of our ignorance (*avidyā*), there are hindrances on the path of yoga, which I group together along with ways to overcome them.

Note the cause of ignorance:

***vitarkāḥ hiṁsā- -ādayaḥ kṛta- -kārita-anumoditāḥ lobha-krodha-moha- pūrvakāḥ-mṛdu- -madhya- -adhimātraḥ duḥkha-ajñāna- -ananta-phalāḥ iti pratipakṣa- -bhāvanam* (II.34)**	Greed, anger and infatuations cause ignorance (*avidyā*), leading to violence, either directly or through temptation. These reactions may be mild, moderate or intense, resulting in endless pain and dubious knowledge.
***tāsām anāditvaṁ ca āśiṣaḥ nityatvāt* (IV.10)**	As this endless pain and ignorance exists from time immemorial, desires (*vāsanā*) also exist from time immemorial. One must develop thoughts cautiously and judiciously through *yaugika* discipline to come out from these seeds of ignorance. This burns the seed of ignorance (*avidyā*) and brings a full stop to the endless pains and desires, sowing the seed of *vidyā* to follow the path of *mokṣa*.

Ignorance (*avidyā*) being the cause of all sorrows (*tasya hetuḥ avidyā* – II.24), *yoga vidyā* or *yaugika* knowledge not only eradicates *avidyā* but also offer ways towards emancipation (*mokṣa*).

Refer to *sūtra* II.25 :

***tad-abhāvāt saṁyoga-abhāvaḥ hānaṁ tad-dṛśeḥ kaivalyam* (II.25)**	This ignorance that binds the seer to the seen is destroyed by breaking the link through direct and right knowledge from experience, filled with wisdom.
***draṣṭṛ-dṛśyayoḥ saṁyogaḥ heya-hetuḥ* (II.17)**	The conjunction of the seen (*prakṛti*) with the seer (*puruṣa*) causes *vṛtti*, *kleśa* and *antarāya*, distorting consciousness. This *sūtra* emphasises that the remedy is to relinquish this conjunction. Though Patañjali says that this is one way, he also suggests another method to make constructive use of *prakṛti* for the evolution of *puruṣa*.

sva-svāmi-śaktyoḥ sva-rūpa-upalabdhi--hetuḥ saṁyogaḥ (II.23) Patañjali shows how the same instruments that cause the conjunction can be used through *yoga vidyā* to perceive the Lord of consciousness. This is achieved by weighing, measuring, balancing the intelligence of consciousness with the awareness of the seer – *prajñā*.

1. The Precipice

The most difficult precipice to walk on comes when one has reached the state of *ekāgratā* or single-focused attention (*dhāraṇā*), where there is neither the emergence nor the termination of thought waves.

tataḥ punaḥ śānta-uditau tulya--pratyayau cittasya ekāgratā-pariṇāmaḥ (III.12) Watching the rising and fading thoughts, and keeping away from them by maintaining the mind, intelligence and consciousness in a steady and stable state with total careful awareness, and without interruption, is *ekāgratā*.

This total attentive awareness may lead one towards intellectual intoxication or the addiction of ego or pride.

tat-chidreṣu pratyaya-antarāṇi saṁskārebhyaḥ (IV.27) This intellectual pride in knowledge grows weeds in the form of intoxication, and scatters and creates cracks in the cultured *buddhi* and *citta*. These cracks become entry points for afflictions.

hānam eṣāṁ kleśavat uktam (IV.28) So with careful attention, one has to protect oneself by renouncing pride. When these weeds are eradicated, one reaches the state of *kaivalya*.

tad-vairāgyāt api doṣa-bīja-kṣaye kaivalyam (III.51) By renouncing the success that comes in the form of *siddhis*, the seed of defects become ineffective and the path towards *kaivalya* is cleared.

sattva-puruṣayoḥ śuddhi-sāmye kaivalyam iti (III.56) For this state of emancipation, the *sādhaka* has to reach perfection in yoga so that the purity of nature's intelligence is made equal to that of the non-changing awareness of the seer (*prajñā*).

From this perfection, he will have *ātma-prasādana* (I.47) and his consciousness will be transformed from *adivya citta* to *divya citta*, or divine consciousness.

XIV

Aṣṭāṅga Yoga Prayoga, Tathā Pariṇāma – The Application of *Aṣṭāṅga* Yoga and Its Effects

Now I would like to share yoga with you as a lifestyle that enables right living by utilising the principles of nature, *puruṣa* and *Īśvara*.

As I mentioned before, *citta* is the bridge that connects the seen and the seer, enabling the seer to realise his own nature. In the same way, *aṣṭāṅga yoga* acts as a bridge for the *sādhaka*s to be liberated from the avenue of sensual pleasures (*bhoga*) and led towards the path of emancipation and freedom (*mokṣa* or *apavarga*).

1. *Śarīra Śarīrī Bhāva*

Before embarking on the path of *aṣṭāṅga yoga*, one has to know that the body (*śarīra*) is a field and that the holder of this body is the seer (*śarīrī*), the *puruṣa* or the *ātman*. As the body is the pillar of the seer, it has to be cared for so that its contents support and uplift the seer and keep him in his own glory.

Before going into the depth of yoga, I would like to present a map of the body, showing its various sheaths as the journey on the *yaugika* path.

The body is a unit with arms, legs, organs and various systems, includng the respiratory, circulatory, nervous, digestive, urinary, excretory and glandular systems. All these systems integrate to form an organism, which has to function harmoniously for good health. Knowledge of the systems and their harmonious functioning is needed for the realisation of the seer.

Yoga darśana created the map of the human body thousands of years ago to enable one to catch sight of the Soul.

2. *Kośas* of the Body

In this *yaugika* journey, we have certain resources at our disposal in the form of the causal body (*kāraṇa śarīra*), subtle body (*sūkṣma śarīra*) and gross body (*kārya śarīra*) or body of action (*sthūla śarīra*).

Like caves within caves, these three bodies of man are enveloped by layers in the form of organs of action, senses of perception, mind, intelligence, 'I'-maker, consciousness, conscience, 'I'-ness (*ahaṁ-ākāra*) and the seer. These again are subdivided into the anatomical sheath, vital-organic sheath, mental sheath, intellectual sheath and the sheath composed of bliss. This way we may fully conceive the body (*śarīra*) and the holder of the body (*śarīrī*) in the right balance.

Each *kośa* is covered with gross, subtle and causal sheaths. Though I often mention the skin, belonging to *vāyu* and *ākāśa tattva*s (the qualities of *vijñānamaya* and *ānandamaya kośas*), on the purely anatomical, musculoskeletal level (*annamaya kośa*), the bones become the causal sheath; muscles, the subtle sheath; and the skin, the gross sheath. In the organic sheath (*prāṇamaya kośa*), the respiratory system is the gross; the blood circulation, the subtle; and the nervous system, the causal. In the mental sheath (*manomaya kośa*), the organs of action are the gross; the senses of perception, the subtle; and the external mind, the causal. In the intellectual sheath (*vijñānamaya kośa*), the internal mind is the gross; intelligence (*buddhi*), the subtle; and the I-maker (*ahaṁkāra*), the causal. And in the sheath of bliss (*ānandamaya kośa*), consciousness (*citta*) is the gross; conscience (*antaḥkaraṇa*), the subtle; and the self, the causal.

As I mentioned before, *aṣṭaṅga yoga* is complete as it covers the art of life (*kalā*), science (*vijñāna*) and *vedānta* (*prajñāna*). They are also interwoven in such a way that each aspect is embedded in all aspects of yoga.

On yoga's journey, one has to interpenetrate the subtle and causal bodies via the gross body or the body of action. One has to go through the inner caves of the body with the intellectual power to develop and live skilfully without allowing the past impressions, which surface from these various caves of the body, to encircle the seer.

Traditionally, the sheath of bliss (*ānandamaya kośa*) is referred to the seer. But I feel the seer is beyond the category of the *pañca bhautika śarīra*, so I feel that this sheath represents the *cittamaya kośa* – just as one experiences a state of bliss from the restraint of consciousness (*citta vṛtti nirodha*).

I feel that yoga covers subjectively the sheath of conscience (*dharmendriya*)[1] along with the seer. On account of this conjunction, each one of us has to pass through these caves to realise the seer who is beyond all these *kośa*s. He is infinitesimally the smallest of the small and the greatest of the great. As it has no *kośa*, *ānandamaya kośa* stands for the conquest of consciousness (*cittajaya*).

Aṣṭaṅga yoga guides us to know, understand and realise the inner mysterious contents of the body from the skin up to the house of the seer.

The *yaugika* journey cleans one from the body up to the seer (*ātman*) and sanctifies all the *kośa*s till the glory of wisdom radiates from the *puruṣa* – the seer.

Look at the next two maps. The first one shows the evolution from causal body to gross body, and the second one the involution from gross body to causal body.

---

1 This classification comes out of my experience and I think it offers a more precise understanding of the mechanism of the human body.

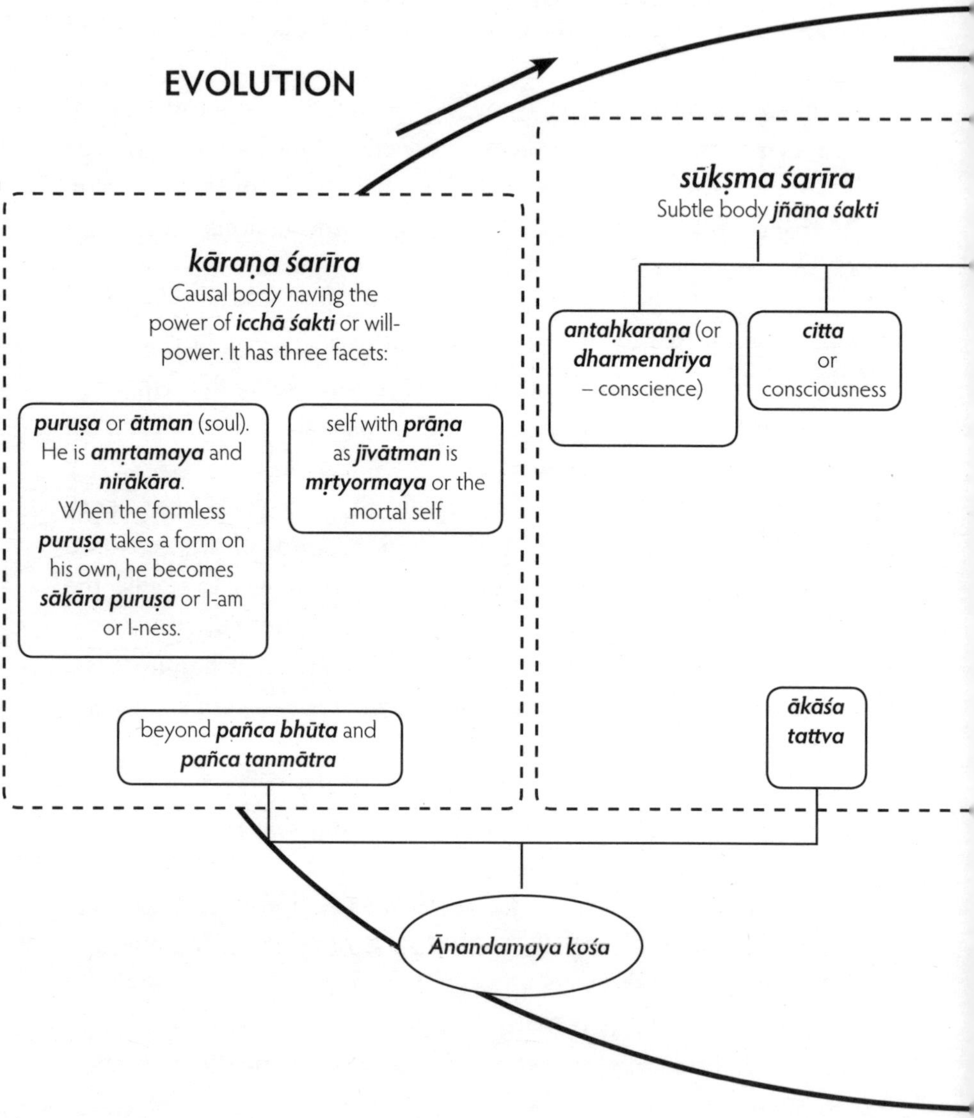
EVOLUTION
kāraṇa śarīra
Causal body having the power of icchā śakti or will-power. It has three facets:
puruṣa or ātman (soul). He is amṛtamaya and nirākāra. When the formless puruṣa takes a form on his own, he becomes sākāra puruṣa or I-am or I-ness.
self with prāṇa as jīvātman is mṛtyormaya or the mortal self
beyond pañca bhūta and pañca tanmātra
sūkṣma śarīra
Subtle body jñāna śakti
antaḥkaraṇa (or dharmendriya – conscience)
citta or consciousness
ākāśa tattva
Ānandamaya kośa

Map of the body (*śarīra*) with its three facets in the process of evolution

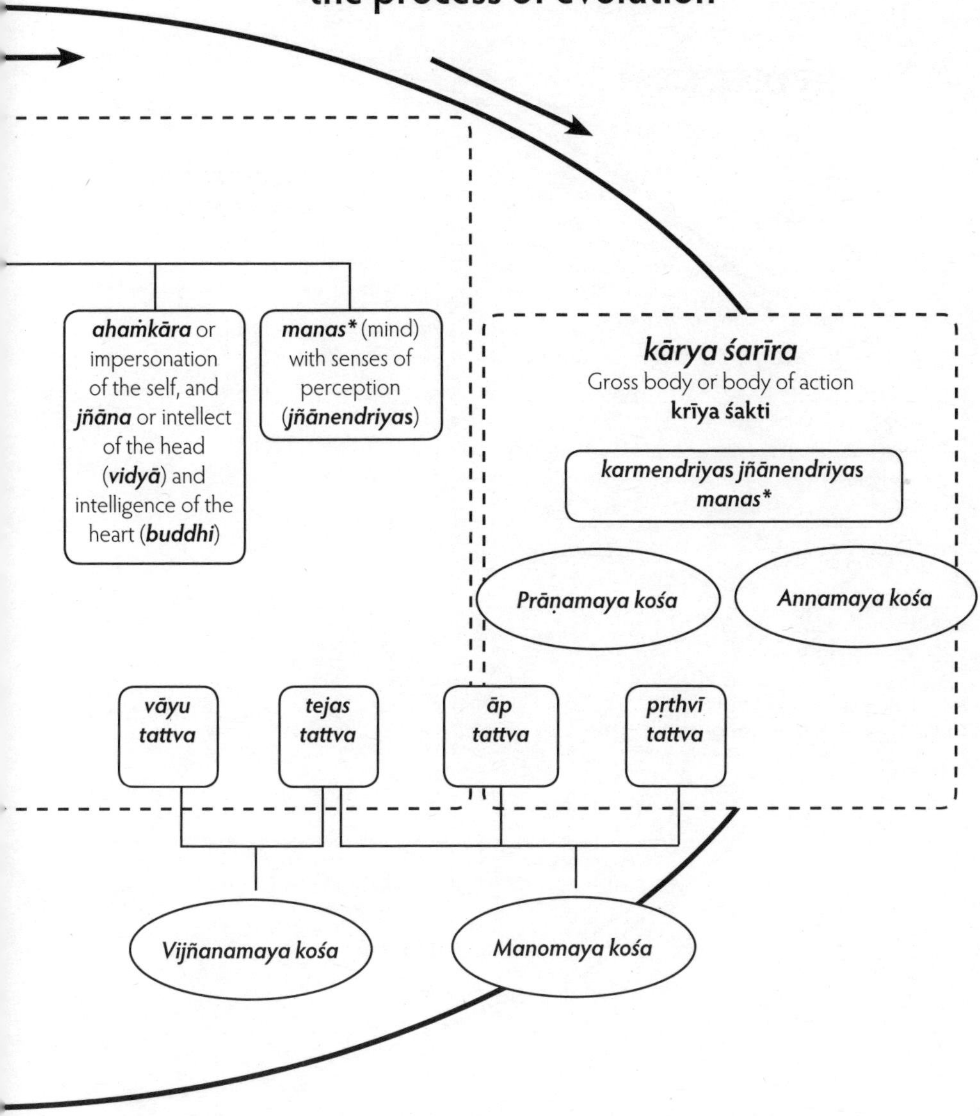

*Note: in the gross body *manas* is the eleventh sense (*ekadaśendriya*), but in the subtle body it acts as the inner mind (*antarendriya*), connecting itself to the finest *indriya*s, such as intelligence (*buddhi*), consciousness (*citta*) and conscience (*dharmendriya*).

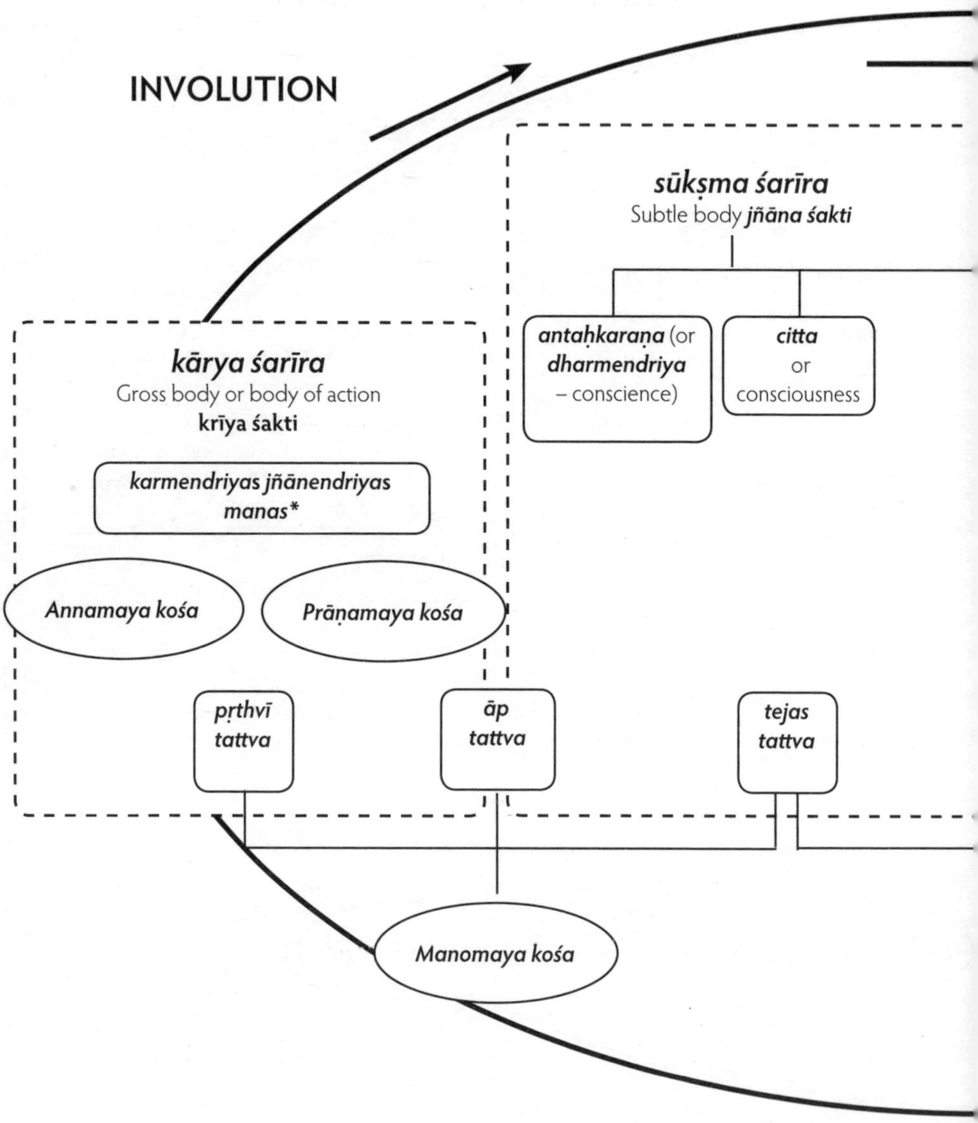

*Note: in the gross body *manas* is the eleventh sense (*ekadaśendriya*), but in the subtle body it acts as the inner mind (*antarendriya*), connecting itself to the finest *indriya*s, such as intelligence (*buddhi*), consciousness (*citta*) and conscience (*dharmendriya*).

Map of the body (*śarīra*) with its three facets in the process of involution

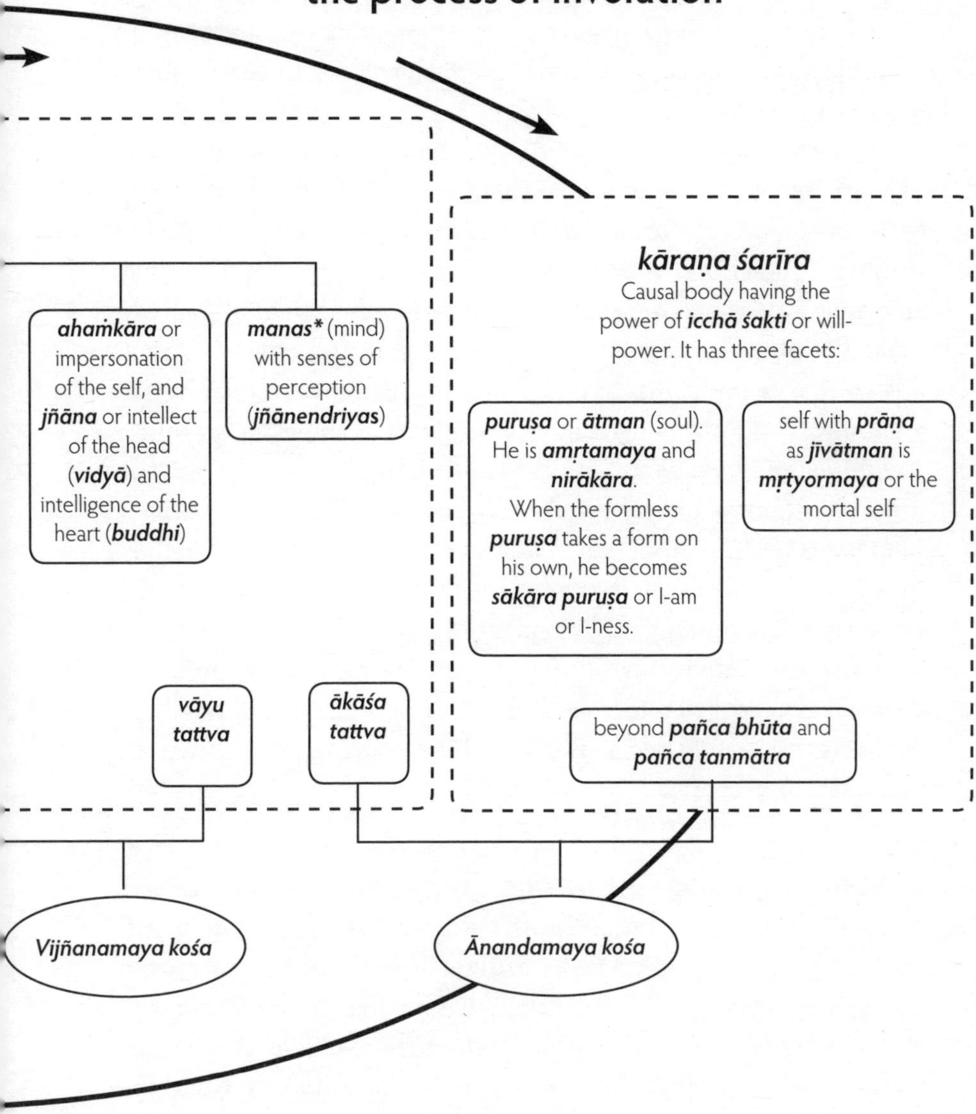

In our ignorance we create our own *kośa*s – namely, *ajñānamaya kośa* (the house of ignorance) and *vāsanāmaya kośa* (the house of desires). Even in these dark houses, there may arise a small desire to begin yoga. Though a person may be considered unfit for yoga (*anādhikārin*) by yoga masters, and though this desire may be *tāmasika*, it is enough to become an *adhikārin* or a fit person to do yoga and gain *yaugika* knowledge.

In *Vibhūti Pāda* (III.4, 7–8), Patañjali demarcates the path of yoga into three aspects for *sādhaka*s to understand according to their intellectual level: *bahiraṅga* (external quest), *antaraṅga* (internal quest) and *antarātman* (interiormost quest). The division into *bahiraṅga*, *antaraṅga* and *antarātman sādhanā* helps to make the notion accessible for a new student. *Bahiraṅga sādhanā* deals with the body of action (*kārya* or *sthūla śarīra*), covering the anatomical and physiological bodies as well as the external mind. *Antaraṅga sādhanā* deals with the subtle body (*sūkṣma śarīra*), the inner mind, intelligence, I-maker and consciousness. *Antarātman sādhanā* is for the causal body (*kāraṇa śarīra*). There is no *sādhanā* for the seer, but since he is involved with the body, yogis coined the word *antarātman sādhanā* to express its depth.

These three divisions of yoga are simply to enable the innocent and ignorant to understand the close connections of the three *śarīra*s (gross, subtle and causal), as all these *śarīra*s are interwoven and interconnected.

3. *Bahiraṅga* and *Antaraṅga Saṁyama*

The word *sādhanā* is often translated as 'quest'. The term 'quest' conveys the idea of a long and arduous search and investigation through practice (*sādhanā*). Patañjali says that *dhāraṇā*, *dhyāna* and *samādhi* together constitute *antaraṅga sādhanā* as an integrated whole (*antaraṅga saṁyama*). This *saṁyama* belongs to the *vijñānamaya*, *cittamaya* and *antaḥkaraṇamaya kośa*s, as these are in close contact with each other. Patañjali connects the *antarendriyas* (*buddhi*, *ahaṁkāra* and *citta*) with *dhāraṇā*, *dhyāna* and *samādhi*. These three *antarendriyas* move close to each other as the last three petals of yoga are close to each other.

trayam ekatra saṁyamaḥ **(III.4)**	These three – *dhāraṇā*, *dhyāna* and *sabīja samādhi* – are together termed *saṁyama*, an integrated whole.

Saṁyama is when the intellect of the head and the intelligence of the heart are united as one (*see* I.17 and I.33). At this time, not only does a vast change happen in consciousness but the extent of knowledge is substantially refined and becomes sensitive. Here one discovers many hidden things under the umbrella of *saṁyama*. For example, *samādhi* is demarcated into *sabīja* and *nirbīja*. In the same way, *saṁyama* too can be demarcated into two parts (*bahiraṅga* and *antaraṅga*). If *dhāraṇā*, *dhyāna* and *samādhi* are *antaraṅga saṁyama*, then *āsana*, *prāṇāyāma* and *pratyāhāra* are *bahiraṅga saṁyama* as they integrate the body with organs of action, senses of perception and the mind.

Let us have a look at what is involved in *saṁyama*. It involves tying up, holding or binding together. More often, it refers to integration. It is a process of absorbing the psychological or mental aspects into the 'object of meditation'. For this to be effective, that object must be magnetic and have an attraction for the meditator (I.39) that encourages him to penetrate deep enough to bring about a transformation both ethically as well as intellectually. This process of deep absorption acts as a tool of cognition for receiving a deeper, subtler and refined intuitive knowledge of the qualities of the object.

In this refined state, one can identify a threefold process, wherein each encases what is enveloped by the other.

The sequence of transformation can be seen in *sūtra*s III.9 to 16, where *nirodha*, *samādhi* and *ekāgratā pariṇāma*s bring about the *dharma*, *lakṣaṇa* and *avasthā pariṇāma* of the elemental body. Handled judiciously, this transformation becomes the conduit for reaching perfection or gaining powers.

A lot of attention is given to the super-normal powers enumerated in the *Yoga Sūtras*. They have a sort of glamour and notoriety.

Dhāraṇā	*Dhyāna*	*Samādhi*
subjugation of intelligence (*buddhi*)	subjugation of the personified self (*ahaṁkāra*)	absorption of *citta* in the *seer* or *ātman*
listening	investigating	Realising
studying	contemplating	Meditating
intent concentration	deep reflection	assimilation and unity
virtuous action	meditative absorption	discerning wisdom
āgama	*anumāna*	*pratyakṣa*
any thoughtful activity	contemplative absorption	deepest level of absorption

But the process of *saṁyama* is not just for these ends. *Saṁyama* is required by the *sādhaka* to vanquish the obscure and cultivate discernment, enabling him to relinquish the small self and realise the true state of the Self, and then to proceed towards *Īśvara praṇidhāna*.

The unit of *dhāraṇā*, *dhyāna* and *samādhi* is the focus for the topic of *saṁyama*, but in fact this unit is relegated to the external when compared to *nirbīja samādhi*. There are levels of *saṁyama* that need not be associated with meditation only, but are a process of integrating one's lifestyle in terms of ethics, correct social observances and self-analysis. These three aspects of integration help to cultivate the whole self. These external aspects are, in fact, vital to enable the refinement of the internal levels of integration. As I mentioned above, a single disturbance in one's moral/ethical conduct sends waves of disturbance, which make it impossible for the *sādhanā*s to reach the zenith but possibly causing a fall.

We can demarcate *aṣṭaṅga yoga* into three parts: *yama* and *niyama* as the art of living (*kalā*); *āsana*, *prāṇāyāma* and *pratyāhāra*, collected together as *bahiraṅga saṁyama*, as science (*vijñāna*); and *dhāraṇā*, *dhyāna* and *samādhi* as *antaraṅga saṁyama*, as *Brahma jñāna* (*prajñāna*) on the *vedāntika* level. This is why I insist that yoga is the integration of art (*kalā*), science (*vijñāna*) and insight (*prajñāna*).

Referring to the art of living, Patañjali uses *vedāntika* language (highly noble words) to build up ethical character by *yama* in the form of *ahiṁsā, satya, asteya, brahmacarya, aparigraha*, and by *niyama* in *śauca, saṁtoṣa, tapaḥ, svādhyāya, Īśvara praṇidhāna*.

The principles of *yama* are universal. They are not meant only for *yaugika* practitioners. *Yama*, the art of living (*kalā*) is for all, whether one moves on the path of *karma, jñāna, bhakti* or yoga. Principles of *yama* are necessary for all paths. As a bird has two wings for flight, so the *sādhaka* of any path needs two wings to reach the goal of *ātma-sākṣātkāra*. If one wing is morality, the other wing is the spiritual understanding and pursuit. Hence *yama* is for all as *ātma-darśana* is for all.

Patañjali uses words in a way that does not alienate the human mind with its instinctive weakness. Men and women may constantly fall prey to destructive instincts and become violent, aggressive, untruthful, libertine and greedy, finding ways to misappropriate another's possessions. Patañjali wants both men and women to live without being caught in these destructive instincts, cultivating constructive thoughts to practise with cleanliness, contentment and passion, and thus gain higher knowledge of the Self and then surrender wholly to God. This is the art of living, in which *jīvanamukti* is hidden. This can be cultivated by following the sublime souls who have lived benevolently.

Āsana, prāṇāyāma and *pratyāhāra* are *bahiraṅga saṁyama*. They integrate the body, organs of action, senses of perception and the external mind through expressions, experiments and experiences. Hence these three aspects of *yaugika saṁyama* come under scientific exploration (*vijñāna śāstra*).

Dhāraṇā, dhyāna and *samādhi* are *antaraṅga saṁyama* of yoga. They enable *sādhaka*s (whether young or old, men or women) to experience directly the state of unalloyed silence in the silence (*prajñāna*) which is beyond words, though many describe this as the state of *satcidānandā*.

***trayam-antar--aṅgaṁ pūrvebhyaḥ* (III.7)**	As the *antaraṅgas* (inner mind, *buddhi, ahaṁkāra, citta, antaḥkaraṇa*) are the inner parts of the seer, so Patañjali considers *dhāraṇā, dhyāna* and *samādhi* to be the internal parts of yoga.

These three petals of yoga (*dhāraṇā, dhyāna* and *samādhi*) are *antaraṅga* (internal) compared to the earlier petals of yoga, namely: *yama, niyama, āsana, prāṇāyāma* and *pratyāhāra*.

Leaving aside *yama* and *niyama*, which are the keys to the art of living, the other six petals actually cover the technical aspects of yoga. As a whole, yoga is *aṣṭāṅga*, but from the technical point of view it is *ṣaḍāṅga yoga*.

I teach the first five petals of yoga, as they are most readily perceived by the mind. When this has been achieved, I make practitioners experience the other three internal petals that can be perceived, so that they become fully integrated, and show them ways to connect the external sheaths with the internal sheaths. This way they cultivate oneness between the body (field) and the seer (fielder).

Patañjali later explains the *antaraṅga saṁyama* of *dhāraṇā, dhyāna* and *samādhi* as *bahiraṅga* (external) compared to the seedless *nirbīja samādhi*. Here the flame of the seer is sighted, indicating the establishment of the *antarātman* aspect of *samādhi*.

The *bahiraṅga* aspects – namely, the organs of action, senses of perception and the external mind – are like the seed that enables further understanding of the internal parts (*antaraṅgas*) – namely, the mind, intelligence, ego and consciousness, which provide the base for recognising the various states of *sabīja*, or seeded *samādhi*. From this state of realisation, one has to move from the seeded *samādhi* to experience the seedless state of *samādhi*, or the absolute state of awareness i.e., the sight of the *puruṣa*.

***tā eva sabījaḥ samādhiḥ* (I.46)**	*Sabīja samādhi* is a *samādhi* with seed or support.
***tadapi bahir-aṅgaṁ nirbījasya* (III.8)**	Patañjali describes this seedless state of *samādhi* (*nirbīja samādhi*) as the finest and the interiormost

(*antarātman*) compared to the *antaraṅga* aspects of yoga.

***tasya api nirodhe sarva-nirodhāt nirbījaḥ samādhiḥ* (I.51)** All the impressions created so far are left behind, and from then on the *sādhaka* remains ever free from all latent impressions (*saṁskāras*).

***taj-jayāt prajñā-ālokaḥ* (III.5)** I feel that this *sūtra* conveys the outcome of *saṁyama* towards *prajñāloka*, the light (*āloka*) of the *ātman* (*prajñāna*).

4. Effects of *Saṁyamas*

***tasya bhūmiṣu viniyogaḥ* (III.6)** With this knowledge, the *sādhaka* changes his awareness and outlook and learns to apply, relay and share this with others according to their physical, moral, mental and intellectual calibre.

What is this knowledge of awareness?

***tasya saptadhā prānta-bhūmiḥ prajñā* (II.27)** There are seven states of awareness of the human consciousness, which are dealt with differently by different traditional authors. For me, the seven states of knowledge (*prajñā*) are either on a perceptible level or on the levels of integration (*saṁyama*).
On a perceptible level are: knowledge of the body, including organs of action and senses of perception (*śarīra*), knowledge of energy (*prāṇa*), knowledge of the mind (*manas*), clarity of intelligence (*vijñāna*), experienced knowledge (*ānubhavika*), absorption of the flavour of experienced knowledge (*rasātmaka*), and the knowledge of the seer (*puruṣa*). On the levels of integration are: the body, senses, energy, mind, intelligence, consciousness and the self.

On a theoretical level, Śrī Vyāsa describes awareness in the following terms: the knowable is known; what must be discarded is discarded; what is attainable is attained; what must be done is done, the aim that must be reached is reached; and independent, self-sustaining, untainted intelligence is built up for the seer to enlighten himself.

Yoga Vāsiṣṭha speaks on a conceptual level and says that right desire and right deliberation make the mind become mindless, ending the duality of the subject/object relationship with external phenomena. This leads to experiencing the state of self-realisation that has no words (and which therefore cannot be related to, even afterwards).

Patañjali explains some effects of *saṁyama* in Chapter III, though one can trace the effects of integration mentioned in each leaf of *aṣṭāṅga yoga*.

***pariṇāma-traya--saṁyamāt atīta--anāgata-jñānam* (III.16)**
By this integration, one gains knowledge of the past and the present.

***śabda-artha--pratyayānām itara-itara--adhyāsāt saṅkaraḥ tat-pravibhāga--saṁyamāt sarva--bhūta-rūta-jñānam* (III.17)**
In this state, no confusion arises in body, mind and speech or in the interplay of word, work and wisdom. They are synchronised and move without any deviations, bringing purity or rightness in mind, speech and body (*trikaraṇa śuddhi*).

***pratyayasya para--citta-jñānam* (III.19)**
This integrated quality of consciousness gives one the ability to grasp what is in the minds of others.

***na ca tat sālambanaṁ tasya aviṣayī bhūtatvāt* (III.20)**
Though the yogi has the ability to read the minds of others, he never wastes his time and energy in exploring the mind and motivations of others, except in helping them towards the right way of living.

***kāya-rūpa-saṁyamāt tad-grāhya-śakti--stambhe cakṣuḥ prakāśa asaṁprayoge--antardhānam* (III.21)**
He develops the power of becoming invisible.

etena śabdā-ādi antardhānam uktam (III.22)	He is able to arrest sound, smell, taste, form and touch.
sattva-puruṣayoḥ atyantā- -asaṁkīrṇayoḥ pratyaya-aviśeṣaḥ bhogaḥ para- -arthatvāt sva-artha saṁyamāt puruṣa- -jñānam (III.36)	He is unified by a pure unmingled intelligence, by contrast to a motivated, mingled intelligence. He lives in communion with the soul.
śrotra-ākāśayoḥ saṁbandha- -saṁyamāt divyaṁ śrotram (III.42)	He acquires the power of hearing sounds from space.
kāya-ākāśayoḥ saṁbandha- saṁyamāt laghu- -tūla-samāpatteḥ ca ākāśa-gamanam (III.43)	He can become as light as cotton and move and fly through space. [I do not think that in recent decades anyone has reached this state.]
kṣaṇa-tat-kramayoḥ saṁyamāt viveka- -jaṁ jñānam (III.53)	By watching the movements of moments without becoming involved in the cycle of movements, he knows and understands time as timeless and space as spaceless.
tārakaṁ sarva- viṣayaṁ sarvathā viṣayaṁ akramaṁ ca iti viveka-jaṁ jñānam (III.55)	The *sādhaka* reaches the exalted state of wisdom wherein he grasps instantly, clearly and wholly the flame of the seer (*ātmāgni*) without undergoing the sequences of transformations or time.

These are the effects of the *saṁyama*s.

When we look through the successive connections of the three bodies, the external quest is for cleanliness of the body, while the inner quest is for cultivating the mind, intelligence and consciousness.

From these one develops clarity for the interiormost seer to live everlastingly in a lively state of benevolence. Though it is not possible to demarcate where the body ends and the mind begins, or where the mind ends and the self begins, these divisions are offered to bring an understanding of this integrated subject of yoga to *sādhaka*s who have inert (*tāmasika*) or scattered minds (*rājasika*). As the seen and the seer are interwoven from the skin to the core, and vice versa, this inter-relationship between the body and the quests (*sādhanā*) might be compartmentalised into *bahiraṅga* (external), *bahiraṅga-antaraṅga* (combination of external and internal), *antaraṅga* (internal), *antaraṅga-antaḥkaraṇa* (combination of internal and interiormost), and *antarātman* (the core of being).

No doubt, there are various paths and practices to experience the benevolence of the seer, but in truth, there is no *sādhanā* such as *antarātman sādhanā*, as *ātman* needs no *sādhanā*. It is we as individuals who as seekers of the seer need the *sādhanā* to feel the seer or the *ātman*.

We are endowed with arms and legs for the path of action (*karma mārga*), head for knowledge (*jñāna mārga*) and the heart's wisdom for devotion to God (*bhakti mārga*) for the total surrender of oneself to God.

In order to progress and evolve in these three paths of *karma*, *jñāna* and *bhakti*, *aṣṭaṅga yoga* acts as a base line and also provides a springboard for further evolution and stability in body, mind and self.

Thus the chapter covers the interlinking of constituents from the body to the seer, and guides one to gain control over the external body in order to explore the inner mind by developing mature wisdom (*buddhi*). From mature wisdom, one has to subjugate the *ahaṁkāra* (I-maker) to sight the flame of the seer. Then on, it is possible to live by the unfading illuminative flame of the seer – the *puruṣa*.

5. Application of Yoga

So far I have dealt with theory. Now let me explain the ways of yoga in turn so that the benefits of yoga can be adopted, adapted and adjusted to as quickly as possible. The practical aspects of yoga begin with *yama* to cleanse the organs of actions; *niyama* for control of the senses of perception; *āsana*s for keeping the body clean; *prāṇāyāma* for right usage of energy; *pratyāhāra* to obtain stability in mind; *dhāraṇā* for clarity and maturity in intelligence; *dhyāna* to cultivate humility by subjugating ego and pride; and *samādhi* for a composed state of equanimity.

I call the aspects of *aṣṭāṅga yoga* petals (*daḷa*s) because just as a flower unfolds all its petals simultaneously, so the eight aspects of yoga have to bloom at the same time. This makes the flame of the soul light the mind, intelligence and consciousness so that they bloom together.

yama-niyama- ***-āsana-prāṇāyāma-*** ***-pratyāhāra-*** ***-dhāraṇā-dhyāna-*** ***-samādhayaḥ aṣṭau*** ***aṅgāni* (II.29)**	This yoga has eight aspects (*aṅga*). These are: a) moral and ethical injunctions, b) observances, c) postures or positions, d) regulation of the breath, e) internalisation of the senses, f) attention, g) meditation and h) absorption.

I feel that these eight petals of yoga are respectively related to the *tri-śārīra* (the three bodies: the causal, subtle and gross bodies, which are a mixture of purity and impurity).

The body of sense and feeling is equally the forum for experiencing sensual pleasures – *bhogasthāna*, as well as *apavargasthāna* or *yogasthāna* (*see* II.15).

We have six *cakra*s, namely *mūlādhāra*, *svādhiṣṭhāna*, *maṇipūraka*, *anāhata*, *viśuddhi* and *ājñā*. The first three *cakras* function on the *bhogasthāna* (seat of pleasure) and the upper three on the *yogasthāna* (seat of unalloyed bliss).

In II.34, Patañjali explains three causes of ignorance (*avidyā*). These are direct action (*kṛta*), complicity (*kārita*) and permissiveness (*anumodita*). These occur due to greed or desire (*lobha*), anger (*krodha*) and delusion or infatuation (*moha*). By thinking carefully, one realises that sensual joys are indirectly caused by *kārita* and *anumodita*, and *apavarga* or liberation comes from direct action (*kṛta*), freeing oneself from the influences of the senses. All aspects of *yaugika* practices help to eradicate this mixture, leading towards sanctity and purity.

When one aspect of yoga is explicitly followed, it does not mean that the other aspects of yoga are overlooked or neglected; they are followed implicitly. When a practitioner pays particular attention to one of the petals of the *yaugika* flower, he cleanses consciousness. This change or transformation refines the relationship of all the petals and transforms them.

yoga-aṅga- ***-anuṣṭhānāt aśuddhi-*** ***kṣaye jñāna-dīptiḥ*** ***aviveka-khyāteḥ*** **(II.28)**	By attentive devotional practice of all the eight aspects of yoga, the impurities of body, mind and intelligence are eradicated and the essence of knowledge and wisdom radiates throughout life.

Patañjali uses the words *aṣṭāṅga yoga*. *Aṣṭa* means eight and *aṅga* means way, manner, mode, limb, member or part of the whole. It also means the root of a word, an expedience or a means to an end.

Now let me explain the eight petals of yoga that begin with *yama*.

6. *Yama*

ahiṁsā-satya- ***-asteya-brahmacarya-*** ***-aparigrahāḥ yamāḥ*** **(II.30)**	To learn to be harmless, truthful, non-covetous, moderate in worldly or material life and to cultivate non-greed verbally, physically and mentally is *yama*.

Patañjali explains *aṣṭāṅga yoga* with its three aspects or divisions, namely external (*bahiraṅga*), internal (*antaraṅga*) and interiormost (*antarātman*). Similarly, *yama* can be divided into three aspects. If *ahiṁsā* and *satya* transform us through contact with external means (*bahiraṅga*), *asteya* and *brahmacarya* are completely subjective or internal (*antaraṅga*), whereas *aparigraha* is purely an instinctive experiential imprint (*saṁskārika*), which continues birth after birth and which has to be handled by the illuminative light of the Self. Hence, it is considered an aspect of *antarātman*. If a mirror is covered with dust, it cannot reflect clearly. Similarly, the *antarātman* cannot be clearly felt due to the dust of ignorance that covers it.

***jāti-deśa- -kāla-samaya- -anavacchinnāḥ sārva-bhaumāḥ mahāvratam* (II.31)**	Ethical developement in life does not depend on class, time or conditions. They are universal principles and are meant to break the destructive instincts of man's mind (verbal, physical or mental).

To improve character, these are to be followed as far as possible. Actions rooted in unskilful or unwholesome mental states disturb the conscientious state, which makes higher practices impossible.

7. Effects of *Yama*

The effects of *yama* are mainly explained in Chapter II. As for many of the miraculous effects described in Chapter III, I believe these are nothing less than the ripeness of what has been acquired through the practice of all the eight *aṅgas*. That is why I include some *sūtras* from Chapter III, which I consider to be closely related to the practice of *yama*.

***ahiṁsā- -pratiṣṭhāyām tat- sannidhau vaira- -tyāgaḥ* (II.35)**	The effect of non-violence makes those who hate each other become friends.
***maitri-ādiṣu balāni* (III.24)**	Similarly, by sticking to the principles of non-violence, one acquires strength and power as well as friendliness.
***baleṣu hasti-bala- -ādīni* (III.25)**	In accordance with the saying 'The pen is mightier than the sword,' words should be judiciously spoken. Otherwise, the words will hurt till the end of life, more so than actions. Yogis with the power to speak wisely have a physical and mental strength like that of an elephant or an eagle.

satya-pratiṣṭhāyāṁ kriyā-phala--āśrayatvam (II.36) For one who lives with genuine honesty, without deviation between actions, thoughts and speech, accuracy and precision are the rewards.

asteya-pratiṣṭhāyāṁ sarva-ratna--upasthānam (II.37) Non-covetousness leads to desirelessness, and this in turn brings worldly and spiritual wealth without a hankering for them.

brahmacarya--pratiṣṭhāyāṁ vīrya--lābhaḥ (II.38) One who controls sensual pleasures develops vigour and energy.

aparigraha-sthairye janma-kathaṁtā saṁbodhaḥ (II.39) One who lives free from possessions and lives without greed reaches the path of knowledge and wisdom, which is real and permanent.

saṁskāra--sākṣāt karaṇāt pūrva-jā-ti-jñānam (III.18) All defective instincts of the past vanish when one has mastery of *aparigraha* (*see* II.39).[1] By this mastery, one gets direct perception of the previous states of birth, and wisdom dawns.

8. *Niyama*

śauca-saṇtoṣa tapaḥ-svādhyāya-Īśvara--praṇidhānāni niyamāḥ (II.32) Practice with a searching mind is meant to purify the body and the mind, bringing satisfaction and contentment. After acquiring purity, one must proceed towards dedicated and devoted practice and study (*tapas* and *svādhyāya*). This guides practitioners to the higher and nobler aspects of life so that they resign to God.

Here too, if *śauca* and *saṅtoṣa* are external quests, *tapas* and *svādhyāya* are internal, and *Īśvara praṇidhāna* is the interiormost aspect.

1 *aparigraha-sthairye janma-kathaṁtā saṁbodhaḥ* (II.39) – Knowledge of past and future lives shines like a mirror when one is free from greed.

9. Effects of *Niyama*

śaucāt sva-aṅga -jugupsā paraiḥ asaṁsargaḥ (II.40)	With purity of body, interest in sensual pleasures or contact with others' bodies fades and the urge towards spiritual knowledge dawns.
sattva-śuddhi- -saumanasya- -eka-agrya-indriya- -jaya-ātma-darśana- -yogyatvāni ca (II.41)	By *śauca*, the wandering mind is transformed, which brings cheerfulness, single-focused attention and control over the senses of perception, which lead towards the realisation of the soul.
saṅtoṣāt anuttamaḥ sukha-lābhaḥ (II.42)	From contentment, one must proceed towards unsurpassable delight.
kāya-indriya-siddhiḥ aśuddhi-kṣayāt tapasaḥ (II.43)	Zealous practice with a single frame of mind leads towards divine perfection.
svādhyāyāt iṣṭa- -devatā- saṁprayogaḥ (II.44)	Self-study from the skin to the Self with the guidance of sacred scriptures leads towards the realisation of God, or communion with the longed-for deity.
samādhi-siddhiḥ Īśvara-praṇidhānāt (II.45)	Samādhi may lead towards the realisation of God; resignation to God leads towards *samādhi*. In this state, the senses of perception develop such qualities that they supersede the mind. There is no longer an inclination to follow the dictates of the mind. Rather, the goal is direct contact with the experience of intellectual wisdom.

Thus, *yama* and *niyama* guide each one in the art of right living to follow the chosen path with grace and honour.

10. *Āsana*

Āsana trains, educates and cultivates the organs of action, senses of perception and the external mind (*bāhyendriyas*) and connects them to the internal organs, which are the inner mind, intelligence and consciousness. By this internalisation, the external senses stop interfering with the objects of the world and get involved with the internal senses to move closer to the seer or the *ātman*. By this practice, the seer (*puruṣa*) is made to come out from his shell to engulf and spread himself all over the body (*prakṛti*).

11. How Should an *Āsana* Be Done?

***sthira-sukham āsanam* (II.46)**	Stability and contentment are just an external definition of the *āsana*. I feel plenty of things are hidden in the words *sthira* and *sukha*. Let us look into their meaning, and into the depth of feeling in the *āsanas*.

Whatever *āsana* one performs, it should not distort the normal or original structure of the anatomical body. Each and every part of the joints and muscles must be kept in their natural shape and form (*svarūpa*). Each one of us must study the distortions that take place while performing the *āsana*s, and at once correct them. For this, the mind and intelligence must be made to involve and to observe by remaining in contact with each and every joint, bone, muscle, fibre, tendon and cell so that the attentive consciousness not only radiates focused awareness but also tastes its flavour. This focused awareness must be felt by every particle of the body, from the skin to the core and from the core to the skin. This is the true meaning of *sthiratā* and *sukhatā* in the *āsana*s.

Actually, the organs of action and senses of perception manifest ego in the form of somatic pride through the musculoskeletal body. Watching and understanding the expressions of this somatic pride, one has to perform the *āsana*s without any expressions of physical ego. This is *sthiratā* in the *āsana*.

Vyāsa explains five states of mind or consciousness of a human being. These are *mūḍha* (dull), *kṣipta* (distracted), *vikṣipta* (scattered), *ekāgra* (single-focused) and *niruddha* (restrained or stable). *Āsanasādhanā* transforms the dull, distracted or scattered mind and consciousness of the *sādhaka*s towards single-focused attention.

In performing the *āsana*s, some parts remain dull while other parts remain contracted or distracted. Some parts are scattered without a sense of direction while others remain with a single-focused grip. Observing and feeling this single-focused grip, one must learn to adjust it on other parts of the body. Then the elements of the body are evenly balanced, making the practitioner experience the feel of ease in the *āsana*s.

In short, while practising the *āsana*s, if one part moves, the whole of the body must co-ordinate and move. Similarly, if the whole body moves, all parts must concur. This is *sukham*.

If, while practising the *āsana*s, the practitioner notices the dull, distracted or contracted parts of the body, he must recharge the battery of his intelligence and alert it to rectify these dull, distracted or contracted parts. Then he can experience all the vestments of the self (the seen) being properly balanced and in unison with the seer. When the single-focused stretch of the somatic body mingles with the association of the self evenly and equally with the conscious energy and intelligence, then it is possible to realise what is *sukha* and what is *sthira* in each *āsana*.

At this state or stage, the *sādhaka* experiences automatically the highest and noblest state of consciousness, which is nothing less than the *niruddha* state.

When the river of energy (*prāṇa*) and focused awareness (*prajñā*) of consciousness flow uniformly and in unison in the presentation of each and every *āsana*, flowing in harmony from the seer to the skin and vice versa, this is the *niruddha* state in the *āsana*. This way of performing the *āsana* is nothing less than perfect precision filled with divinity. When the *āsanas* are practised with effort for years, then the *sādhaka* reaches a non-dual state of body, mind, intelligence and consciousness, where effort seems effortless. This is my experience regarding the definition of '*sthira sukham āsanam*'. For me *sthiram* stands for *satyam* (truth), *śivam* (goodness), *sukham* (contentment), and *āsana* (position) for *sundaram* (beauty).

Unfortunately, practitioners today misread the *sūtra* and from the very beginning seek comfort and ease when performing the *āsana*s. This means that, in their practices, they surrender their discerning mind to the dictates of the body and become slaves of convenience.

This type of comfortable presentation becomes *bhogāsana*. In this *bhogāsana* way of practice, they allow their minds to follow the motions of the body without any sensitivity or the use of their discerning powers. Instead the *āsana*s must be done using the body as an instrument to sensitise the mind and intelligence. While practising the *āsana*s, one has to explore and investigate the veiled, concealed or hidden weaknesses of the body, mind and intelligence. This requires action and reflection along with further study so that disparities are constructively removed to experience parity in body, mind, intelligence and consciousness.

If the *āsana*s are done from the source (the core of being), they are termed *yogāsana*s. If the same *āsana*s are done by the senses for the senses, they are called *bhogāsana*s.

pravṛtti-āloka-
-nyāsāt-sūkṣma-
-vyavahita-
-viprakṛṣṭa-jñānam
(III.26)

The perfect practitioner of *āsana*s develops a supersensory perception when performing the *āsana*s, which enables him to direct the flame of awareness to trace those parts where the light of awareness does not penetrate or where awareness is hidden, veiled or concealed or remains in darkness for ever. For me, studying all the above points and achieving a careful alignment of body, senses, nerves, mind, intelligence and consciousness is a sign of the perfect presentation of an *āsana*. If the alignment of every sheath in the body is rightly and precisely adjusted, this is enlightenment. Such precise alignment leads one towards illuminative intelligence.

For this, one must develop super-sensitive perception in the senses while practising, so that one earns knowledge and wisdom to bring parity from the centre into either side of the body.

jāti-lakṣaṇa deśaiḥ
anyatā anavacchedāt
tulyayoḥ tataḥ
***pratipattiḥ* (III.54)**

By knowledge born from discernment, the *sādhaka* is able to distinguish with clarity the differences within his own body, as well as between similar objects, which normally cannot be distinguished by rank, creed, quality, place or space.

First of all, we must learn and adjust what we can both see and perceive in order to develop this quality of observation. For example, our eyes can perceive the front body and correct its movements. However, the back body cannot be seen, but is only felt and conceived by the mind, so it must be adjusted and corrected by the mind. The key to doing this is to balance the senses of perception with the senses of conception – the mind and intelligence – so that they observe together the changes that take place while adjusting the various facets of the body.

This means that the *sādhaka* must use the fire of vision (*darśanāgni*) together with the fire of the intelligence of the mind (*jñānāgni*) to co-operate and co-ordinate, and, by by utilising the fire of the seer (*ātmāgni*), to witness and correct whenever and wherever such corrections are needed. Such presentation establishes harmony, removing the disparities between the front, back and the right and left sides of the body, and the nerves, mind, intelligence and consciousness. By 'nerves', I mean the *prāṇa* or energy flows in the nervous system.

As *praṇava* has three letters *ā*, *u* and *ś*, which stand for generation, continuation and culmination in words or actions, *āsana* too has three movements. The first is going into position – *akāra* (the first letter) of the *praṇava*. The second is stabilising and staying in the *āsana* – *ukāra* (the second letter) of the *praṇava*. The third is coming out of the position – *makāra* (the third letter) of the *praṇava*. In this way, an *āsana* mentally expresses the *praṇava mantra* of *āuṁ*, without uttering it. If a practitioner with a clear intention retains the significance of *āuṁ* and practises the *āsanas*, observing the three syllables of *āuṁ*, he becomes involved silently in the awareness of *āuṁ*.

This way of practice diffuses the flame of the seer so that it radiates throughout the body. The *sādhaka*s then experience stability in the physical, physiological, psychological, mental and intellectual bodies. In short, the seer abides and feels each and every cell with unbiased attention.

***prayatna-śaithilya-ananta-samāpattibhyām* (II.47)** [1]This is *antaraṅga* (internal) in *āsanas*.

In the beginning, all the scattered vestments of the seer struggle to reach the exalted state of equanimity, stability, concord and bliss. When this state of unison is reached, then comes the inner quest, wherein the feeling of effort disappears and a boundless joy is experienced. The seer spreads throughout his own vestments just as if he were practising the *āsanas*, occupying the body and sublimating his agents to assume the shape of the body as self.

***tataḥ dvandvāḥ-anabhighātaḥ* (II.48)** [2]This is the *antarātman* (the interiormost) aspect of the *āsanas*. I have spoken previously of *satī* (wife) and *pati* (husband). Without *pati*, there cannot be *satī* – and vice versa. In the beginning each must be dependent upon the other. In *āsana* practice, evolution of the seer and involution of the senses and mind have to go together.

If *prakṛti* (body) is *satī* (wife), *puruṣa* (the seer) is *pati* (husband). If the family is to be happy and contented, there must be a good understanding between husband and wife.

In the same way the seer and the seen must work in unison with a thorough understanding, because both are needed to experience sensory pleasures (*bhogārtha*) or emancipation (*apavarga* or *kaivalya*).

Patañjali explains beautifully the union of *prakṛti* (*satī*) with *puruṣa* (*pati*), presenting the *āsanas* with such a perfect precision that the identities or differences (*bheda*) between *prakṛti* and *puruṣa* vanish – just like the union of husband (*pati*) and wife (*satī*) (*abheda*).

---

1 When the effort to perform becomes effortless, perfection in an *āsana* is achieved.

2 From then on, the practitioner is undisturbed by dualities and is fit to begin *prāṇāyāma*.

12. Effects of *Āsanas*

Here I would like to bring together from different chapters the *sūtra*s that clearly convey the depth of feeling to be observed in each *āsana*.

parama-aṇu- -parama- -mahattva-antaḥ asya vaśīkāraḥ **(I.40)**	The *paramāṇu* refers to the microscopic cells covering the length, width and depth of the visible body. The presentation of the *āsana*s must be such that they cultivate these millions and trillions of cells and then subjugate them to the seer's command.
kūrma-nāḍyāṁ sthairyam **(III.32)**	The nervous system of the alimentary canal (*kūrma nāḍī*) controls it from the throat to the anus. It is kept clean through *āsana*s and *prāṇāyāma*s so that the faculties of hearing, touch, vision, taste and smell remain healthy and able to experience the faculty of spiritual perception without hindrance.
rūpa-lāvaṇya- -bala-vajra- -saṁhananatvāni kāya-saṁpat **(III.47)**	The perfect presentation of *āsana*s brings out grace, loveliness, liveliness, strength and power. According to circumstance, this is like the hardness and brilliance of a diamond or the softness and fineness of a flower.

Note that the mind plays a dual role since it is placed between the senses of perception and the organs of action on one side and intelligence, ego, consciousness and conscience on the other. The mind wants to satisfy the senses of perception, and at the same time to please its Lord – the seer. A simple example is that it acts like a Public Relations officer, trying to please the customers and, at the same time, the boss.

Here the mind plays the same role. It wants to satisfy its customers – namely, the mind, the senses of perception and the organs of action on one side – and at the same time it wants to satisfy its master – the seer. Hence, the main effect of the practice of *āsana*s is the extinction of the dual function of the mind. I consider this non-dual state of mind to be the *antarātman* (the interiormost) *sādhanā* of the *āsana*s (*see sūtra* II.48).

āsanāni ca tāvanti yāvanto jīva-rāśyaḥ (*H. P.*, I.33).

*Āsana*s are innumerable. It is said that there are as many *āsana*s as there are species in the universe. To put it another way, we have hundreds and hundreds of joints and muscles, miles and miles of avenues for the blood and energy to flow. In order to keep all of these in a perfect state of health and freedom, the practice of a few *āsana*s is not enough. This is why so many *āsana*s were mapped out by the ancient yogis.

Modern medicine investigates the new diseases that afflict millions of people and also discovers new drugs to combat them. Yogis knew of diseases too and discovered various *āsana*s to combat them. I believe that by performing the various *āsana*s accurately and precisely, each particle of the body is nourished with fresh blood and energy. This increases our defences to combat even today's new diseases. Each *āsana* has a certain function wherein the mind and intelligence are made to reach with ease the least accessible areas of the body.

Besides all their psycho-spiritual benefits, the *āsana*s filter the blood and enable it to reach even the unattainable areas of the body to keep it clean and healthy. All these reactions from *āsana*s help to soak the body in freshly oxygenated blood. There is a vitalizing action between muscles and mind, which creates space in the body for the seer to look within and enter the body without obstructions. *Āsana*s help in unifying the body with the mind and seer, to make a single unit. This is *saṁyama: trayam ekatra saṁyamaḥ* (III.4).

Extending the thought of this *sūtra*, we can demarcate the organs of action, senses of perception and external mind as one unit; the internal mind, intelligence and *ahaṁkāra* as another unit; and consciousness, conscience and seer as the third unit. One must practise *āsana*s by reference to the map of these three triangles, which form a bigger triangle; doing so will clear the external unit, the internal unit and the interiormost unit.

13. Differences between *Āsana* and *Dhyāna*

I would like to bring the attention of *sādhaka*s to the differences between *āsana*s and *dhyāna* (meditation). In the correct presentation of *āsana*s, the seer is made to come out and evolve, spreading himself in the body. By contrast, in *dhyāna* the senses, mind and intelligence are involuted to journey towards the site of the seer (*see* the diagrams on evolution and involution on pages 130–3).

While practising *āsana* or *prāṇāyāma*, it is essential for one to maintain a singular uninterrupted flow of energy and awareness in each cell of the body to and from the seer.

14. *Prāṇāyāma*

***tasmin sati śvāsa- -praśvāsayoḥ gati-vicchedaḥ prāṇāyāmaḥ* (II.49)**	When elasticity and freedom in the muscles and fibres of the torso are acquired through perfection in the *āsana*s, the *sādhaka* is said to be fit to practise *prāṇāyāma*.

Our breath is interrupted and flows in a zigzag manner. Patañjali suggests the *sādhaka*s to regulate the in-breath and out-breath by listening to and maintaining a smooth, steady sound (*nādānusaṇdhāna*) along with a soft flow.

Here, two points are to be noted by *sādhaka*s. One is that while we must hold the correct *tāḍāsana*, it is essential to place the feet on the floor, spreading the bottom feet of the skin evenly without crumbling in any part of it. In the same way, throughout *prāṇāyāma* practice, it is also important to hold the seat (the buttock bones) as if the tail of the spinal column itself is performing *tāḍāsana*. Correct positioning of the spine enables the torso to function without distraction, contraction or refraction in the flow and rhythmic movements of breath. The entire spine must be kept alert and steady, as *prāṇāyāma* deals mostly with the subtle body.

While performing the *āsana*s, the eyes (*tejas tattva*) must be alert and attentive to perceive defects that occur in presentation and correct them at once. In *prāṇāyāma*, the ears (*ākāśa tattva*) must be alert and receptive to catch disharmony in the sound of in-breath and out-breath and correct it.

***bāhya-abhyantara-staṃbha-vṛttiḥ deśa--kāla-saṁkhyābhiḥ paridṛṣṭaḥ dīrgha--sūkṣmaḥ* (II.50)**	This *sūtra* explains the internal aspect of *prāṇāyāma*. It refers to the aspects of the outgoing breath, incoming breath and the restraints between them. These are to be regulated by prolongation, refinement and precision, depending on the anatomical and physiological condition of the torso and its capacity.

As such it is the *antaraṅga* aspect of *prāṇāyāma*.

Patañjali expresses in *Samādhi Pāda* another aspect of *prāṇāyāma* in the form of passive exhalation and retention (*recaka* and *kuṁbhaka*).

***pracchardana--vidhāraṇābhyāṁ va prāṇasya* (I.34)**	A pensive state of mind (*manolaya*) arises through slow, soft, subtle and steady exhalation, which helps consciousness to become silent.

This *prāṇāyāma* is suggested as a way to silence the fluctuations of the thought waves without resort to any technique, whereas the *sūtras* attributed here on *prāṇāyāma* offer a methodology and technique. This *prāṇāyāma* makes one experience a passive, pensive and alert state of mind. It indicates an interaction between the method of *prāṇāyāma* (given later) and the expected change in the state of consciousness.

This *prāṇāyāma*, with the soft release of breath and passive retention without strain, is suggested for gaining *citta prasādana* – a peaceful state of consciousness where the restless and oscillating mind gains a certain measure of stability and quietness.

Having laid out the right disposition of the *citta* in the form of friendliness, compassion, gladness and cultivating indifference to vice or virtue (I.33), Patañjali indirectly likens the concept of *vairāgya* (renunciation) in *prāṇāyāma* to the experiences of non-attachment, a stepping stone for renunciation.

Patañjali explains four types of *prāṇāyāma* in three *sūtras*. The first three are:

1) rhythmic deep inhalation (*pūraka*) and exhalation (*recaka*) without retention;
2) inhalation retention (*antara kuṁbhaka*) and exhalation retention (*bāhya kuṁbhaka*); and
3) a *prāṇāyāma* that is regulated and measured with minute precision, with long in-breaths and out-breaths, bringing them to exquisite fineness.

Having noted three types of *prāṇāyāma* in two *sūtras* (II.49–50), he moves on to the fourth type in II.51:

bāhya-abhyantara- -viṣaya-ākṣepī caturthaḥ (II.51)

This *prāṇāyāma* is beyond effort and deliberation. It transcends the regulation of in-breath, out-breath and retention, as well as place, duration and minute precision. It is without effort or deliberation. It represents the *tūriya* state, which is beyond wakeful, dreamy or sleepy states.

This *prāṇāyāma* is from *citta*. When *citta* automatically and non-deliberately remains still, breath does not move. This retention has no reference, sphere or realm but transcends the above three types of *prāṇāyāma*, which follow a certain methodology. I call this *manovṛtti nirodha* without *prāṇavṛtti nirodha*. Instead of stilling the mind indirectly through the instrument of breath, here the mind controls and holds the breath directly. This is why it is called non-deliberate *prāṇāyāma*.

15. Effects of *Prāṇāyāma*

viśeṣa-darśinaḥ ātma-bhāva- -bhāvanā-nivṛttiḥ (IV.25)

In this fourth state (II.51), the feel of the seer and of the seen both fade, and awareness (*prajñā*) spreads all over the body. Is it not then the state of *turīya* or *kaivalya* or *mokṣa*?

See how Patañjali explains the finest and the highest type of *prāṇāyāma* in its *antarātman* aspect, where all movements of thought waves are stilled on their own without depending upon the external and internal movements of the breath.

At this level, a few parallels can be made to some concepts of yoga theory, which may help us understand the depth of the *prāṇāyāma* practices.

Following what Patañjali says in I.34, I feel that retention after exhalation (*bāhya kuṁbhaka*) is *nivṛtti mārga* (going towards the source), whereas retention after inhalation (*antara kuṁbhaka*) is the way of evolution from the source towards the periphery (*pravṛtti mārga*). This type of *prāṇāyāma* is nothing less than total absorption (*laya*). If exhalation is a state of void (*śūnya*), inhalation is a non-void (*aśūnya*) state. Beyond these two states there is a void and non-void (*śūnyāśūnya*) state, where the seer glows like a full moon.

***tataḥ kṣīyate prakāśa--āvaraṇam* (II.52)**	The effect of *prāṇāyāma* is that it disperses the veils that cover the seer.
***dhāraṇāsu ca yogyatā manasaḥ* (II.53)**	Its practice helps the mind, intelligence and consciousness to become fit instruments to move towards the next step, i.e. *dhāraṇā*.

NOTE

As I described how each *āsana* has *akāra*, *ukāra* and *makāra* of *praṇava mantra*, so too *prāṇāyāma* represents *āuṁ mantra*. If the inhalation (*pūraka*) is *akāra*, retention of breath in inhalation (*antara kuṁbhaka*) is *ukāra*, whereas exhalation (*recaka*) and retention after exhalation (*bāhya kuṁbhaka*) are *makāra*. Actually *akāra* stands for **G**eneration or creation (Brahma), *ukāra* for **O**rganisation and protection (Viṣṇu) and *makāra* for **D**estruction of vice or evil in one (Maheśvara).

As we normally direct pupils to exhale before inhalation, some yogis, like Brahmānanda in his commentary on *Haṭhayoga Pradīpikā* known as *Jyotsnā*, take *recaka* as *akāra*. As we release the breath before *prāṇāyāma*, this does not accord with the techniques and philosophy of *prāṇāyāma*; exhalation is done to prepare the lungs for *prāṇāyāma*. As *prāṇāyāma* begins after the release of the residual breath, *akāra* of *āuṁ* begins with *pūraka*.

This *mantra japa* in *prāṇāyāma* teaches one to recognise the core of the being. If a cup is empty, it is filled with air, and when the cup is filled with water, the air comes out. This gave me the idea to investigate what allows room for the in-breath (*pūraka*) to enter and the out-breath (*recaka*) to exit.

As the breath moves in, the seer moves or evolves from his residence to embrace the external frontier of his torso (the seen). Then in retention, the seer is made to associate (*saṁyoga*) with the torso, to experience and integrate (*saṁyama*) with the seen. Similarly exhalation leads to an experience of the seen (torso) moving, involuting towards the residence of the seer. The torso or the seen is *prakṛti* and the seer, the *puruṣa.*

This means that, in inhalation, the seer evolves and moves towards the torso (the seen), while in inhalation-retention (*antara kuṁbhaka*) the seer and the seen mingle and are merged or united. In exhalation-retention (*bāhya kuṁbhaka*), the seen moves towards the seer, and surrenders to rest in the residenc of the seer.

This also taught me to feel the *viśva cetana śakti* or the Supreme Being in the form of *puruṣa* moving out from his abiding place for *caitanya śakti* (*vāyu*) to enter, and as I exhale I feel the *caitanya śakti* moving out and *puruṣa* moving back to his residence. In *antara kuṁbhaka* I feel the union of *puruṣa* with *prakṛti* (body); and, in *bāhya kuṁbhaka*, *prakṛti* embracing the *puruṣa.* This Supreme Being takes three forms to command the world. I mentioned that these forms are known as Brahmā, Viṣṇu and Maheśvara. These attributes of *Ādi Puruṣa* are represented as *trimūrti*s, the three main divinities of our pantheon. These *trimūrti*s can be felt in the practice of *prāṇāyāma:* inhalation (*pūraka*) represents the **G**enerative energy of the creator (Brahmā); retention (*kuṁbhaka*) is **O**rganiser for survival (Viṣṇu), and the release of the polluted breath in exhalation (*recaka*) is the force of **D**estruction (Maheśvara). If the contaminated breath is held, and not let out, it eats away the life force. Hence for me the three functions of *prāṇāyāma* – inhalation, retention and exhalation – represent the three main functions of God.

I would also like to describe one more sensation in *prāṇāyāma*. This is the union of macrocosm (*brahmāṇḍa*) and microcosm (*piṇḍāṇḍa*). We all know that the macrocosm (*brahmāṇḍa*) is found in the microcosm (*piṇḍāṇḍa*), and vice versa. *Prāṇāyāma* practices make us understand and realize how these two meet together and become one.

For example, in *prāṇāyāma* inhalation, macrocosm (*brahmāṇḍa*) is made to move towards microcosm (*piṇḍāṇḍa*). In internal retention, both are made to unite and become one; whereas in exhalation, the microcosm is made to involute towards macrocosm, and in external retention, microcosm is made to mingle with macrocosm. Thus *prāṇāyāma* is nothing less than an instrument of the *sādhaka* to bring and to feel the integration and union of these two, *brahmāṇḍa–piṇḍāṇḍa and piṇḍāṇḍa-brahmāṇḍa saṁyama.*

Before concluding, I would like to remind readers of the importance of *āsanas.* These are said to be essential to *prāṇāyāma* practice. Please note that they are just as essential to practise after *prāṇāyāma.*

All of us know that the practice of *prāṇāyāma* stores energy. But what about its use? The water in a lake is still and without energy, whereas the water in a river expresses energy. In the same way, *āsana* practice is as essential after *prāṇāyāma* as before.

It is only the practice of *āsanas* that takes the energy from the lungs to supply the needy parts in the land of the body, kinetically generating energy in each and every cell. So do not underestimate the role of *āsana*s even though you may be in an evolved state of consciousness.

16. *Vāyu*

Since *prāṇāyāma* is dependent on *viśva caitanya śakti*, which governs the element of *vāyu* (air), let me introduce this element so that you can understand the importance of *prāṇāyāma.*

Just as the body is divided into five sheaths or caves (*kośa*), *viśva caitanya vāyu* (or *śakti*) is divided into five *vāyus* or energies, representing the five elements in the five sheaths of the body.

See the following table:

Pañca vāyus	*apāna*	*prāṇa*	*samāna*	*udāna*	*vyāna*
Pañca bhūtas	*pṛthvī*	*āp*	*tejas*	*vāyu*	*ākāśa*
Pañca kośas	*annamaya*	*prāṇamaya*	*manomaya*	*vijñānamaya*	*ānandamaya*

(*See also* the characteristics of the five *bhūtas* in Chapter VIII)

***udāna-jayāt jala--paṅka-kaṇṭaka--ādiṣu asaṅgaḥ utkrāntiḥ ca* (III.40)**

Udāna makes one levitate. It uplifts. Those who have complete control of *udāna* can walk over water.

***samāna-jayāt jvala-nam* (III.41)**

Samāna being the element of *tejas* (fire), it makes life shine and glow with spiritual light. The presence of *samāna* in abundance gives the appearance of lustre, or a glowing sheen. With the help of this *vāyu*, he may even begin to perceive a special glow, or 'spiritual aura', in others also, if there is any.

***śrotra-ākāśayoḥ saṁbandha--saṁyamāt divyaṁ śrotram* (III.42)**

Through the control of *vyāna*, one can move in space and listen to the divine sounds. The quality of *vyāna* is that it spreads throughout and everywhere in the body. Hence *vyāna* is associated not only with the skin but also with the blood circulation. As *vyāna* is connected to the skin and circulation, both of these extend all over the body. When the *sādhaka* cleanses and refines the *vyāna vāyu* through *yaugika* practices, he acquires the ability to move everywhere throughout space. The inner channels of the body, including those of hearing (*śabda*), open that faculty to the supremely refined vibration of the divine.

***rūpa-lāvaṇya-bala-vajra-saṁhananatvāni kāya-saṁpat* (III.47)**	[1]*Apāna vāyu*, corresponding to *pṛthvī*, makes the *annamaya kośa* shine like a diamond.

In *prāṇāyāma*, the inhalation (*prāṇa*) is done with the help of *apāna* and *samāna*; *antara kuṁbhaka* (retention after inhalation) with the support of *samāna* and *vyāna*; while retention after exhalation (*bāhya kuṁbhaka*) is done with the help of *udāna* and *vyāna*. Thus, these *pañca vāyu*s are closely interconnected in the practice of *prāṇāyāma*.

Similarly, there is a close connection between the *āsana* and *prāṇāyāma*, as both work on the spinal column (*merudaṇḍa*).

17. *Cakras*

Many think that *cakra*s are the subject of *Haṭha Yoga* and that Patañjali does not speak of *cakra*s. I would like to bring to your attention that Patañjali does, in fact, deal with the *cakra*s.

In Chapter III, there is an important passage describing different *cakra*s and their effects on a perfect yogi. Some of these he describes as *cakra*s, and some he describes differently, but their locations are identical to the other *yaugika* texts that deal with *cakra*s.

Medical scientists relate *cakra*s to plexuses since the locations of *cakra*s and plexuses are very nearly at identical places. These are often treated in equivalent terms. The plexuses belong to the anatomical sheath and nervous system (*kārya śarīra* and *sūkṣma śarīra*), whereas the *cakra*s are connected to the subtlest of the subtle body (*kāraṇa śarīra*). The *cakra*s are located inside the spine, whereas the plexuses are outside the spine.

Plexuses and glands work on psycho-physiological levels, whereas *cakra*s work on the level of spiritual enlightenment. In the following table I present the relevant *sūtra*s where Patañjali

---

1 He acquires unsurpassed beauty, grace, strength and lustre.

describes the *cakra*s and the effects of *saṁyama* on them. Though Patañjali does not speak of the *devatā*s of the *cakra*, I mention the names of the *devatā*s of each *cakra* according to *Śaṭ Cakra Nirūpaṇa*.

Sūtra:	**It represents:**	***Ādidevatā:***
***kūrma-nāḍyāṁ sthairyam* (*Y. S.*, III.32)** *By **saṁyama** on **kūrma nāḍī**, which covers the nervous system of the alimentary canal, the **yogi** can make his body and mind firm and immobile like a tortoise.*	*mulādhāra*	*Brahma with Sarasvatī*
***prātibhāt vā sarvam* (*Y. S.*, III.34)** *Through the faculty of spiritual perception, the **yogi** becomes the knower of all knowledge.*	*svādhiṣṭhāna*	*Viṣṇu with Lakṣmī*
***nābhi-cakre kāya-vyūha-jñānam* (*Y. S.*, III.30)** *This **cakra** of the navel helps one to understand the entire structure and function of the body*	*maṇipūraka*	*Rudra*
***hṛdaye citta-saṁvit* (*Y. S.*, III.35)** ***Saṁyama** on the region of the heart brings thorough knowledge of consciousness.*	*anāhata*	*Īśvara with Ādiśakti or Ambikā*
***kaṇṭha-kūpe kṣut-pipāsā-nivṛttiḥ* (*Y. S.*, III.31)** *By **saṁyama** on the pit of the throat, one overcomes hunger and thirst.*	*viśuddhi*	*Sadāśiva with Pārvati*
***mūrdha-jyotiṣi siddha-darśanam* (*Y. S.*, III.33)** *By performing **saṁyama** on the light of the middle of the eyebrows (**ājñā cakra**), one has visions of perfected beings.*	*ājña*	*Ātmadevatā or Ādidevatā*
***tataḥ prātibha-śrāvaṇa-vedanā-ādarśā-āsvāda--vārtāḥ jāyante* (*Y. S.*, III.37)** *Through **saṁyama** on the light of the crown of the head (**sahasrāra cakra**), one acquires the divine faculties of hearing, touch, vision, taste and smell. He can even generate these divine emanations by his will.*	*sahasrāra*	*Parabrahma*

18. *Pratyāhāra*

Pratyāhāra is a state where the scattered thoughts and thinking processes that motivate the organs of action, senses of perception and the outgoing mind are braided together to co-ordinate and become one. It is a unity, as external thoughts and objects are associated as one.

In short, *pratyāhāra* is the way of silencing all functions of the brain. With this, the discerning mind becomes free from fluctuations and temptations. Living in the house of consciousness is *pratyāhāra*.

Training in *pratyāhāra* begins with quietening the mind and withdrawing the senses of perception and the intellect of the brain from objects. This gives one time to establish fully what has been learnt so far. Without a firm base in the first four petals of yoga, one cannot move towards the other petals. Hence, this fifth petal offers a firm grip on what has been learnt so far. It is a pause enabling all that has been learnt to be absorbed, so that the experiences and their effects cascade through consciousness, preparing the ground for *saṁyama*.

Pratyāhāra acts as a bridge to cross from the external sheaths of investigation (*bahiraṅga anveṣaṅa*), cleansing (*śodhana*) the inner sheaths for further investigation (*antaraṅga anveṣaṇa*) and then re-filtering to dry out all the impurities (*mala śoṣaṇa*) where passivity and pensiveness of both body and mind can be experienced and noted. *Pratyāhāra* is a space to establish stability in *yama*, *niyama*, *āsana* and *prāṇāyāma* and then to move with attention towards *dhāraṇā*, *dhyāna* and *samādhi*.

Just as between *sabīja* and *nirbīja samādhis* there is a pause in the form of *virāma pratyaya*, *pratyāhāra* is a meaningful pause between *bahiraṅga* and *antaraṅga saṁyamas*. This pause indicates the crucial standard of the *sādhaka*. These two pauses in the form of *virāma pratyaya* in *samādhi* and *pratyāhāra* in *aṣṭāṅga yoga* may cause one to be caught in the net of success. This in turn may cause one to fall into the trap of *avirati* (carelessness in practice), leading towards the unsettled state (*anavasthitatva*).

Alternatively, one may practise without interruption, to sustain and maintain the *sādhanā* without caring about success. Take for example King Viśvāmitra, who wanted to reach the level of asceticism of Sage Vaśiṣta. He began rigorous *tapas* and at the height of his success, Menakā tempted him and made him succumb to her charms (read the story of *Śakuntalā*). He realised his fault and with determination restarted *tapas* and became a *brahmaṛṣī*.

This story is enough for the *sādhaka* to know the effect of *virāma pratyaya* in *samādhi* and of *pratyāhāra*, as they are the bridge between *bahiraṅga* and *antaraṅga sādhanās*.

Pratyāhāra, too, has three stages. These are as follows:

***viṣayavatī vā pravṛttiḥ utpannā manasaḥ sthiti--nibandhanī* (I.35)**

This is the external aspect of *pratyāhāra*. In order to control the fluctuations of consciousness, one needs to follow and stick to *ekatattva abhyāsa* – adherence to a single-minded effort to achieve the graceful diffusion of consciousness (*citta prasādanam*). This *sūtra* relates to the senses of perception and mind, which must be used with devotion to make progress, so that the mind is engrossed to accomplish stability.

Out of the eight aspects of yoga, whatever aspect of yoga that the *sādhaka* chooses, he should stick to it steadfastly, keeping the end goal in sight – making the mind a single unit (*eka manas*). By this approach, all his senses and mind are involved to develop a single state of mind.

***sva-viṣaya--asaṁprayoge cittsya sva-rūpa-anukāra iva indriyāṇāṁ pratyāhāraḥ* (II.54)**

This is the internal aspect of *pratyāhāra*. Here the *bahiraṅga*s (external garments or vestments) of the seer, which go for outward objects or thoughts (*bhogārtha*) are turned inwards (*apavargārtha*) towards the *antaraṅga*s, namely intelligence, I-maker (*ahaṁkāra*) and consciousness. I think we should understand this word *'svarūpānukāra'* as the disciplining of the constituents of the human being (limbs, *indriya*s, *citta*, *ahaṁkāra*, *manas*) to remain in their positions during the practice of *āsana*, *prāṇāyāma* or *dhyāna*. When all these constituents stay in their positions in whatever *āsana* or *prāṇāyāma* one does, their *rūpa* disappears, and only *prajñā* remains. That is how the state of *pratyāhāra* is felt during the practice of *āsana* or *prāṇāyāma*.

***tataḥ paramā vaśyatā indriyāṇām* (II.55)** This is the *antarātma* aspect of *pratyāhāra*, wherein the mind, which was close to the senses as external mind (*ekādaśendriya*), is made to become an inner mind (*antarendriya*) so that this inner mind is connected with *buddhi* and *citta*, enabling it to come in close proximity with the *ātman*.

19. Effects of *Pratyāhāra*

Pratyāhāra is the culmination of the process of *indriyajaya*, the mastery over the 11 *indriyas* (the five organs of action, five senses of perception, and the external functioning of mind).

***grahaṇa-svarūpa--asmitā-anvaya--arthavattva--saṁyamāt indriya-jayaḥ* (III.48)** As the powers of the senses of perception and external movements of the mind turn inwards towards the interior intellectual senses, they are freed from *bhogārtha* (sensual pleasures) and made to move towards emancipation (*apavarga*), as is explained in *sūtra* II.18.

***tataḥ mano-javitvaṁ vikaraṇa-bhāvaḥ pradhāna-jayaḥ ca* (III.49)** This is the innermost aspect of *pratyāhāra*. The individual mind, which was pleasing the senses on one side and the seer on the other, transforms into a single state of attention (*eka citta*). This *eka citta* transfigures into cosmic mind (*mahat*), the first principle of *mūla prakṛti*. When this single mind is submerged in the root of nature (*mūla prakṛti*), the seer shines on his own.

20. *Dhāraṇā*

Dhāraṇā, *dhyāna* and *samādhi* are the internal or *antaraṅga* aspects of yoga, and as such Patañjali brackets them together as *saṁyama*.

The mind that remains closer to the organs of action and senses of perception is made to take a U-turn through *yama*, *niyama*, *āsana*, *prāṇāyāma* and *pratyāhāra* to become associated with the inner senses - namely the intelligence, the 'I', consciousness and the conscience. Out of the eight aspects of *samādhi* - *savitarka*, *nirvitarka*, *savicāra*, *nirvicāra*, *sānanda*, *sāsmitā*, *virāma pratyaya* and *nirbīja* or *dharmamegha samādhi*[1] - the first seven states of *samādhi* are *sabīja* (with seed). *Nirbīja* or *dharmamegha samādhi* is an entirely individual experience and no words can express this state.

As the *dharma* of clouds releases rain, the *nirbīja* or *dharmamegha samādhi* releases the rain of virtues (*śīlatā*) from the seat of the *antarātman*.

21. Definition of *Dhāraṇā*

Dhāraṇā has three aspects.

deśa-bandhaḥ cittasya dhāraṇā **(III.1)**

This *dhāraṇā* is external. Here *deśa* stands for a place for attention. This place is nothing less than the body within which *citta* dwells. Śri Vyāsa's comment on this *sūtra* confirms my view. Also, I use the word body for *deśa*, as the senses, mind, intelligence, consciousness and the seer dwell in it. As the body is impermanent and non-eternal, it has its own limitations. Its contents (organs of action, senses of perception, *manas*, *buddhi* and *ahaṁkāra*) are charged through yoga *sādhanā* towards refinement and involution.

As such, this *sūtra* is very interesting for *sādhaka*s to make their minds penetrate towards the spiritual world and capture the self (as a camera captures an image), rather than capturing the external postures of the senses. Methods like the study of scriptures or gazing at the flame of a candle deal with matter outside the body,

---

1 Some *haṭha yoga* texts name *aṣṭa-samādhi* differently. *See Aṣṭadaḷa Yogamāḷā*, vol. VIII, p. 299.

but Patañjali does not discard them as they are external props for meditation.

vīta-rāga-viṣayaṁ vā cittam (I.37)	Contemplating on enlightened souls or divine objects is internal *dhāraṇā*.
viśokā vā jyotiṣmatī (I.36)	[1]This is the interiormost *dhāraṇā*. In life, we have experienced at certain times, knowingly or unknowingly, a sudden sorrowless state that makes the mind a shining mind, serene and tranquil. One can recollect such conditions as *jñāna jyoti* and concentrate on them. By keeping the mind and consciousness in this state of stillness and silence, the *sādhaka* has to enhance his time on *dhāraṇā*. All of us have experienced a state of grace and serenity while listening to a beautifully played concerto or *rāga*, or watching the sunset over the horizon of a vast ocean, hearing the far cries of migrating birds, high in the vast blue sky, as they fly to lands in far-off places. Recollection of this state keeps the mind tranquil.

22. Effects of *Dhāraṇā*

Maintaining a thoughtful attention (*dhāraṇā*), then prolonging that attention leads in time to total absorption (*dhyāna*).

Let us now move on to understand the *dharma* of *dhyāna*.

23. *Dhyāna*

Actually for me, the very first *sūtra* of Patañjali covers contemplation or meditation or total absorption.

atha yogā-anuśāsanam (I.1)	I translate this as: Total attentive and contemplative practice on the described discipline of yoga is a path towards yoga, as yoga is nothing but meditation (*dhyāna*).

1 And/or by meditating on a sorrowless, luminous, effulgent light.

***svapna-nidrā-jñāna--ālambanaṁ vā* (I.38)**	The recollection of experiences of dream-filled or dreamless sleep in the wakeful state is also a part of *dhyāna*.
***yathā-abhimata--dhyānāt vā* (I.39)**	Total involvement on any agreeable thing or idea within the frame of *yamas* and *niyamas* is *dhyāna*.

I consider the above two *sūtras* to be external aspects of *dhyāna*.

***dhyāna-heyāḥ tad--vṛttayaḥ* (II.11)**	This *sūtra* and the next are connected to the internal aspects of *dhyāna*. *Dhyāna* is what guides and helps one to see and identify clearly dubious actions and thoughts. By this we eliminate all obscurity, leaving the intelligence and consciousness clean and pristine. Then they become fit to reflect on the light of the seer. Total focused awareness leads towards total absorption.
***tatra pratyaya--eka-tānatā dhyānam* (III.2)**	This is the innermost aspect of *dhyāna*. Patañjali defines *dhyāna* as a method for bringing the senses, mind and intelligence to think and reflect through a continuous, single flow of attention and awareness.

Actually when a continual, single-focused attention is maintained, this attention transforms itself both centripetally and centrifugally. It extends and expands over the entire sheath of the *sādhaka* as awareness (*prajñā*) without the feel of I or me; this is meditation, or *dhyāna*.

Dhyāna is completely subjective. The experience cannot be expressed in words.

24. Effects of *Dhyāna*

Ahaṁkāra is subdued through *dhyāna* and, when it is subdued, one experiences the effects of *dhyāna*.

***tatra dhyāna-jam anāśayam* (IV.6)**	*Dhyāna* frees the *sādhakas* from all thoughts, impressions, afflictions, psychic or mental *antarāyas* or impediments, which arise on account of

fluctuating thoughts and afflictions. This includes *saṅkara vṛttis* (mixed impressions) and *saṁskāra vṛttis* (latent impressions). *Dhyāna vṛtti* makes the *sādhakas* move closer to the core of the being.

***citeḥ apratisaṁkramāyāḥ tad-ākāra-āpattau sva-buddhi--saṁvedanam* (IV.22)**

This means that consciousness, having understood its position, identifies the seer. Then the seer's true form (*svarūpa*) is assumed.

This means that the *pariṇāma citta* or *nirmita citta* (created consciousness) transforms and unites with *kūṭastha citta* as *nirmāṇa citta* (absolute consciousness).

I said in relation to *āsanas* that they make the seer or *puruṣa* evolve from his hidden residence and come out to embrace the entire frontier of the body. This is nothing less than *dhyāna*. In *āsana* practices, the seer is made to come out from his residence towards the body, whereas in *dhyāna* it is the body that moves closer to be associated with the seer. In *dhyāna* the senses, mind, intelligence and consciousness are made to involute and move towards the seer, whereas in the practice of *āsanas*, the seer is made to evolute and move towards the body.

In *prāṇāyāma* practice the seer is made to move from his residence towards the body in inhalation, and unite in *antara kuṁbhaka*, while in exhalation the contents of the body are made to move towards the seer, and in *bāhya kuṁbhaka* both mingle together. In slow, soft inhalation of *prāṇāyāma*, the seer moves out, giving room for the breath or *prāṇa* to occupy the torso, and in slow, soft exhalation the contents of the body recede towards the seer.

To put it another way, in *āsana* and *prāṇāyāma* the seer is made to come out from his dwelling to conjoin with the contents of the body; and in *dhāraṇā* and *dhyāna*, it is the contents or elements of the body which move towards the seer to embrace him.

The seer is a witness when he is in a *nirākāra* state. Yet he has the ability to take form when *āsanas* and *prāṇāyāmas* are done with total attention and awareness. The seer takes the form of participant (actor) and witness, both at the same time.

In the beginning, one has to harness the power of recollection through conditioned mental impressions and mirror-like observation, taking care not to let the mind wander. Some say that conditioning or training the mind is not a feasible way to reach *dhyāna*. But my experience says it is possible to reach that level.

A final, but cardinal, point to understand about *dhyāna* is that it helps each of us shed completely the veil of ego as *dhyāna* neutralises the *kleśas* (*avidyā, asmitā, rāga, dveṣa* and *abhiniveśa*) as well as *vṛttis* (*pramāṇa, viparyaya, vikalpa, nidrā* and *smṛti*), and acts as an instrument of *Īśvara*.

25. *Antarātman* Aspect of Yoga

The *antarātman* aspect of yoga resembles the relationship between *prakṛti* and *puruṣa*. If the universe is the playground for *Īśvara* or *Ādi Puruṣa*, this individual body becomes the playground for *puruṣa*, for his own amusement (*līlā*). Actually the seer (*antarātman*) has no *sādhanā*. But to reach the *antarātman* and the sight of the seer, the sages of yore gave us the eight aspects of yoga.

To encounter the seer is *samāpatti* or *samādhi*.

26. *Samādhi* or *Samāpatti*

The difference between *samādhi* and *samāpatti* is that *samādhi* is the perfect natural absorption of oneself with the seer, and *samāpatti* is a method of transformation to assume the natural and original state of the seer.

Samādhi has two states – *sabīja samādhi* (with its seven stages) and *nirbīja samādhi*.

Patañjali first explains the seven states of *sabīja samādhis* as *savitarka, nirvitarka, savicāra, nirvicāra, sānanda, sāsmita* and *virāma pratyaya samādhi*. Out of these seven states, he mentions *virāma pratyaya* as a different state of *samādhi*, as this state acts as a bridge to cross over from the first six states of *samādhi* towards *nirbīja samādhi.*

The first six *sabīja samādhis* (*saṁprajñāta samādhis*) have a *rūpa*, whereas in *virāma pratyaya*, there is no room for *rūpa* (though there is 'seed' in the form of hidden impressions). This is why the term *asaṁprajñāta samādhi* has been coined. I identify *dharmamegha samādhi* (IV.29) with *nirbīja samādhi* (I.51), as both convey the showering rain of virtues. *Nirbīja samādhi* is the experiencing state of *puruṣa*, and can be equated to *kaivalya*.

While commenting on the first six *samādhis*, Vyāsa speaks of *sāttvika ahaṁkāra*. In the *virāma pratyaya* state, there is no existence of *ahaṁkāra*. Here *citta* loses its *rūpa*. Until consciousness reaches the absolute state of intelligence, which is equal to the seer, it is not possible to reach the state of *nirbīja samādhi*. Please note that the moment *ahaṁkāra* appears, the *sādhanā* falls from the grace of yoga.

In his *Vedānta sūtra* Śrī Rāmānuja identifies *sabīja* as *savikalpa* and *nirbīja* as *nirvikalpa samādhi*, and divides them into *savitarka, nirvitarka, savicāra, nirvicāra, Sānandā, nirānanda, sāsmita* and *nirāsmita samādhis*. These terms assist us only in the study of *samādhis*.

27. Effects of *Samādhi*

samādhi-bhāvanā- -arthaḥ kleśa- -tanū-karaṇa- -arthaḥ ca **(II.2)**	*Samādhi* helps in eradicating all types of afflictions. If this is not possible, it can at least minimise them. This is the external effect of the *bahiraṅga* state of *samādhi*.

In the practice of yoga, it is true that what can be cured is bound to be cured. Yoga also gives the power and strength to endure what cannot be cured.

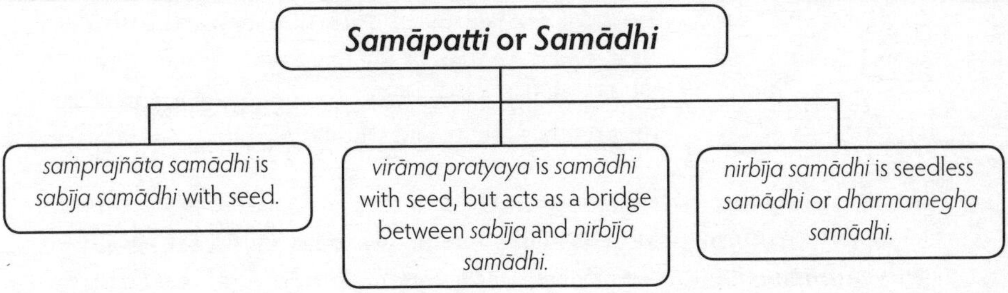

Samāpatti or Samādhi
saṁprajñāta samādhi is sabīja samādhi with seed.
virāma pratyaya is samādhi with seed, but acts as a bridge between sabīja and nirbīja samādhi.
nirbīja samādhi is seedless samādhi or dharmamegha samādhi.

28. *Antaraṅga Samādhi*

In *vitarka, vicāra samādhis* (*see sūtra* I.17), the feel of 'I' and 'me' is present, whereas in *sānanda* the 'I' and 'me' are neutralised. As 'I' and 'me' fade out, one comprehends and experiences the illuminative (*sāttvika*) state of 'I'.

***kṣīṇa-vṛtteḥ abhijātasya iva maṇeḥ grahītṛ--grahaṇa-grāhyeṣu tat-stha-tad-añjanatā samāpattiḥ* (I.41)**

In this state, consciousness feels its source on account of the dissolution of all its movements. As such, consciousness is transformed into a flawless gem (*abhijātamaṇi*) and therefore at this stage the seeker, the seer and the seen are felt to be one and the same.

***tatra śabda-artha--jñāna-vikalpaiḥ saṅkīrṇā savitarkā samāpattiḥ* (I.42)**

When the *trikaraṇa śuddhi* or the purification of body, speech and mind takes place and consciousness remains single-focused without deviations, this is *savitarka samādhi.*

***smṛti-pariśuddhau sva-rūpa-śūnyā iva artha-mātra-nirbhāsā nirvitarkā* (I.43)**

As the memory ripens, consciousness does not create or fabricate *vṛttis*. In this state one stays without refractions or reflections. This is *nirvitarka samādhi.*

***etayā eva savicārā nirvicārā ca sūkṣma--viṣayā vyākhyātā* (I.44)**

The *savicāra* and *nirvicāra samādhis* connect investigation and reflection on the level of the subtlest of the subtle, or the finest of the fine. Knowledge hitherto unknown is explored in detail.

***nirvicāra-vaiśāradye adhyātma-prasādaḥ* (I.47)**

As consciousness spreads in the entire body as *citta prasādanam*, if the seer spreads in the entire body, it becomes the *nirvicāra* state of *samādhi* or *ātman prasādanam*. For this, the practitioner has to learn to spread the *ātman* or the seer evenly in the body while practising the *āsana*s and *prāṇāyāma*, and feel his presence totally and wholly.

sūkṣma-viṣayatvaṁ ca aliṅga-paryavasānam (I.45)

Consciousness being the subtlest part of *prakṛti*, it loses its marks and merges in nature. (*See* II.19 on the principles of nature.)

samādhi-siddhiḥ Īśvara-praṇidhānāt (II.45)

In the dissolution of all marks and signs of separateness, one experiences *samādhi* and surrenders oneself to God.

prayatna-śaithilya-ananta-samāpattibhyām (II.47)

On dealing with *āsana*s, Patañjali says that when the effort of performing comes to an end, then that effortful mind loses all resistance and changes into an effortless state, and finds solace in experiencing its real state and status. This means that when the effortless state is reached in practice, the movements take place from the source and cover the entire body as if body were the self. The self can be the smallest of small and the greatest of great, and so by the assuming of *āsana*s, the finest self engulfs the body as the greatest Self. From this angle, *āsana*s transform one from the finite state to experience the infinite (*ānanta*) state as well.

tad eva artha-mātra-nirbhāsaṁ svarūpa-śūnyam iva samādhiḥ (III.3)

Profound reflection in meditation (*dhyāna*) makes *sādhaka*s forget their own form (*svarūpa*), as they lose their identity in the object on which they are meditating, and become one with it.

sarva-arthatā-ekāgratayoḥ kṣaya-udayau cittasya samādhi-pariṇāmaḥ (III.11)

Moving from scattered attention towards single-focused attention helps one to gain total absorption (*samādhi*) as one loses the awareness of 'I'.

All these states of *samāpatti*s or *samādhi*s are sequential stages in experiencing the state of *samādhi*. They show the internal evolution of consciousness from the grossest to the finest state.

29. *Virāma Pratyaya*

This is the last stage in *sabīja samādhi*. There is a possibility here of losing the identity of *asmitā rūpa* (as it is formless, though not seedless). Vyāsa mentions it as *asaṁprajñāta samādhi*. But the text explains later that this *samādhi* is *sabīja*, which leads towards *nirbīja* or *dharmamegha samādhi*. It does not imply a negative state (*a* = not; *saṁprajñāta* = awareness of the self), but a qualified state of a non-oscillating and non-vacillating state of consciousness. There is no self-conceit or self-centredness in this state.

This *virāma pratyaya* is an essential state in moving towards the seedless (*nirbīja*) state of *samādhi*.

30. Effects of *Virāma Pratyaya*

***bhava-pratyayaḥ videha-prakṛti--layānām* (I.19)** Past impressions remain dormant in this state, and one may feel a state of bodilessness and of merging in the root nature (*mūla prakṛti*). This is a state of *manolaya* and not *manojaya*. If one constructively builds up this focused awareness in oneself, then it is possible to move from *manolaya* to *manojaya* and emancipation (*kaivalya*). Otherwise one may be submerged in nature, losing the path towards *nirbīja samādhi*.

I would like to underline this difference between *manolaya* and *manojaya* states. *Manolaya* (I.19) is the rhythmic silent state of the mind. I speak about rhythm, as the stability of silence is needed in order to overcome the vibrations of the mind. *Manojaya* (III.44) is the mastery over the mind which corresponds to the higher levels of *samādhi*. It becomes an universal, cosmic mind. *Manolaya* is the prerequisite for the conquest of the mind (*manojaya*).

This *virāma pratyaya* state is no less than a state of passive alertness.

See:

***tā eva sabījaḥ samādhiḥ* (I.46)** All the seven states of *samāpatti* or *samādhi* come under *sabīja samādhi*. Though *virāma pratyaya* is said to be different (*anyaḥ*: I.18), it is a form of *sabīja samādhi*. Here the feeling of being with oneself fades, though there remains the lustre of wisdom and insight, which can be tapped for furthering spiritual growth. Hence, this *samādhi* is a precursor for *nirbīja samādhi*.

31. Cautions to *Sādhakas* on *Samādhi*

In *nirbīja samādhi* the *puruṣa* shines with liveliness and loveliness.

***te samādhau upasargāḥ vyutthāne siddhayaḥ* (III.38)**

Here practitioners are cautioned that accomplishments act as impediments in the long run for those who want to proceed towards emancipation. If they cultivate indifference to such successes, yoga itself makes them experience *ātma-prasādanam* (*see* I.47), leading them towards emancipation (*kaivalya*).

***sattva-puruṣa-anyatā-khyāti-mātrasya sarva-bhāva-adhiṣṭhātṛtvaṁ sarva-jñātṛtvaṁ ca* (III.50)**

From the insight of the seer comes an understanding of all manifestations, but at the same time, one must be careful that *ahaṁkāra* does not entice and pull him back, causing the downfall of *sādhanā*.

***tad-vairāgyāt api doṣa-bīja-kṣaye kaivalyam* (III.51)**

Patañjali again emphatically cautions with all his might that one must spurn and forgo accomplishments. Otherwise they act as defective seeds generating *ahaṁkāra*-causing afflictions.

***sthāni-upanimantraṇe saṅga-smayā-akaraṇaṁ punar-aniṣṭa-prasaṅgāt* (III.52)**

In this state of accomplishments, one may be enticed by celestial beings or good-looking women or men, to fall into the trap of temptations.

32. *Samādhi Phala*

***ṛtaṁbharā tatra prajñā* (I.48)**

When the practitioner liberates himself from the attraction of the senses towards the world and moves towards illuminative emancipation, he gains the faculty of insight. He feels what is 'real', crosses the bridge of accomplishments and moves towards freedom and beatitude.

***śruta-anumāna-prajñābhyām anya-viṣayā viśeṣa-arthatvāt* (I.49)**

When he is well established in the 'real', the faculty of insight and wisdom becomes subjective. Then he needs neither books nor testimonies because he lives in the 'real'. From this insight and wisdom, he reaches the seedless *samādhi* (*nirbīja samādhi*).

33. *Nirbīja Samādhi*

This is the innermost state of *samādhi*, called *ātma saṁyama* state.

***taj-jaḥ saṁskāraḥ anya-saṁskāra-pratibandhī* (I.50)**

In order to reach *nirbīja samādhi* and to live in that seedless state of *samādhi*, one has to leave behind both old and new experiences (*see sūtras* I.48–49).

***tasya api nirodhe sarva-nirodhāt nirbījaḥ samādhiḥ* (I.51)**

In this state of seedless (*nirbīja*) *samādhi*, no impressions enter the mind, intelligence or consciousness. Here, the seer spreads evenly in his vestments, and the feeling of separateness between the seen and the seer is extinguished and only awareness (*prajñā*) stands.

The search for the seer ends. Even the feel of *ātma* fades and only *prajñā* occupies and engulfs its frontiers.

***puruṣa-artha-śūnyānāṁ guṇānāṁ pratiprasavaḥ kaivalyaṁ sva-rūpa-pratiṣṭhā vā citi-śaktiḥ iti* (IV.34)**

At this state, the *guṇa*s recede and merge in nature, and then the yogi lives devoid of aims. From this point onwards, the *puruṣa* that shines in him lives in his own power (*śakti*) like the lotus flower, which grows out of the mud of the swamp with a flower that does not touch the swamp.

34. *Yogaphala* (Effects of *Aṣṭāṅga* Yoga)

On the way to the final destination, some deeper and profound transformations arise in *sādhanā*, which must be considered as only partial effects. With these partial effects, the *sādhaka* must further his *sādhanā* to bring all of them together to form a whole so that he reaches the main effect of yoga: to establish consciousness in its own original purity so that it is on par with the seer (*citi*).

***heyaṁ duḥkham anāgatam* (II.16)**

Pains that are dormant may manifest at a later time and can be prevented through the regular practice of yoga. The practice of yoga helps also in building up strength and power to endure the pains which cannot be cured.

On the gross level, Patañjali says that yoga acts as a preventive art and science in healing. It enables one to start working, as a curative method, culminating in divine health and divine wisdom.

This explains that the practitioner, having worked to prevent impediments, should proceed in building up an enduring power and strength to keep at bay the obstacles that arise in *sādhanā*. He should also proceed in generating skill in thought and action to establish wholesomeness in all the layers of the seer.

Sūtra II.34 explains that physical (*ādhibhautika roga*), mental (*ādhidaivika roga*) or spiritual (*ādhyātmika roga*) pains and sufferings are due to dubious understanding, violent nature, anger and greed, whether *kṛta* or done directly (*ādhyātmika*), *kārita* or permitted to be done (*ādhidaivika*) and *anumodita* or caused to be done (*ādhibhautika*). These create fissures in body, senses, mind, intelligence and consciousness. He guides us not to fall prey to these traps but to use the achievement as a guideline for the cultivation of right thoughts and actions in the form of *aṣṭāṅga yoga*.

***sūkṣma-viṣayatvaṁ ca aliṅga-paryavasānam* (I.45)**

The subtlest particle of nature is consciousness (*citta*). One has to learn to merge the *citta* through *yaugika sādhanā* into the cosmic consciousness (*mahat*), so that these together are merged in the root nature or *mūla prakṛti* for the seer to shine from his dwelling: *tadā draṣṭuḥ svarūpe avasthānam* (I.3).

Having understood the relationship between the individual consciousness (*citta*) and the universal consciousness (*mahat*), the *sādhaka* uses his body, organs of action, senses of perception, mind, intelligence and consciousness to reach a conscientious state of consciousness; returns the *guṇa*s to their state of perfect equilibrium; and puts an end to all painful actions (IV.30).

***prakāśa-kriyā--sthiti-śīlaṁ bhūta--indriyā-ātmakaṁ bhoga-apavarga--arthaṁ dṛśyam* (II.18)**

Due to uninterrupted, focused practice with observation and absorption, one will no longer be swept by the pleasures of the senses, but will turn towards the unalloyed sight of the soul. *See, tad--arthaḥ eva dṛśyasya ātmā* (II.21); the principles of nature are solely there for serving the seer to live in the state of emancipation.

***prayatna--śaithilya-ananta--samāpattibhyām* (II.47)**

When all resistance dissolves and effortful efforts are transformed into effortless efforts, the *sādhaka* becomes alert at once and experiences changes and transformations. Besides this, he also experiences the infinite or immortal *puruṣa*, who resides inside as *citi śakti* (*ātma śakti*), transforming the dual mind into a single, simple and innocent mind without ignorance or arrogance.

This is how yoga practice brings conjunction between *prakṛti* and *puruṣa*, as *yaugika* practice acts as an instrument to peel the inner layers:

***sva-svāmi-śaktyoḥ sva-rūpa-upalabdhu--hetuḥ saṁyogaḥ* (II.23)**

The conjunction of the seer with the seen is essential for the seer to discover his own true nature. One can reach this state through *yaugika* knowledge and practice, where the 24 principles of nature are made to merge in the root nature for the seer to establish on his own.

See, viveka-khyātiḥ aviplavā hāna-upāyaḥ (II.26).

***dṛg-darśana-śaktyoḥ eka-ātmatā iva asmitā* (II.6)** The seer is ever pure. When this pure seer is connected to *prāṇa*, he as individual self identifies himself with *vṛttis*, whereas *citta* believes that this identification is from the pure seer who is dwelling within.

***bhuvana-jñānaṁ sūrye saṁyamāt* (III.27)** When one reaches purity in the body and freedom from fluctuations of thought waves, the *puruṣa* or the seer residing in the body shines like a Sun that never fades.

***tasya bhūmiṣu viniyogaḥ* (III.6)** By gaining experiential knowledge through yoga, the *sādhaka* must use this wisdom in his daily life, in day-to-day activities, as well as in sharing it with his fellow beings.

My own yoga path is neither the approach of monks nor for householders. It is for all.

I am a dedicated and vehement practitioner committed to living in the world and sharing my knowledge with you all. I live in the world, fulfilling and meeting the demands and expectations of family and society. Yet, I remain dedicated to my *sādhanā*, from my interiormost core of being.

***ṛtaṁbharā tatra prajñā* (I.48)** When one is absorbed in practice, inner action and refinement take place, leading towards matured and measured wisdom. Observe the closeness of this *sūtra* with the following one:

***prasaṁkhyāne api akusīdasya sarvathā viveka-khyāteḥ dharma-meghaḥ samādhiḥ* (IV.29)** The person who is free from aversions and ailments maintains constant focused awareness from the musculoskeletal body towards the spiritual kingdom. When this is achieved, he lives with the shower of virtues. See the similarity between *ṛtaṁbharā prajñā* (I.48) and *dharma-megha samādhi* (IV.29).

***tataḥ kleśa-karma--nivṛttiḥ* (IV.30)** He covers all types of actions (*karmas*). *Karma* is general action. Actions with motivation are *vikarma*. Auspicious and good actions are *sakarma*, and actions without ambitions or motivations are *niṣkāma karma*. He says that, from now on, actions with perfect precision help people to be free from all destructions, distractions, refractions and afflictions. Their actions afflict neither themselves nor others.

***yoga-aṅga--anuṣṭhānāt aśuddhi-kṣaye jñāna-dīptiḥ aviveka-khyāteḥ* (II.28)**	This way of dedicated practice with all aspects of yoga destroys all impurities, radiating the crown of wisdom in glory, introducing the seven states of *prajñā* or awareness.

He speaks of the greatest effect of yoga in the simplest of words. These are:

***tasya saptadhā prānta-bhūmiḥ prajñā* (II.27)**	To gain the ceaseless flow of attentive awareness, one must know and have full knowledge and understanding of the various sheaths of the seer: *śarīra-jñāna, indriya-jñāna, prāṇa-jñāna, manojñāna, buddhi paripakva-jñāna* (ripened intelligence), *citta-jñāna* and *ātma-jñāna*. *Yoga Vāsiṣṭa* and Vyāsa interpret these *prajñās* differently.[1]

35. *Prakṛti Puruṣa Jaya*

In *Vibhūti Pāda*, besides a detailed list of *yaugika* accomplishments, Patañjali describes, in sequence, the conquest of *prakṛti* and *puruṣa*:

a. *Bhūta jaya* – mastery over the elements

***sthūla-svarūpa--sūkṣma-anvaya--arthavattva--saṁyamāt bhūta-jayaḥ* (III.45)**	[2]Inner pervasiveness, along with knowing the purposefulness of the conjunction of the inner body with the outer body, brings mastery over the elements (*bhūtas*).

1 See *Light on the Yoga Sūtras of Patañjali*, table 10, page 131.
2 He knows in full the gross and subtle mutations of nature.

b. *Tanmātra jaya* – mastery over the infrastructural qualities of the elements

tato' ṇima-ādi-
-prādur-bhāvaḥ
kāya--saṁpat
tad-dharma-
-anabhighātaḥ ca
(III.46)

[1]As I have already explained, many link this *sūtra* to *aṣṭa-siddhi* (eight supernatural powers). But I feel it conveys the mastery of the infrastructural (*aṇu*) qualities of the elements (*tanmātra*), or *tanmātra jaya*, because it clearly speaks of the wealth of the body (*kāya saṁpat*) and mastery over the senses of perception.

c. *Śarīra jaya* – mastery over the body

rūpa-lāvaṇya-
-bala-vajra-
-saṁhananatvāni
kāya-saṁpat (III.47)

Perfection of the body lies in the quality of its beauty, grace, strength, compactness and brilliance.

d. *Indriya jaya* – mastery over the organs of action and senses of perception

grahaṇa-
-svarūpa-asmitā-
-anvaya-arthavattva-
-saṁyamāt
indriya-jayaḥ (III.48)

[2]Integration of the *indriya* in *āsana* and *prāṇāyāma* brings mastery over the organs of action, senses of perception and mind.

e. *Manojaya* – mastery over the mind and consciousness

tataḥ mano-javitvaṁ
vikaraṇa-bhāvaḥ
pradhāna-jayaḥ ca
(III.49)

[3]Since mind is the outer layer of consciousness, when it is mastered, then consciousness is mastered. By mastery over the mind and consciousness, the individual mind transforms into a universal or cosmic mind or cosmic intelligence (*mahat*).

---

1 He can reduce himself to the size of an atom or expand himself. He can become light or heavy. He has access to everything. He can pierce rocks, control anything and be a Lord of everything.

2 He has mastery over nature and recognises the purpose of the conjunction without involving himself.

3 He subdues nature and moves faster than light and sound.

f. Realising the seer

sattva-puruṣa-anyatā-khyāti-mātrasya sarva-bhāva-adhiṣṭhātṛtvaṁ sarva-jñātṛtvaṁ ca **(III.50)**

[1]When the difference between the knowledge of nature and that of the seer is realised, the wisdom of the seer surfaces.

g. *Ātmajaya* – sight of the seer

puruṣa-artha-śūnyānāṁ guṇānāṁ pratiprasavaḥ kaivalyaṁ sva-rūpa-pratiṣṭhā vā citi-śaktiḥ iti **(IV.34)**

[2]Then the illuminative soul or seer surfaces, subjugating the *mahat* and establishing himself in his own natural purity.

The effect of yoga is to give one a grasp of all the 24 principles of nature to lead the rest of life illuminated by the flame of the soul.

From this supreme knowledge and wisdom and with the flame of the soul, he imparts knowledge (*viniyoga*) by guiding those who come for help.

Today yoga universities offer Diploma, Degree and Master's courses and even a Doctorate (PhD) in yoga. Patañjali, though a great *ātma-darśin*, speaks academically of gaining diplomas, degrees or doctorates in yoga.

Reading carefully from III.45 onwards, one will see that the founder of the yoga system suggests there are various stages of qualifications to gain a 'doctorate' in yoga. In *sūtra*s 45 and 47 he suggests qualification for diploma. The *sūtra*s 46 and 48 are meant for a Degree course, sutras 49 and 50 are meant for a Master's in yoga, while 55 and 56 are meant for a Doctorate. Do any universities follow these academic descriptions suggested by Patañjali in their syllabus? I am not sure.

---

1 He gains lordship over all things; he becomes omnipresent, omnipotent and omniscient.

2 From now on, the yogi is devoid of all aims of life. He is free from the qualities of nature and lives in the state of *kaivalya* (emancipation).

Thus yoga begins with an explanation of the fluctuations of thought waves, and shows ways to develop stability and silence in consciousness in order to live by the flame of the soul, surrendering the entire being to *Sṛṣṭi-kartā* – the Lord of All.

XV

Samādhi-Kaivalya Bheda – The Difference between *Samādhi* and *Kaivalya*

In the state of *sabīja samādhis*, one loses awareness of oneself as well as a connection with the world (*sva-rūpa-śūnya-avasthā*) (I.43 and III.3).

Kaivalya corresponds to *nirbīja samādhi*. This is the highest state of profound establishment of the seer (*svarūpa-pratiṣṭhā*), in which the seer shines in his own glory. In this state 'nature' (*prakṛti*) is exiled and the coronation of the *ātman*, *citi-śakti*, takes place.

samādhi-bhāvanā--arthaḥ kleśa-tanū--karaṇa-arthaḥ ca **(II.2)**	Patañjali explains in *Sādhanapāda* on *kriyā yoga* that *samādhi* attenuates the afflictions or eradicates them at the level of gross and subtle bodies (*kārya* or *sthūla śarīra* and *sūkṣma śarīra*).

Kaivalya

tad eva artha--mātra-nirbhāsaṁ svarūpa-śūnyam iva samādhiḥ **(III.3)**	The destruction and eradication of ignorance and of arrogance through right knowledge and right approach in yoga cuts the link between *prakṛti* and *puruṣa*, bringing about the experience of *kaivalya*.

samādhi-siddhiḥ Īśvara-praṇidhānat **(II.45)**	Perfection in *samādhi* leads one to surrender to God.
tad-abhāvāt saṁyoga-abhāvaḥ hānaṁ tad-dṛśeḥ kaivalyam **(II.25)**	[1]One loses the awareness of the world in *samādhi* and as such one loses self-awareness. Here stands the main difference between *samādhi* and *kaivalya*. Self-awareness is lost through absorption in *samādhi*, whereas in *kaivalya* one lives in a state of being a pure seer (*puruṣa*), which is alone and independent from the vestments (*prakṛti*) of thc Self. This means that *samādhi* is a state without an individual awareness of identity. In *kaivalya* all identities are subsumed with the Universal and Supreme Being.

The zenith in yoga is not only the eradication of *ahaṁkāra* (the impostor of the Self) and the feeling of emptiness (*svarūpa-śūnya*), but also the consecration in the Self (*svarūpa-avasthā*).

tad-vairāgyāt api doṣa-bīja-kṣaye kaivalyam **(III.51)**	Non-involvement as well as total detachment from the so-called super-normal or supernatural powers helps to burn out the defective seed in the intelligence which causes attachments and desires. This state of consciousness makes the Self live in its original state, which is nothing less than the eternal state of perfect divinity.
sattva-puruṣayoḥ śuddhi-sāmye kaivalyam iti **(III.56)**	Then consciousness becomes absolute and experiences the exalted subjective state of aloneness. This is *kaivalya*.
tadā viveka-nimnaṁ kaivalya-prāgbhāraṁ cittam **(IV.26)**	[2]When the fruit is ripe, the fruit falls to the ground due to the change in the relationship of two forces – the gravitational force and the force attaching

1 The merging of the meditator and the object of meditation is absorption (*samādhi*).

2 On account of this purity, consciousness inclines the seer to experience the state of indivisible existence.

the fruit to the tree. In the same way, the absolute consciousness (*kūṭastha citta*) rests on the lap of the soul due to its ripeness and to the altered balance between the pull of the seer and attachment (I.41 and IV.26). From here on, the *puruṣa* lives alone. This is *kaivalya*.

And lastly:

***puruṣa-artha--śūnyānāṁ guṇānāṁ pratiprasavaḥ kaivalyaṁ sva--rūpa-pratiṣṭhā vā citi-śaktiḥ iti* (IV.34)**

This way the *yoga sādhanā* culminates with the establishment of *puruṣa* without any contact with *prakṛti*.

Thus, the treatise of yoga ends with the expression '*citi śakti*' or the power of the soul.

Once the four aims of life (*puruṣārthas – dharma, artha, kāma, mokṣa*) are fulfilled, the only purpose that remains for the *sādhaka* is the maintenance of *sādhanā*. The *sādhaka* has learnt and earned merit upon merit, and acquired the treasure of *siddhis*. The only remaining act is self-surrender and transference of merit to the pure stainless Lord – *Īśvara*. Though Patañjali concludes with the power of *citi* (the seer), I feel that the implicit and hidden fifth *puruṣārtha* (*Īśvara praṇidhāna* in I.23) is the finality of *yoga sādhanā*.

Śrī Rāmānuja speaks of *Īśvara-praṇidhāna* as the fifth *puruṣārtha*. Patañjali has already dealt with this fifth *puruṣārtha*, which is untold and unnamed – that is, the total surrender of oneself to *Ādi-puruṣa*:

***Īśvara-praṇidhānāt vā* (I.23)**

From *citi-śakti*, the *yogi* has to move from the four established aims towards the realisation of the *ātman*, to surrender totally to God. His journey moves him from *citta-prasādana* to *ātma-prasādana* and from *ātma-prasādana* to *Īśvara-praṇidhāna*.

Here culminates *yoga-mārga*.

// ĀUṀ TAT SAT //

Glossary of *Sanskṛta* Words

This glossary contains all the *Saṅskṛta* terms and expressions in this book. It is meant particularly for those who are not familiar with the terminology of the *yaugika* tradition, to help them to grasp the contents of the text with ease. To that end, some words and phrases have been hyphenated.

To help readers who are not acquainted with *Saṅskṛta*, the words are arranged according to Latin alphabetical order.

abheda: Extinction of the differences.
abhijāta-maṇi: Flawless gem.
abhiniveśa: Clinging to life, fear of death. The fifth of the five *kleśas*.
abhyāsa: Practice, effort, repetition. Along with *vairāgya*, they are the first means advised by Patañjali to restrain the fluctuations of consciousness.
ācārya: A spiritual guide, one who preaches and teaches what he practises.
adhaḥpatana rekhā: The razor edge.
ādhibhautika roga: Disease produced due to the disturbance or imbalance in the elements of the body; physical disease. The third of the three types of *roga*.
ādhidaivika roga: Disease produced by genetic factors or diseases over which humans have no control, disease due to fate or destiny. The second of the three types of *roga*.
adhikārin: Fit person, privileged to do yoga.
adhimātra: Ardent, intense, keen. The third of the four types of practitioner, along with *mṛdu*, *madhyama* and *tīvra*.

adhimātrātma: In *Śiva Saṁhitā*, corresponding to *tīvra* of the *Yoga Sūtras*.

adhyātma prasādana: Tranquillity, serenity pertaining to the presence of the real self.

ādhyātmika roga: Self-inflicted disease. Physical or mental disease induced by one's own behaviour. The first of the three types of *roga*.

Ādi-daiva: Primal God.

Ādi-devatā: The Primal God or the Creator.

Ādi-puruṣa: Primal *puruṣa*, God

Ādi-śakti: Primal energy, primal *śakti*.

adivya citta: Non-divine, the opposite to *divya citta* (divine, brilliant and intelligent).

āgama: Authoritative scriptures or testimony of realised masters. One of the three means of *pramāṇa* or right knowledge.

āgāmi karma: *Kriyamāṇa karma*.

āgāmi: Yet to come, next life.

ahaṁ: The pure 'I', the self as form of the soul.

ahaṁ-ākāra: I-ness. Term introduced to mean the form taken by *puruṣa* to come in contact with *prakṛti*. It is a mediated form of the seer to be in contact with *citta* or consciousness.

ahaṁkāra: Making of self, the I-maker, ego, haughtiness, principle of individuality. One of the three constituents of *citta*, along with *buddhi* and *manas*. It impersonates the self and acts as an impostor of the self. But it can also be transformed through practice to reach the sublime. One of the categories of *Sāṁkhya Darśana*, corresponding to the *aviśeṣa* stage of evolution of *prakṛti*.

ahiṁsā: Non-violence (in action, word and thought). The first of the five principles of *yama*.

ājñā cakra: *Cakra* located between the two eyebrows, at the base of the brain. It rules over *ānandamaya kośa*.

ajñānamaya kośa: The sheath of ignorance. Created by one's ignorance, it disturbs one's evolution.

ā-kāra: Letter 'Ā'. The first of the three components of the syllable *ĀUṀ*.

ākāra: Form, shape.

akarma: Action totally free from any expectation or reward.

ākāśa: Ether or space. The fifth of the *bhūtas* or elements of nature.

akliṣṭa: Non-painful, commonly applied to the fluctuations of consciousness, which may be *kliṣṭa* (painful or perceptible) or *akliṣṭa* (non-painful or imperceptible).

alabdha-bhūmikatva: Missing the point, failure to reach the goal, lack of perseverance. One of the nine *antarāyas* or obstacles.

ālasya: Physical laziness, idleness. One of the nine *antarāyas* or obstacles.

aliṅga: Noumenal. The first of the four stages of the evolution of *prakṛti* or nature. It corresponds to *mūla prakṛti*.

āloka: Light, lustre, looking, seeing, beholding.

Ambikā: An aspect of the Mother Goddess Śakti.

amṛtamaya: Immortal, imperishable.

anādhikārin: Unfit, not worthy of doing yoga.

anāhata cakra: *Cakra* situated in the heart region, the abode of the soul. It rules over *manomaya kośa*.

ānanda: Bliss, joy.

ānandamaya kośa: Sheath of bliss, of joy. The fifth of the five *kośas*.

ananta: Infinite, endless. Sometimes equated to the Seer, the Self. One of the epithets of Lord Viṣṇu, as He is difficult to know even for His devotees, on account of his infinity. In addition, the great thousand-headed serpent on whom Lord Viṣṇu rests is named Ananta or Śeṣa, as he represents cosmic time, which is infinite and endless. We invoke his blessings as the giver of yoga, who incarnated himself as Patañjali.

anavasthi-tattvā: Inability to maintain progress, backsliding, inability to maintain steady practice. One of the nine *antarāyas* or obstacles.

aṅga: Limb, part, aspect, member. Commonly, each one of the eight limbs or petals of *aṣṭāṅga yoga*.

aṇimā: The power of becoming very small. One of the eight *siddhis* or one of the supernatural powers.

aṇimādi: Eight supernatural powers.

annamaya: Anatomical. Literally, 'built on food'.

annamaya kośa: Physical or anatomical sheath. The first of the five *kośas*. It constitutes the gross body.

anta: Culmination, end.

antaḥkaraṇa: Conscience or *dharmendriya*, the organ of duty.

antaḥkaraṇamaya kośa: The sheath of the conscience.

antaḥkaraṇa śuddhi: Purification of the conscience, purity.

antar or **antara**: Internal.

antara kuṁbhaka: In *prāṇāyāma*, retention of breath after inhalation.

antara manas: Inner mind, the part of the mind that is closer to the intelligence or directed towards the intelligence.

antaraṅga: Concerning the inner aspect or inner part of the referred concept; internal.

antaraṅga anveṣaṇa: Investigation of the internal aspects.

antaraṅga sādhanā: Internal level of practice, including the limbs of *aṣṭāṅga yoga* from *pratyāhāra* to *dhyāna*, and dealing with the subtle body or *sūkṣma śarīra*.

antaraṅga saṁyama: Integration of the three internal limbs (*dhāraṇā*, *dhyāna* and *samādhi*) as a unit.

antaraṅga śarīra: Inner body. It corresponds to the subtle body or *sūkṣma śarīra*, and is formed by the inner mind, intelligence, I-ness, consciousness and conscience.

antarātma sādhanā: Interiormost level of practice, consisting of the eighth limb of yoga or *samādhi*, and dealing with the causal body or *kāraṇa śarīra*. I must mention that this expression may seem contradictory, as *ātma* has no practice.

antarāyas: Obstacles. They are nine: *vyādhi*, *styāna*, *saṁśaya*, *pramāda*, *ālasya*, *avirati*, *bhrāntidarśana*, *alabdhabhūmikatva* and *anavasthitatva*. They are also called *citta-vikṣepas* (the distractions of consciousness).

antarendriya: The innermost organ connecting the intelligence and I-ness to the soul; conscience.

antaryāmin: The Universal Soul dwelling within the human being; God in us.

aṇu: Literally, tiny, minute. Atom, infrastructure.

ānubhāvika: Felt, experienced.

ānubhavika jñāna: Knowledge earned through experience.

anukūla. Favourable.

anukūla vṛtti: Favourable modifications of consciousness, conducive to spiritual progress, helping the practitioner on the path of Self-realisation.

anumāna: Inference, investigation, logical reasoning. One of the three means of *pramāṇa*, or right knowledge.

anumodita: Abetted, consented, allowed to be done. One of the three types of actions mentioned by Patañjali in *sūtra* II.34.

anusandhāna: Re-arrangement, re-investigation.

anuśāsanam: Setting in order, connecting, congruous, code of conduct traditionally followed, something to be followed from ancient times.

anvaya: All-pervasiveness, association, conjunction or interpenetration.

anveṣaṇa: Investigation.

āp: Water. The second of the elements of nature, one of the five *bhūtas*.

apāna: One of the five *prāṇas* or *vāyus*. It is located in the lower abdominal region and rules over the excretory and reproductive functions.

aparigraha: Non-possessiveness, greedlessness, non-covetousness, non-receiving of gifts. The fifth of the five principles of *yama*.

apātra: Not destined for, unfit, unworthy.

apavarga: Liberation, emancipation, enlightenment, spiritual bliss.

apavargārtha: Means towards emancipation.
apavargasthāna: Seat or place for emancipation.
apuṇya: Wrong action, vice.
ārambha. Commencement. The first of the four stages of evolution in practice or *avasthā*.
Arjuna: Hero of the *Mahābhārata*, to whom Lord Krishna teaches the *Bhagavad Gītā*.
artha: Means. Acquisition or the means of livelihood, the second of the four aims of life or *puruṣārthas*.
arthavatva: Means and purposes.
āsana: Posture, positioning of the body as pose and repose. The third of the eight petals of *aṣṭāṅga yoga*.
asmitā: Individual pure self. Pure state of being. It also stands for pride, egoism. The second of the five *kleśas*.
asmitā prajñā: Awareness of the pure individual self.
asmitārūpa citta: Consciousness with the form of the pure state of being.
āśrama: Stage of life. The four stages covering the span of life. These are: *brahmacaryāśrama*, *gṛhasthāśrama*, *vanaprasthāśrama* and *sannyāsāśrama*.
Aṣṭadaḷa Yogamālā: Collected Works. A compendium in eight volumes in which this author has theorised and explained his own experience in the field of yoga.
aṣṭāṅga yoga. Yoga of eight limbs. Related to yoga explained by Lord Patañjali as composed of eight parts, limbs or petals. These are: *yama*, *niyama*, *āsana*, *prāṇāyāma*, *pratyāhāra*, *dhāraṇā*, *dhyāna* and *samādhi*.
aṣṭa siddhi: The eight powers or *siddhis*. They are: *aṇimā*, *mahimā*, *garimā*, *laghimā*, *prāpti*, *prākāmya*, *vaśitva* and *īśatva*.
asteya: Non-stealing, non-covetousness. The third of the principles of *yama*.
aśūnya: Non-void.
aśūnya-avasthā: State of non-void, passive alertness.
atha: Now. First word of the *Yoga Sūtras* of Patañjali.
ātmā, ātman: Soul, self, *puruṣa*, seer.

ātma-agni: Flame of the seer, flame of the soul.
ātma-darśana: Sight of the soul, vision of the Self, spiritual enlightenment.
ātma-devatā: Divinity of the soul.
ātma-jaya: Sight of the seer.
ātma-jñāna: Knowledge of the Self, Self-realisation.
ātmamaya kośa: Concept introduced to refer to the sheath or layer of the Self, the spiritual kingdom.
ātma-prasāda or ***ātma-prasādanam***: Expansion and diffusion of the soul. Quietness, evennesss and stability in this diffusion, where each part and each cell of the body is permeated by the self.
ātma-sākṣātkāra: Opening the gates of the Self, perception of the Self, Self-realisation.
ātma-śakti: The energy or power of the soul.
ātma-saṁyama: Union of the soul, the innermost state of *samādhi*.
āuṁ: The sacred syllable, also called *praṇava*.
auṣadha *or* ***auṣadhi***: Herbs, elixirs, drugs.
avasthā: State, condition, position. Stages of evolution in practice. Traditionally, there are four stages: *āraṁbha*, *ghaṭa*, *paricaya* and *niṣpatti*.
avasthā-pariṇāma: The third type of change in the process of transformations (*pariṇāma*) of consciousness, where it reaches the zenith of its refinement.
avidyā: Ignorance. The first of the five *kleśa*s and the ground for all of them.
avirati: Sense-gratification, self-indulgence, incontinence, indiscipline of the senses. One of the nine *antarāya*s or obstacles.
aviśeṣa: Non-distinguishable. The third of the four stages of the evolution of *prakṛti* or nature. It corresponds to the five *tanmātra* and *ahaṁkāra*.
avyakta: Unmanifested.
avyapadeśya: Latent.

bādhanā: Pain, sorrow.
bahiraṅga: Concerning the outer aspect or the outer part of the referred concept; external.
bahiraṅga anveṣaṇa: Investigation of the external aspects.
bahiraṅga sādhanā: External level of practice, including the limbs of *aṣṭāṅga yoga* from *yama* to *pratyāhāra*, and dealing with the body of action or *kārya śarīra*.
bahiraṅga saṁyama: Integration of the three external practices (*āsana*, *prāṇāyāma* and *pratyāhāra*) as a unit.
bahiraṅga śarīra: External body. It corresponds to *kārya śarīra* or gross body.
bāhya-indriya: External organs.
bāhya kuṁbhaka: In *prāṇāyāma*, retention of breath after exhalation.
bāhya manas: Outer mind, the part of the mind that is closer to the senses and receives impressions from them.
Bhagavad Gītā: Lord Krishna's song, one of the most important sacred scriptures in the *Mahābhārata*, considered a main text of yoga, which presents the dialogue between Lord Krishna and Arjuna, in which the Lord explains to Arjuna the right attitude in life.
bhakta: Devotee.
bhakti: Devotion, love.
bhakti-mārga: Path of devotion and love. One of the four *mārgas* or paths for Self-realisation.
bhāvanā: Feelings, sensations, conceptions.
bheda: Difference.
bhoga: Pleasures of the material world, material joy, enjoyment in life.
bhoga-artha: Means for obtaining pleasures, worldly joy.
bhoga-āsana: *Āsana* practised in the gravity of the pleasure of the senses.
bhoga-sthāna: Place to experience pleasures.
bhrānti-darśana: Mistaken notion, erroneous view, living in the world of illusion. One of the nine *antarāyas* or obstacles.

bhūmi: Ground, soil, abode, land.

bhūta: Elements. Commonly understood as the five elements of nature, namely *pṛthvī*, *āp*, *tejas*, *vāyu* and *ākāśa* (earth, water, fire, air and ether). They are categories of *Sāṁkhya Darśana* and they correspond to the *viśeṣa* stage of evolution of *prakṛti*.

bhūtādika ahaṁkāra: Principle of individuality related to the five elements and the five subtle qualities.

bhūta-jaya: Mastery over the elements.

biṁba: Mirror. It is applied to the reflection of the self in the mind or in the I-ness. It is related to *pratibiṁba*, the re-reflection of the image of a mirror in a second mirror.

bindu: Dot, seed, drop.

Brahmā: The Creator, the Generator. One of the three main Gods of the Hindu pantheon, along with Viṣṇu and Śiva.

brahmacarya: Continence, control of sensuality, celibacy. The fourth of the five principles of *yama*. Synonymous with *brahmacaryāśrama*.

brahmacarya-āśrama: The first of the four stages of life or *āśramas*. It is the stage of learning, of studentship, previous to marital life.

brāhmaṇa: Literally, 'one who knows *Brahman*' or the *Vedas*. Priest class. The first of the four *varṇas* or castes, formed by those who pursue a life of spiritual study and practice, and who attend to the spiritual needs of the people.

brahma-aṇḍa: Macrocosm, universe, always mentioned in reference to *piṇḍāṇḍa*.

brahma-ṛṣi: A *ṛṣi* of very high rank. Each one of the seven principal *ṛṣis* of each age.

buddhi: Intelligence. One of the three constituents of *citta*, it is the faculty for creating concepts. It is also the main instrument for guiding the mind and the organs to turn towards the objects of the senses or towards the seer. The refined intelligence is our closest faculty to the self.

buddhi-paripakva-jñāna: Mature intelligence.

caitanya-śakti: Energetic force, animating energy.
cakra: Wheel, disc. In the esoteric anatomy of yoga, they are energy centres located inside the spine, belonging to the causal body or *kāraṇa śarīra*, and not to the anatomical body. The principal *cakra*s are: *mūlādhāra, svādhiṣṭhāna, maṇipūraka, anāhata, viśuddhi, ājñā* and *sahasrāra*.
cakṣu: Eye.
chidra-citta: Consciousness with pores or fissures. This fissured or split consciousness is the sixth of the *citta śreṇis*, or stages in the transformations of consciousness. Fissures appear in consciousness as a result of pride cultivated in the stage of *ekāgra citta*.
cid-ākāśa: Synonymous with seer.
cintana: Thinking, reflecting upon, analysis, objective thinking.
citi: The eternal *puruṣa*, seer, soul, Self.
citi-śakti: The energy or the power of the Self. The eternal *puruṣa* that resides within; one experiences him when one is ripe in intelligence. It is the last word of the *Yoga Sūtra*s of Patañjali.
citta: Consciousness. Central concept in yoga, defined by Patañjali as the restraint of the fluctuations of the *citta*. It is composed of *ahaṁkāra* (I-maker), *buddhi* (intelligence) and *manas* (mind). *Ahaṁ-ākāra* (I-ness) connects the seer with the principles of nature existing in the body; a bridge between nature and the eternal soul.
citta-bhūmi. The ground, the soil, the land of consciousness.
citta-jaya: Conquest of consciousness.
citta-lakṣaṇa: Characteristics of consciousness.
cittamaya kośa: The sheath of consciousness. It corresponds to *ānandamaya kośa*, and replaces it when we consider that *ānandamaya kośa* belongs to the seer and thus it is out of the five elemental sheaths.
cittan: The holder of the *citta*.
citta-nirodha: Restraint of consciousness.
citta-nirūpaṇa: Definition of consciousness.
citta-parivartana: Transformation of consciousness.

citta-prabhu: Master of consciousness.

citta-prajñā: Awareness of consciousness.

citta-prasādanam: Expansion and diffusion of consciousness. Quietness, evenness and stability in this diffusion, in which consciousness equates itself with each part, each cell of the body, and in which the body is no less than consciousness.

citta-śreṇi: Ranges or provinces of consciousness, successive transformations of consciousness from the wandering consciousness to the divine consciousness. The seven ranges are: *vyutthāna*, *nirodha*, *śānta*, *ekāgra*, *nirmāṇa*, *chidra* and *divya*.

citta-staṃbha-vṛtti: Stable state of consciousness, synonymous with the restraint of the fluctuations of consciousness.

citta-stambhana-vṛtti: Pause that takes place between *vyutthāna* and *nirodha-citta*.

citta-svabhāva: Natural state of consciousness.

citta-vṛtti: Modifications, movements, fluctuations of consciousness. They constitute the different types of the normal functioning of consciousness and they must be restrained to reach yoga. They are five: *pramāṇa*, *viparyaya*, *vikalpa*, *nidrā* and *smṛti*.

citta-vṛtti-nirodha: Restraint of the modifications of consciousness. This is the definition of yoga given by the *Yoga Sūtras* in *sūtra* I.2.

daḷa: Petal. Each one of the eight limbs of yoga that constitute the flower of yoga.

darśana: Sight, vision, manifestation, reflection, mirror. Also the six classical systems of Hindu philosophy.

darśana-agni: Fire of vision.

deśa: Place, region, territory.

devadatta: One of the five subsidiary energies, or *upavāyus*. It causes yawning and induces sleep.

devatā: Deity, God.

dhanaṁjaya: One of the five subsidiary energies or *upavāyus*.

It produces phlegm to lubricate the entire system and remains in the body even after death, inflating and degenerating the corpse.

dhāraṇā: Concentration, focus of one's attention. The sixth of the eight petals of *aṣṭāṅga yoga.*

dharma: Duty, science of duty, performance of duty. The first of the four aims of life or *puruṣārtha*s.

dharma-indriya: Conscience, the organ of righteous duty, conscientiousness.

dharma-indriya-kośa: The sheath of conscience.

dharma-megha-samādhi: The highest type of *samādhi*, in which virtuousness pours like rain from a cloud. Synonymous with *nirbīja samādhi.*

dharma-pariṇāma: The first type of change in the process of transformations (*pariṇāma*) of consciousness, in which it cultivates its potential states.

dharmin: Literally, 'form possessor'. Virtuous, just, pious, characteristic, substratum.

Dhruva*:* Literally, 'fixed, firm, immovable'. The pole star.

dhyāna: Meditation. The seventh of the eight petals of *aṣṭāṅga yoga.*

divya citta: Pure, flawless, divine consciousness, experience of the divine state of evolution. The seventh of the *citta śreṇis*, or stages, in the transformation of consciousness.

divya citta karma: Actions of the pure divine consciousness, which have no reactions at all.

doṣa bīja: Defective seed, seed of blemish, destructive seed.

draṣṭā: Seer, *puruṣa*, soul.

dvandva: Literally, 'two-two-two..., pair'. Duality, pair of opposites; dual.

dveṣa: Aversion. The fourth of the five *kleśas.*

eka-citta: Single state of attention.

ekādaśa-indriya: The 11th sense, the external mind – i.e., the part of the mind which is in contact with outer objects.

ekāgra or ***ekāgratā:*** Single-focused, attentive, steady, concentrated. One of the five states of consciousness.

ekāgra or ***ekāgratā citta:*** Single-focused consciousness, with the power to hold on to single-focused attention, attentive. The fourth of the *citta śreṇis* or stages in the transformation of consciousness. If lived with humbleness, it transforms the *citta* into *nirmāna citta*; if lived with arrogance, it leads to *chidra citta*.

ekāgratā-pariṇāma: The third of the transformations of consciousness, in which the practitioner learns to maintain single-focused attention without interruption to rest in the house of the Self.

eka-manas: Mind as a single unit.

ekatattva-abhyāsa: Single-minded effort, single-minded practice.

gandha: Odour. One of the five *tanmātras* or infrastructural qualities of the five elements, corresponding to the element earth.

gariman: The power of becoming heavy. It is one of the eight *siddhis* (supernatural powers).

ghaṭa. Intent endeavour. The second of the four stages of evolution in practice or *avasthā*.

gṛhastha-āśrama: The second of the four stages of life or *āśramas*. It is the stage of a house-holder.

guṇa: Quality, attribute, qualities of nature. The three modes of being that create the movement of the phenomenal world, that stir the world from its essence to its phenomenal existence. The three *guṇa*s are: *sattva, rajas* and *tamas*.

guṇa-atīta: One who is free from the influences of the *guṇa*s.

guṇa-karma: Quality of actions, of work.

guṇa-parvāṇi: Specific transformations, characteristic divisions, stages in evolution. See *prakṛti*.

guru: Preceptor, master. One who enlightens, who brings his pupil from ignorance towards light and wisdom.

Haṭhayoga Pradīpikā: The most famous classical text on *haṭha yoga*, written by Svātmārāma in the 14th century.

indriya: Organ, sense. Classically they are considered to be 10 (five *karmendriyas* and five *jñānendriyas*) or 11 (when the external mind is added to them).
indriya-jaya: Mastery over the 11 *indriya* or organs.
indriya-jñāna: Knowledge of the organs and senses.
indriyamaya kośa: The organs of action and senses of perception as a whole.
īśa: Lord, the one who commands.
īśatva: Supremacy over all. One of the eight *siddhis*.
Īśvara: God, the Supreme Lord, the Almighty.
Īśvara-praṇidhāna: Surrender of all actions to God, devotion to the Lord, surrender of one's self to God. The fifth of the five principles of *niyama*, as well as the third of the three components of *kriyā-yoga*.
itihāsa: The two major epics of India: *Mahābhārata* and *Śrīmad Rāmāyaṇa*.

janma: Birth
janma-mṛtyu-cakra: Wheel of birth and death.
japa: Literally, 'recitation'. Continued repetition of *mantras* or the name of the Lord, with devotion and following the prescribed rules; a prayer.
jaya: Mastery, victory, conquest, success.
jihvā: Tongue.
jīvana-mukti: Emancipated life, liberated while living in the physical body.
jīvātman: Individual self, individual soul, which is a part of the Universal Self. Core of being, embodied soul.
jñāna: Knowledge.
jñāna-agni: Fire of knowledge, fire of intelligence.
jñāna-indriya: Senses of perception. The five senses of perception are: ears, nose, tongue, eyes and skin. They are the categories of *Sāṁkhya Darśana* and they correspond to the *viśeṣa* stage of evolution of *prakṛti*.
jñāna-jyoti: Light of knowledge.

jñāna-mārga: Path of knowledge. One of the four *mārga*s or paths for Self-realisation, in which the seeker learns to discriminate between the real and the unreal.

Jyotsnā: The most authoritative commentary on *Haṭhayoga Pradīpikā*, written by Brahmānanda.

kaivalya: Aloneness, emancipation, absolute freedom, the zenith of the spiritual path, in which the yogi lives independently from the vehicles of the Self.

***Kaivalya Pāda*.** The fourth chapter of the *Yoga Sūtras* of Patañjali, describing absolute liberation. It deals with the state of aloneness, in which the yogi realises and experiences the emancipation of the Self from its vehicles or vestures.

kalā: Art, art of living, art of life.

kāla: Time, duration, timing.

kalyāṇa-guṇa: Auspicious character, prosperous quality.

kāma: Enjoyment of life, gratification of desires. The third of the four aims of life or *puruṣārthas*. Lust, sensual desire. One of the six *ṣaḍripus*, or emotional disturbances.

kāraṇa: Cause, factor.

kāraṇa-śarīra: Causal body, primordial body. One of the three *śarīra*s, or bodies. It is the abode of the ever-existing force, and it covers the self as *jīvātman* and *puruṣa* or *ātman*.

kārita: Provoked, induced, caused to be done by someone else. One of the three types of action mentioned by Patañjali in *sūtra* II.34.

karma: Action. Action in general. Concerning the wheel of life and death, they are three types of actions*: saṁcita*, *prārabdha*, and *kriyamāṇa* or *āgāmi*.

karma-indriya: Organs of action. The five organs of action are: arms, legs, mouth, generative and excretory organs. They are the categories of *Sāṁkhya Darśana* and they correspond to the *viśeṣa* stage of evolution of *prakṛti*.

karma-mārga: Path of action. One of the four *mārgas* or paths for Self-realisation, where the seeker acts without looking for the benefits of their actions.

karma-phala: Effect of actions, fruits of actions.

karṇa: Ear.

karuṇā: Compassion to all, compassion towards those who are in sorrow. One of the devices advised by Patañjali in *sūtra* I.33 for the development of a favourable mental disposition.

kārya-śarīra: Gross body, physical body. One of the three *śarīras*, or bodies. It is the house of action, and it covers the organs of action, the senses of perception and the external mind. It is also called *sthūla śarīra*.

kāvya: Poem. In Sanskṛta literature, a poetical composition distinguished for its erudition.

kāya-saṁpat: The wealth of the body.

kleśa: Affliction, defect or suffering that impedes progress on the spiritual path. They are five in number: *avidyā*, *asmitā*, *rāga*, *dveṣa* and *abhiniveśa*.

kleśa-karma: Actions following the pull of any of the afflictions.

kleśa-nivṛtti: Cessation of the afflictions.

kliṣṭa: Painful, commonly applied to the fluctuations of consciousness, which may be *kliṣṭa* or *akliṣṭa*.

kośa: Sheath, layer, cover. Each one of the five sheaths of the human being that envelope the in-dweller, the seer, the *puruṣa* in us. The five sheaths are: *annamaya*, *prāṇamaya*, *manomaya*, *vijñānamaya* and *ānandamaya kośa*s

krama: Structure, method, sequence, progressive classification, sequential order.

Krishna*:* One of the most celebrated deities of the Hindu pantheon. The eighth incarnation of Lord Viṣṇu. He participated in the war related in the *Mahābhārata*, and offered to Arjuna and to the whole of humanity the wonderful gift of the *Bhagavad Gītā*.

kriyā: Action.

kriyamāṇa-karma: Synonymous with *āgāmi-karma*. Third type of *karma* or action, consisting of actions from this life having their effects in the next lives.

kriyā-yoga: Yoga of action. The way of practice indicated by Lord Patañjali in the first *sūtra* of Chapter II of the *Yoga Sūtras*. It is composed of three components: *tapas*, *svādhyāya* and *Īśvara-praṇidhāna*.

kṛkara: One of the five subsidiary energies or *upavāyus*. It does not allow unwanted matter to enter through the nose or throat, making one sneeze or cough it out.

krodha: Anger. One of the *ṣaḍripus* or six emotional disturbances.

kṛṣṇa: Black.

kṛta: Directly done, done by oneself. One of the three types of actions mentioned by Patañjali in *sūtra* II.34.

kṣatriya: Belonging to the martial class. The second of the four *varṇas* or castes, formed by those who defend the country and govern.

kṣetra: Field, ground. In yoga, nature or body.

kṣetra-jña: Fielder, the owner, the master or the knower of the field. In yoga, *puruṣa*, the Self.

kṣipta: Neglected, distracted, lazy, in disarray. One of the five states of consciousness.

kuṁbhaka: Retention.

kuṁbhaka-vṛtti: Steadiness in the fluctuations of energy during retention.

kuṇḍalinī śakti: The energy of nature, the power of *prakṛti*, when it becomes divine.

kūrma: One of the five subsidiary energies, or *upavāyus*. It controls the movement of the eyelids, preventing foreign matter entering, and adjusts the muscles of the eyes according to the intensity of light.

kūrma nāḍī: Nerve in the esoteric body covering the alimentary canal and going from the throat to the genito-excretory organs.

kūṭastha: Immovable, perpetually unchangeable, universal.

kūṭastha-citta: Absolute consciousness, unchangeable. It represents the seer, the soul.

laghiman: The power of becoming weightless, one of the eight *siddhis* (the supernatural powers).

lakṣaṇa: Refinement.

lakṣaṇa-pariṇāma: The second type of change in the process of transformations of consciousness, in which it reaches its refinement.

Lakṣmī: Goddess of wealth, fortune, prosperity and the embodiment of loveliness, beauty, grace and charm. She is the consort and power of Lord Viṣṇu.

laukika-jnāna: Knowledge of the material world, worldly knowledge.

laya: Total absorption, rhythmic silence, dissolution in the object of devotion.

Light on the Yoga Sūtras of Patañjali: A book about the *Yoga Sūtras*, in which this author has translated and commented extensively on all the *sūtras*.

līlā: The entire creation as a play of God, amusement.

liṅga: Phenomenal. The second of the four stages of the evolution of *prakṛti*, or nature. It corresponds to *mahat*.

lobha: Greed, desire, miserliness. One of the six *ṣaḍripus* or emotional disturbances.

mada: Pride. One of the *ṣaḍripus* or six emotional disturbances.

madhyama: Moderate, average. The second of the four types of practitioner, along with *mṛdu*, *adhimatrā* and *tīvra*.

Mahābhārata: One of the two main epics (*itihāsa*) of India, considered the fifth *Veda* and composed by the sage Vyāsa. It narrates the great war between the Pāṇḍavas and Kauravas. The text is a wonderful treatise on human behaviour, with all its qualities, defects, aspirations and limitations.

mahat: Cosmic intelligence. The first evolution of nature, resulting from the union of *puruṣa* and *prakṛti*, and provoking *prakṛti* into action. It is one of the categories of *Sāṁkhya Darśana* and corresponds to the *liṅga* stage of evolution of *prakṛti*.

mahat-ākāśa: Great space, universal sky, macrocosm.

Maheśvara*:* Another name for Lord Śiva, the Lord of dissolution and reproduction.

mahiman**:** The power of increasing one's own size, of waxing in magnitude. One of the eight *siddhis* (the supernatural powers).

maitrī: Friendliness. One of the devices advised by Patañjali in *sūtra* I.33 for the development of a favourable mental disposition.

ma-kāra: Letter 'ṁ'. The third of the three components of the syllable ĀUṀ.

mala: Impurity, toxins, excretions.

mala śoṣana: Filtering or drying out impurities.

maṇas: Mind. One of the three constituents of *citta*, it is the one which is closer to the senses of perception and forms the representation of reality by arranging the information given by the senses. One of the 25 categories of *Sāṁkhya Darśana*, corresponding to the *viśeṣa* state of evolution of *prakṛti.*

maṇgala-āśāsana: Benediction.

maṅgaḷamaya-puruṣa: Full of auspiciousness and prosperity, God.

maṇipūraka-cakra: *Cakra* situated slightly below the navel region. It is the foundation for *prāṇamaya kośa.*

manojaya: Conquest of the mind, mastery over the mind, corresponding to the higher levels of *samādhi.*

manojñāna: Knowledge of the mind.

manolaya. Total absorption of the mind, pensive state, rhythmic silent state of mind. It is a pre-requisite for *manojaya.*

manomaya-kośa: Mental or psychological sheath. The third of the five *kośas.*

manovṛtti-citta: Consciousness of mental modifications.

manovṛtti-karma: Actions following the pull of any mental fluctuations.

manovṛtti-nirodha: Cessation, stillness of the movements of mind. It is the result of the practice of *pratyāhāra.*

mantra: Literally, 'spell'. Sacred prayer, magic formula, incantation.

mantra-japa: Continuous recitation or repetition of a *mantra* or prayer.

mārga: Path for Self-realisation. Traditionally, they are considered to be four: *jñāna*, *karma*, *bhakti* and *yoga*.

mastiṣka: Brain.

mātsarya: Jealousy, malice, hatred. One of the *śaḍripus* or six emotional disturbances.

Menakā: Celestial nymph of extraordinary beauty. Instructed by Indra, she enticed sage Viśvāmitra and broke the continuity of his penance. She succeeded in seducing him at her first attempt, destroyed his power of penance and gave birth to the famous Śakuntalā. After living with her for 10 years, Viśvāmitra realised his mistake, left her and went back to his penance.

meru-daṇḍa: Literally, 'rod of gems, central rod'. Spinal column.

mithyā-jñānam: Illusory knowledge.

moha: Infatuation, delusion. One of the *ṣaḍripus* or six emotional disturbances.

mokṣa: Emancipation, liberation from worldly life. The fourth of the four aims of life or *puruṣārtha*s.

mṛdu: Mild, soft, casual, feeble. The first of the four types of practitioner, along with *madhyama*, *adhimātra* and *tīvra*.

mūḍha: Dull, stupid, ignorant, forgetful. One of the five states of consciousness.

muditā: Joy, gladness. One of the devices advised by Patañjali in *sūtra* I.33 for the development of a favourable mental disposition.

mūlādhāra-cakra: *Cakra* situated between the anus and genitals. It is the base of *annamaya kośa*.

mūla-prakṛti: Root nature, unevolved matter. One of the categories of *Sāṁkhya Darśana*. It corresponds to the *aliṅga* stage of evolution of *prakṛti*.

mūla-puruṣa: Primordial *puruṣa*, God.

mūla-vigraha: Basic idol, the idol permanently installed in a temple. Its replica (*utsava*) is taken out in procession, but *mūla vigraha* never changes its place.

Muṇḍakopaniṣad. One of the main *Upaniṣads* or philosophical texts in *Vedas*, in which the Universal Self and the individual self are represented as two birds abiding in the same tree.

nābhi-cakra: Name used by Patañjali for *maṇipūraka cakra*.
nāda: Sound, vibration.
nāda-anusaṇdhāna: Literally, 'cultivation of the inner sound'. It is considered to be the means of accomplishing *manolaya* (*H. P.*, IV.66).
nāga: One of the five subsidiary energies or *upavāyus*. It relieves pressures of the abdomen by belching.
nava-antarāya: The nine *antarāyas* or obstacles.
nidrā: Sleep, state of void. The fourth of the five *cittavṛttis*, or modifications of consciousness.
nirākāra: Formless, shapeless, beyond dimension.
nirākāra-ātman: Formless self, shapeless soul.
nirānanda-samādhi: Type of *samādhi* mentioned by Vācaspati Miśra, taking the practitioner beyond the experience of bliss.
nirāsmita-samādhi: Litterally, '*samāpatti* beyond bliss'. Type of *samādhi* mentioned by Vācaspati Miśra (I.41) and denied by Vijñāna Bhikṣu, taking the practitioner beyond the experience of the depth of pure being. Synonymous with *nirbīja samādhi*.
nirbīja: Without seed, without support.
nirbīja-samādhi: *Samādhi* without seed, without support. The highest type of *samādhi*, where I-ness is not only absent but has been expunged for ever. It is synonymous with *dharmamegha samādhi*.
nirguṇa: Without qualities or *guṇas*, beyond the expression of *guṇas*.
nirguṇa-upāsaka: (God) without form and attributes.
nirmāṇa-citta: Sprouted, established, steady state of consciousness of being one within oneself. Auspicious state of 'I'. The sixth of the *citta śreṇis* or stages in the transformation of consciousness.

nirmita-citta: Created or fabricated consciousness. Consciousness that follows its inbuilt tendencies. Equivalent to *pariṇāma citta.*
nirodha: Restraint, control, cessation.
nirodha-citta: Restraining consciousness. The second of the *citta śreṇis*, or stages, in the transformation of consciousness.
nirodha-kṣaṇa: Pause between the raising thought waves and the restraining thought waves.
nirodha-pariṇāma: The first of the transformations of consciousness, in which it switches between fluctuations and restraint. Transformation of consciousness towards restraint.
niruddha: Restrained, stable, beyond the feeling of 'I' and 'mine'.
nirvicāra-samādhi: The fourth type of *sabīja samādhi*, taking the practitioner beyond reasoning.
nirvikalpa-samādhi: Name given in *haṭhayoga* texts for *nirbīja samādhi.*
nirvitarka-samādhi: The second type of *sabīja samādhi*, taking the practitioner beyond analysis.
nispatti-mārga: Path of involution, going from the periphery towards the source, involutionary method.
nivṛtti: Becoming one with the body, mind and self.
niyama: Individual ethical discipline, universal moral commandments for the individual. The second of the eight petals of *aṣṭāṅga yoga*, being composed of five principles: *śauca, saṅtoṣa, tapas, svādhyāya* and *Īśvara-praṇidhāna.*

pāda: Leg, chapter.
pakṣa-bhāvanā: Going with the current. It is always associated with *pratipakṣa-bhāvanā.*
pañca: Five.
pañca-bhautika-śarīra: Body made out of the five elements.
pañca-bhūta: Five elements of nature. See *bhūta.*
pañca-kośas: Five sheaths of the body, which correspond to five *bhūtas* (elements). *Annamaya* is connected to *pṛthvī*, *prāṇamaya* to *āp*, *manomaya* to *tejas*, *vijñānamaya* to *vāyu* and *ānandamaya* to *ākāśa.*

pañca-tanmātra: Five subtle qualities of the elements. See *tanmātra.*

pañca-vāyu: Five energies. See *vāyu.*

pāpa-saṁskāra: Unfavourable imprints, unmerited impressions.

parā: Transcending, beyond.

parābhakti: Utter devotion.

parabrahma: Supreme God.

parajñāna: Knowledge beyond the boundaries of discernment.

paramāṇu: Infinitesimally small, atom.

parama-puruṣa: Supreme *puruṣa*, God.

paramātma-darśana: Sight of the Supreme Self, vision of God.

paramātman: Supreme Soul, Supreme Self, God.

paraṁparā: Lineage, link from teacher to pupil, tradition.

pāribhāṣika-prajñā: Awareness that is universally common.

paricaya: Intimate knowledge. The third of the four stages of evolution in practice or *avasthā.*

parigraha: Hoarding, collecting; possessiveness, covetousness.

pariṇāma: Transformation. Transformations are of two types:

1. From *sūtra* III.9 to III.12, Patañjali mentions three phases of transformation or *pariṇāma: nirodha, samādhi* and *ekāgrata.*

2. In *sūtra* III.13, he indicates three types of changes or *pariṇāma* produced in consciousness by these transformations: *dharma, lakṣaṇa* and *avasthā.*

pariṇāma-citta: Alternating consciousness, changeable. It sprouts as *ahaṁkāra* to impersonate the *kūṭastha citta.* It is the individual consciousness, which oscillates and vacillates.

paripakva: Mature, fully ripened.

paripakva-asmitā: Mature individual self.

paripakva-citta: Mature, ripe consciousness. Synonymous with *divya citta.*

paripakva-karma: Mature, ripe action.

Pārvati*:* Literally, 'the daughter of the mountain'. Goddess, consort and power of Lord Śiva, a benevolent form of the Goddess, often depicted as a good wife and a devoted mother.

Pātañjala-Yoga-Sūtras: The *Yoga Sūtras* of Patañjali. See *Yoga Sūtras.*

Patañjali: (Fourth to third century BCE). The compiler and codifier of the science of yoga, author of the *Yoga Sūtras*, the main reference on the subject, to whom we salute and pray before our daily practices.

pati: Husband.

patra: Leaves.

phala: Effects, fruits.

piṇḍāṇḍa: Microcosm, individual. It is always mentioned in reference to *brahmāṇḍa.*

pīṭhikā: Definition, description.

prajnā: Awareness, penetrating discernment, conscious intelligence.

prajñāloka: Light of awareness, light of insight.

prajñāna: Distinctive intelligence accompanied by prudence and wisdom, pinnacle of experienced, illuminative wisdom.

prākāmya: The power of attaining every wish. One of the eight *siddhis* (the supernatural powers).

prakāśa: Light, illumination. A quality of *sattva.*

prakṛti: Nature. According to *Sāṁkhya Darśana*, one of the two foundational categories of the entire existence, along with *puruṣa*. It has four stages in its evolution: *aliṅga*, *liṅga*, *aviśeṣa* and *viśeṣa.*

prakṛti-jaya: Mastery over matter, conquest of nature. It is synonymous with *kaivalya.*

prakṛti-laya: Dissolution in nature, merging in the elements of nature, quietening of the fluctuations of nature or *guṇa*s.

prakṛti-puruṣa-jaya: Conquest or mastery over the entire existence with all its constituents.

prakṛti-śakti: Energy of nature. It is another name for *kuṇḍalinī śakti.*

pramāda: Negligence, carelessness, callousness, heedlessness. One of the nine *antarāyas*, or obstacles.

pramāṇa: Right, valid, correct knowledge or perception. The first of the five *cittavṛtti*s, or modifications of consciousness. It is constituted of *pratyakṣa*, *anumāna* and *āgama*.

prāṇa: Energy, bio-energy, vital energy, breath. In human beings, it takes five different aspects, called *vāyu*s. These are: *prāṇa*, *apāna*, *samāna*, *udāna* and *vyāna*. One of the five *prāṇa*s or *vāyu*s. It is located in the head and the region of the chest, controls the movement of breath and absorbs vital atmospheric energy.

prāṇa-jñāna: Knowledge of energy or breath.

prāṇamaya-kośa: Physiological sheath. The second of the five *kośas*, connected to the element of *āp* (water).

prāṇa-pratiṣṭhā: Literally, 'infusing life'. Ceremony to consecrate an idol before worshipping it; the rites of bringing life into an idol.

prāṇa-staṃbha-vṛtti: Stable state of energy or breath, restraint of breath.

praṇava: Name of the sacred syllable ĀUṀ.

prāṇavṛtti-nirodha: Cessation of the movements of energy or breath.

prāṇāyāma: Control of *prāṇa* or energy, rhythmic control of the breath. The fourth of the eight petals of *aṣṭāṅga yoga*.

prāpti: The power of obtaining everything. One of the eight *siddhi*s (the supernatural powers).

prārabdha-karma: *Karma* or action which manifests in this life as an effect of many previous lives.

pratibhā: Effulgent light, spiritual perception, brilliant conception.

prātibha-jñāna: Knowledge of spiritual perception, divine knowledge.

pratibiṁba: Re-reflection of a mirror that reflects the image received by another mirror. It applies to the re-reflection by the mind or the I-ness of the image of the self reflected on them.

pratikūla: Adverse, contrary, unfavourable.

pratikūla-vṛtti: Unfavourable or adverse modifications of consciousness, moving the practitioner away from progress on the spiritual path, not helpful for spiritual development.

pratipakṣa-bhāvanā: Literally, 'cultivating the opposite'. Going against the current. Counteraction, force against the wrong feelings, tendencies and thoughts.

pratyāhāra: Withdrawal of the senses, mind-control, emancipation of the mind from the domination of the senses. The fifth of the eight petals of *aṣṭāṅga yoga*. It constitutes a bridge to connect the external or *bahiraṅga* and internal or *antaraṅga* practices.

pratyakṣa: Direct knowledge from experience, direct perception. One of the three means of *pramāṇa*, or right knowledge.

pravṛtti-mārga: Path of evolution, going from the source towards the periphery, evolutionary method.

pṛthivī: Earth. The first of the elements of nature, one of the five *bhūtas*.

puṇya: Right action, virtue.

puṇya-saṁskāra: Favourable imprints, merited impressions.

pura: Fort, house, city, dwelling place.

pūraka: Inhalation, in-breath; filling-up.

purāṇa: Legend, belonging to ancient times. A class of Sanskṛta literature, giving a legendary account of ancient times. On account of their importance, they come immediately after the *itihāsa*.

puruṣa: Self, pure witness, ever changeless, eternal soul, God. According to *Sāṁkhya Darśana*, one of the two foundational categories of the entire existence, along with *prakṛti*.

puruṣa-artha: Aims of life. There are four: *dharma*, *artha*, *kāma* and *mokṣa*.

puruṣa-śakti: The power or the energy of the self. It is another name for *ātman*.

puruṣa-svarūpa: Natural condition of the soul or *ātman*, its own natural form.

Puruṣa-Viśeṣa: Supreme Being, name given by Patañjali to God.

pūrva-saṁskāra-vṛtti: All the latent impressions of past experiences.

rāga: Literally, 'that which colours'. Attachment. The third of the five *kleśa*s. A particular musical mode or order of sound of Indian classical music, on which melodies are improvised.

rajas: Vibrancy, activity. One of the three *guṇa*s or modes of nature.

rājasika: Adjective related to *rajas*.

Rāmānujācārya: (Traditionally, 1017–1137 CE). One of the two greatest saint philosophers of Hinduism, founder of one of the principal philosophical doctrines, known as 'qualified monism', in which he holds that the individual self and the Absolute (God) are not completely identical, as in 'monism'. Rather, individual selves and material world are both real and, at the same, modes of the Absolute.

rasa: Taste. One of the five *tanmātra*s or infrastructural qualities of the five elements, corresponding to the element water.

rasātmaka-jñāna: Essence of experienced knowledge that is filtered repeatedly; fragrance relished from experienced awareness.

recaka: Exhalation, out-breath; emptying.

roga: Disease. Classified as *ādhibhautika*, *ādhidaivika* and *ādhyāmika*.

ṛṣi: Sage, patriarch, enriched with extraordinary power and wisdom.

ṛtaṁbharā prajñā: Truth-bearing knowledge, seasoned awareness, matured wisdom, state of direct spiritual perception.

Rudra: Name of Lord Śiva.

rūpa: Form. One of the five *tanmātra*s or infrastructural qualities of the five elements, corresponding to the element fire.

śabda: Sound. One of the five *tanmātra*s, or infrastructural qualities of the five elements, corresponding to the element ether.

sabīja: With seed, with support.

sabīja-samādhi: *Samādhi* with seed or with support. This type of *samādhi* corresponds to *saṁprajñāta samādhi*. It includes seven types: *savitarka, nirvitarka, savicāra, nirvicāra, sānanda, sāsmita* and *virāma pratyaya*.

ṣaḍāṅga-yoga: Yoga of six limbs, six aspects, six petals.

Sadā-śiva: Literally, 'the ever-auspicious one'. One of the aspects and names of Lord Śiva. In some texts, Sadāśiva is the supreme Godhead, absolutely formless, all-pervading, extremely subtle and incomprehensible.

sadguṇa: Righteous and virtuous qualities or *guṇas*.

sādhaka: Seeker, searcher, aspirant, practitioner.

sādhanā: Quest, practice, effort in the path, discipline, pursuit, spiritual endeavour.

sādhanā-krama: Method, structure or sequence of practice, sequential ascension in practice, particularly considered as *tapas, svādhyāya* and *Īśvara praṇidhāna*.

sādhanā-kriyā: The actions of practice, dynamic actions in the quest. They can be classified according to three angles: *sādhanā traya, sādhanā krama* and *sādhanā stambha*.

Sādhana-pāda: Chapter on practice. Second chapter of the *Yoga Sūtras* of Patañjali, dealing with the means of yogic practice. It is a chapter on the ways to uplift the beginner towards the internal practices.

sādhanā-stambha: The pillars of practice, particularly with reference to the eight petals of *aṣṭāṅga yoga* and to surrender to God.

sādhanā-traya: The three tiers of practice – i.e., *bahiraṅga, antaraṅga* and *antarātma sādhanās*.

ṣaḍripu: The six enemies of consciousness, emotional disturbances, the spokes of turmoils, toxins and poisons of the mind. They are: *kāma, krodha, lobha, moha, mada* and *mātsarya*.

saguṇa: With qualities or *guṇas*.

saguṇa-upāsaka: One who prays and meditates on God with form or with attributes.

sahaja: Natural.

sahaja-pravṛtti: Natural, skilful tendencies, *svabhāva-pravṛtti.*

sahasrāra-cakra: The most sacred of the *cakras*, where *prakṛti* and *puruṣa* unite. It is the *cakra* signifying emancipation, represented by a lotus of one thousand petals. It rules over *ātmamaya kośa.*

sahavāsa-guṇa: Qualities of nature developed through good companionship.

sakāra: With form, with shape, with dimension.

sākāra-ātman: Self or soul with form, personified self.

sakarma: Auspicious and good actions.

sākṣātkāra: Realisation, perception, experience.

śakti: Energy, power, vital power, strength.

Śakuntalā: Daughter of sage Viśvāmitra and the celestial nymph Menakā.

sālokya: Literally, 'entering the house of Viṣṇu'. The first of the states of relationship with God, where one feels God. The others are: *sāmīpya*, *sārūpya* and *sāyujya.*

samādhi: Absorption, experience of the grace of the soul, experience of unalloyed bliss. The eighth of the eight petals of *aṣṭāṅga yoga*. It can be *sabīja* or *nirbīja.*

Samādhi Pāda: Chapter on total absorption. First chapter of the *Yoga Sūtras* of Patañjali, dealing with the means to reach *nirbīja samādhi*. It is a chapter for those who are already at a high level of evolution.

samādhi-pariṇāma: The second of the *pariṇāmas* or transformations of consciousness, in which the practitioner begins to lengthen the pause between the fluctuations and restraint. In this state there is a feeling of tranquillity.

samādhi-prajñā: Awareness in reaching the soul, complete absorption with full awareness. The fourth of the four qualities required to reach perfection in practice and mentioned by Patañjali in *sūtra* I.20.

samāhita-citta: Equipoise in consciousness, state of equilibrium, stability, balance and harmony, wholesome state of consciousness.

samāna: One of the five *prāṇas* or *vāyus*. It is located in the stomach and intestines, controls digestion and helps assimilation.

śamana: Pacifying, soothing, appeasing, quenching.

śamana-kriyā: In Indian medicine, the action, process or technique of appeasing, soothing or pacifying.

samāpatti: Consummation, completion, conclusion. Method of transformation, transforming state to assume the original form of the seer, to be one with the Infinite within. Though it is not exactly the same, it is usually equated to *sabīja samādhi*.

samatvam: Equanimity, evenness.

saṁcita: Accumulated (from previous lives).

sāmīpya: Literally, 'proximity to God'. The second of the states of relationship with God, where one lives with closeness or proximity to God. The others are: *sālokya*, *sārūpya* and *sāyujya*.

Sāṁkhya: Literally, 'enumeration' or 'discerning knowledge'. One of the six orthodox systems of Hindu philosophy. It explains the world as constituted by 25 basic categories. The theory of yoga is built up on the base of this philosophy.

saṁprajñāta-citta: Full awareness of consciousness that comes with *sabīja samādhi*.

saṁprajñāta-samādhi: *Samādhi* of self-awareness. It is also called *sabīja samādhi*. This self-awareness is of four types: *vitarka*, *vicāra*, *ānanda* and *asmitā rūpa*.

saṁśaya: Doubt, indecision. One of the nine *antarāyas* or obstacles.

saṁskāra: Imprints, subliminal or latent impressions, imprints from previous lives.

saṁskāra-vṛtti: Modifications due to latent impressions, imprints of previous actions.

saṁskārika: Adjective related to *saṁskāra*.

saṁyama: Integration, integrated whole. Integration or union of the individual soul with the Universal Soul. In *sūtra* III.4, integration or blending of the three last limbs of *aṣṭāṅga yoga*.

saṁyoga: Union, association, conjunction. Conjunction of body, mind and self.

sānanda: Auspicious joy.

sānanda samādhi: One of the four *saṁprajñāta-samādhis* indicated in *sūtra* I.17. The fifth type of *sabīja samādhi*, taking the practitioner to experience a state of bliss.

sañcita-karma: Second type of *karma*, which manifests in this life as an effect of the immediate past life.

saṅkara-citta: Confused consciousness due to admixture of thoughts.

saṅkara-citta-vṛtti: Admixture of thoughts acting against evolution.

saṅkara-vṛtti: Mixed imprints.

sannyāsa-āśrama: The fourth of the four stages of life or *āśrama*s. It is the stage of detachment from the affairs of the world and attachment to the service of God.

Saṅskṛta: Classical language of India, the language of the *Yoga Sūtras*.

śānta: Calm, tranquil, free from passion, meditative.

śānta-citta: Calm, quiet, silent, tranquil consciousness. It is the pause between the wandering and the restraining consciousness, which is increased for a longer period of time. The third of the *citta śreṇi*s, or stages, in the transformation of consciousness.

saṅtoṣa: Contentment. The second of the five principles of *niyama*.

śaraṇāgati: Excellence in devotion, total self-surrender.

Sarasvatī: Goddess of knowledge, wisdom, speech, poetry, music, all sciences and crafts and learning, consort of Lord Brahmā.

śarīra: Body. According to the anatomy of yoga, the human being is a compound of three bodies: gross, subtle and causal, known as *kārya* (or *sthūla*) *śarīra*, *sūkṣma śarīra* and *kāraṇa śarīra*.

śarīra-jaya: Mastery over the body.

śarīra-jñāna: Knowledge of the body.

śarīra-śarīri-bhāva: The relation subsisting between body and soul.

śarīrin: The holder of the body, the seer, *puruṣa*, soul.

sārūpya: Literally, 'having the form of God'. The third of the states of relationship with God, where God is considered as free from the powers of yoga. The others are: *sālokya*, *sāmīpya* and *sāyujya*.

sārva-bhauma: Universal, of the entire universe.

sāsmitā: Auspicious and pure individual self or *asmitā*.

sāsmita-citta: Auspicious and pure state of consciousness or the individual self, synonymous with *nirmāṇa citta*.

sāsmita-samādhi: (*sāsmita* = auspicious self). One of the four *saṁprajñāta-samādhi*s indicated in *sūtra* I.17, mentioned by Vācaspati Miśra. The sixth type of *sabīja-samādhi*, in which the intellect itself becomes the object of concentration, taking the practitioner to experience the depth of being, which is closer to 'I'-consciousness.

Ṣaṭ-Cakra-Nirupaṇa: Literally, 'the description of the six vital centres'. A medieval text on *cakra*s and other components of the causal body, composed in 55 verses by Pūrṇānanda.

sat-cid-ānanda: State of eternal truth, knowledge and bliss.

sat-cit: Knowledge of the eternal truth, pure existence of the soul.

satī: Wife.

sattva: Luminosity, illumination. One of the three *guṇa*s, or qualities of nature.

sāttvika: Adjective related to *sattva*.

satya: Truthfulness. The second of the principles of *yama*.

satyam: True. One of the attributes of God, along with *śivam* and *sundaram*.

śauca: Cleanliness, purity. The first of the five principles of *niyama*.

savicāra-samādhi: (*savicāra* = right reflection). The second of the four *saṁprajñāta-samādhi*s indicated in *sūtra* I.17, and mentioned by Vācaspathi Miśra. The third type of *sabīja samādhi*, taking the practitioner towards reasoning.

savikalpa-samādhi: Name given to *sabīja-samādhi* by Rāmānuja in his *Vedānta-sūtra*.

savitarka-samādhi: (*savitarka* = right analysis). The first of four *saṁprajñāta-samādhi*s indicated in *sūtra* I.17, mentioned by Vācaspati Miśra. The first type of *sabīja-samādhi*, taking the practitioner towards analysis.

sāyujya: Literally, 'united to God'. The fourth of the states of relationship with God, where one mingles with God. The first three are: *sālokya*, *sāmīpya* and *sārūpya*.

siddhi: Supernatural powers, coming to the practitioner as a result of mastery over the five elements (*bhūta*) and the five subtle qualities of the elements (*tanmātra*). *See also aṣṭa siddhi.*

śīlatā: Virtue, virtuous life, virtuosity.

Śiva*:* Literally, 'the auspicious one'. The Destroyer, the remover of evil and ignorance. One of the three main deities of the Hindu pantheon, along with Brahmā and Viṣṇu.

śivam: Auspicious, pure. One of the attributes of God, along with *satyam* and *sundaram*.

Śiva-Saṁhitā: One of the most authoritative medieval texts on yoga, along with *Haṭhayoga Pradīpikā*.

śloka: Verse.

smṛti: Memory. The fifth of the five *cittavṛttis*, or modifications of consciousness. Recollection and permanent imprints. The third of the four qualities mentioned by Patañjali in *sūtra* I.20 and required to reach perfection in practice.

śobhana: Auspicious presentation, brilliance.

śodhana: Purificatory, cleansing action.

śoṣana: Desiccation and absorption, drying out.

śoṣaṇa krama: Sequential order of absorption.

sparśa: Touch. One of the five *tanmātra*s, or infrastructural qualities of the five elements of nature, corresponding to the element air.

śraddhā: Faith, ripened revelation through experience, confidence, reverence. The first of the four qualities mentioned by Patañjali in *sūtra* I.20 and required to reach perfection in practice.

śreṇi: Range, classification, stage. It is mainly used for the stages in the transformation of consciousness or *citta śreṇi*.

Śrīmad-Rāmāyaṇa or ***Rāmāyaṇa:*** One of the two main epics (*itihāsa*) of India, composed by the sage Vālmīki, and treating the relationship between Rāma and Sītā, the abduction of Sītā by Rāvana, and her discovery and liberation by Rāma, helped by Hanuman. The text can be read as a relationship between the Universal Soul and the individual self.

sṛṣṭi-kartā: Creator of the universe, God.

sṛṣṭi-krama: Structure of the universe.

staṃbha-vṛtti: State of stability, steadiness.

sthira: Firm, steady and stable.

sthiratā: Firmness, steadiness and stability.

sthiti: Position, remaining in a position. Inert state, dormancy.

sthūla: Gross.

sthūla-śarīra: Gross body, physical body. See *kārya śarīra*.

styāna: Mental laziness, sluggishness, inertia, lack of interest. One of the nine *antarāyas* or obstacles.

śuddhi: Purification, rightness, sanctity, cleanliness.

śūdra: Labouring class. The fourth of the four *varṇas*, or castes, formed by those who provide service and manpower for the growth of society.

sujñāna: Acquisition of auspicious spiritual knowledge, matured knowledge.

sukarma: Good actions with auspicious motivations.

sukha: Pleasure, happiness.

sukham: Pleasant, contented, with poise of mind, comfortable.

sukhatā: Delightfulness, perfect balance.

śukla: White

sūkṣma: Subtle.

sūkṣma-śarīra: Subtle body. One of the three *śarīras*, or bodies. It is the house of thinking and it covers the *prāṇa*, mind, I-maker, intelligence, consciousness and conscience.

sundaram: Beautiful. One of the three attributes of God, along with *satyam* and *śivam*.

śūnya: Void, emptiness.
śūnya-āśūnya: Void yet non-void.
śūnya-avasthā: State of void, passive emptiness.
sūrya: Sun.
sūtra: Aphorism, concise sentence. Etymologically, thread, which gives consistency and sense to the pearls woven together in a necklace. The *Yoga Sūtras* of Patañjali contains 196 *sūtras*.
sva: Self, considered as individual self or as Universal Self. *Prakṛti* or nature, as related to *svāmi* or the seer.
svabhāva: Natural state, inherent natural disposition.
svabhāva-pravṛtti: See *sahaja pravṛtti*.
svabuddhi: One's own intelligence. Nature's intelligence.
svādhiṣṭhāna-cakra: *Cakra* situated between the genitals and hypogastric plexus. It rules over *annamaya* and *prāṇamaya kośas*.
svādhyāya: Study of the self. When it is considered as individual self, it is the study of oneself, the observation of ourselves. When considered as universal, it is the study of the Supreme Self – i.e., the study of sacred scriptures. It is the fourth of the five principles of *niyama*, as well as the second of the three components of *kriyā-yoga*.
svāmi: *Puruṣa* or the seer, as related to *sva* or nature. The inner Lord.
svāmi-buddhi: Intelligence of the seer, as related to *svabuddhi* or intelligence of nature.
svarūpa: One's own form, essential form, natural state.
svarūpa-anukāra: Staying in one's own position, remaining in one's own nature, following one's natural state.
svarūpa-avasthā: State of being established in its own nature, in the Self.
svarūpa-pratiṣṭhā: Establishment in one's own nature.
svarūpa-śūnya: Void of one's own form.
svarūpa-upalabdhi: Recognition of one's own status or stature, obtaining one's own natural state.
svastha: Self-abiding, being in the self.

tāḍāsana: Basic standing position, in which one stands firm from the bottom of the feet, which are placed together, with legs straight and arms by the side of the trunk.

tamas: Inertia, dormancy. One of the three *guṇa*s or qualities of nature.

tāmasika: Adjective related to *tamas*.

tanmātra: Subtle or infrastructural qualities of the five elements, their subtle counterparts. They are categories of *Sāṁkhya Darśana* and they correspond to the *aviśeṣa* stage of evolution of *prakṛti*. The five *tanmātra*s are: *śabda*, *sparśa*, *rūpa*, *rasa* and *gandha*.

tanmātra-jaya: Mastery over the subtle qualities of the elements.

tapaḥ, tapas: Ascetic practice, zeal, austerity, penance, determination, self-discipline. The third of the five principles of *niyama*, as well as the first of the three components of *kriyā yoga*.

tattva: Category. Each one of the 25 principles of the *Sāṁkhya Darśana* philosophy.

tej, tejas: Fire, light. The third of the elements of nature, one of the five *bhūta*s.

tej-ahaṁkāra: Principle of individuality related to the mind.

tejomaya: Related to the quality of fire.

tīvra/tīvra-saṁvegin: Supremely intense, intensely intense, vehement. The fourth of the four types of practitioner, along with *mṛdu*, *madhyama* and *adhimātra*.

toyam: Water.

tridaṇḍa: Three rods, three pillars.

triguṇa: Three qualities of nature or *guṇa*s.

trikaraṇa-śuddhi: Cleanliness, rightness or purification in body, speech and mind.

trimūrti: The three main Gods of the Hindu pantheon: Brahmā, Viṣṇu, and Śiva or Maheśvara.

tri-śārīrika: Related to the three bodies or *śarīra*.

tūriya: The fourth state of consciousness, beyond the wakeful, dreamy or sleepy states.

tvak: Skin.

udāna: One of the five *prāṇa*s or *vāyu*s. It is located in the region of the throat and chest, and controls the intake of air and food as well as the functioning of the vocal cords.

udita: Manifesting.

ukāra: Letter 'u'. The second of the three components of the syllable ĀUṀ.

Upaniṣad: Philosophical and meditative texts, attached to the *Vedas*, conveying the mystical and esoteric doctrines of *Vedānta*, one of the classical Hindu philosophies.

upavāyu: Subsidiary energies, completing the functions of the five *vāyus*. They are also five: *nāga*, *kūrma*, *kṛkara*, *devadatta* and *dhanaṁjaya*.

upekṣā: Indifference, neutrality towards those who are full of vices. One of the devices advised by Patañjali in *sūtra* I.33 for the development of a favourable mental disposition.

utsava-vigraha: Replica of *mūla vigraha*, or the basic idol of a temple, which is taken out in procession on festival days.

vaidika jnāna: Spiritual knowledge, knowledge related to the *Vedas*.

vaikārika-ahaṁkāra: Principle of individuality related to the organs of action and senses of perception.

vairāgya: Renunciation, detachment. Along with *abhyāsa*, they are the first means advised by Patañjali to restrain the fluctuations of consciousness.

vaiśya: Merchant class. The third of the four *varṇa*s, or castes, formed by those who look after the economic growth and prosperity of the society.

vānaprastha-āśrama: The third of the four stages of life or *āśrama*s. It is the stage of learning to detach from worldly matters and living as a guide for one's children and surrounding youngsters.

varṇa: Community, social division, caste or class. They were established according to the division of labour. The four *varnas* are: *brāhmaṇa*, *kṣatriya*, *vaiśya* and *śūdra*. Nowadays, this division of castes is ceasing to exist.

vāsanā: Desires, the impression of anything remaining unconsciously in the mind that may stir up desires.

vāsanāmaya-kośa: Sheath of desires, the house of desires.

vaśitva: The power of subjugation over anyone or anything. One of the eight *siddhi*s.

vāyu: Air. The fourth of the elements of nature, one of the five *bhūtas*. Generic name given to the five energies or *prāṇas* in the human being.

Veda: Literally, 'knowledge'. The most sacred texts of Hinduism, the source of Hindu religion, having been revealed to humanity by Gods. The main *Veda*s are four in number.

vedānta: Consummation or culmination of all knowledge. Etymologically, the end or culmination of the *Veda*s. One of the six orthodox systems of Hindu philosophy, discussing the Ultimate Principle and Final Reality of existence. It is based on the *Upaniṣads*.

vedāntika: Adjective related to *vedānta*.

Vibhūti-Pāda: Chapter on the wealth of yoga. It is the third chapter of the *Yoga Sūtras* of Patañjali, dealing with the accomplishments or effects of practice.

vicāra: Synthesis, reflection.

vicāra-jñāna: Knowledge of the discriminative intellect.

vidyā: Acquired knowledge, knowledge earned through intellect, science or art.

vidyā-śakti: Power of the intellect.

vijñāna: Scientific enquiry, investigation through experiment, specialised knowledge attained by investigation and discrimination.

vijñāna-śāstra: Instruction, treatise on a subject with scientific experimentation, scientific exploration.

vijñānamaya: Intellectual, related to the objective intelligence.

vijñānamaya-kośa: Intellectual sheath. The fourth of the five *kośas*. It belongs to the subtle body connected to the element of *vāyu* (air).

vikalpa: Misconception, imaginative or fanciful knowledge, wrong conception, imagination, delusion. The third of the five *cittavṛttis*, or modifications of consciousness.

vikarma: Actions with pleasant motivations.

vikṣipta: Oscillating, agitated, scattered. One of the five states of consciousness.

vimala: Stainless.

viniyoga: Application of knowledge, utilisation.

vipāka: Result, fruition, fructification, ripening process; cooked.

viparyaya: Misperception, perverse or illusory knowledge, wrong perception, illusion. The second of the five *cittavṛttis* or modifications of consciousness.

virāma-pratyaya: The seventh type of *sabīja samādhi*, where there is a complete suspension of movements of consciousness. It is a 'spiritual desert', where emptiness emerges. By remaining firm in the effort and full of faith in this empty state, the practitioner may reach the ultimate stage (*nirbīja* or *dharmamegha-samādhi*).

vīrya: Vigour, potency, valour, courage; physical, moral, mental power and spiritual strength. The second of the four qualities mentioned by Patañjali in *sūtra* I.20 and required to reach perfection in practice.

viśeṣa: Distinguishable. The fourth of the four stages of the evolution of *prakṛti* or nature. It corresponds to the body, with the five *karmendriyas* and the five *jñānendriyas*, the mind and the five *bhūtas*.

Viṣṇu*:* Literally, 'the all-pervader'. The Protector, the Organiser. One of the three main Gods of the Hindu pantheon, along with Brahmā and Śiva.

viśuddhi-cakra: *Cakra* situated in the pit of the throat, at the base of the neck. It rules over the intellectual sheath or *vijñānamaya-kośa*.

viśva-caitanya-śakti / viśva-caitanya-vāyu: Universal source of life energy, cosmic energy, the power of God. Cosmic breath.

viśva-cetana-śakti / viśva-cetana-puruṣa / viśva-puruṣa: Supreme Being, Supreme Soul, Universal Self, God.

vitarka: Analysis, analytical thinking.

vivekaja-jñāna: Exalted knowledge, exalted intelligence, shining wisdom.

viveka-khyāti: Crown of wisdom, glory of knowledge, discernment, real insight that is beyond intuition.

vṛtti: Fluctuations, modifications, waves, movements.

vṛtti-nirodha: Restraint; controlling fluctuations or movements (of consciousness).

vyādhi: Physical or psycho-physiological disease. One of the nine *antarāya*s or obstacles.

vyakta: Manifest.

vyāna: One of the five *prāṇa*s or *vāyu*s. It controls the entire body and the heart, moves through the blood and nerves, and distributes energy all over the body.

vyavasāyātmikā buddhi: Determined, resolute, decided intelligence.

vyutthāna citta: Wandering, fluctuating, raising consciousness. Its tendency is outgoing. The first of the *citta śreṇi*s, or stages, in the transformation of consciousness.

yama: 1. Social ethical disciplines, universal moral commandments for the healthy functioning of society. The first of the eight petals of *aṣṭāṅga yoga*, being composed of five principles: *ahiṁsā*, *satya*, *asteya*, *brahmacarya* and *aparigraha*. 2. God of death.

yaugika: Adjective related to yoga, i.e., yogic.

yoga: Union. One of the six orthodox systems of Hindu philosophy, searching; involves restraining the movements of consciousness, to unite the individual self with the Universal Soul.

yoga-mārga: The path of union. One of the four *mārga*s or paths for Self-realisation, where the practitioner reaches the zenith by controlling the activities of consciousness.
yoga-māyā: Power of God.
yoga-phala: Fruits of yoga, effects of yoga.
yoga-sādhanā: Practice of yoga, discipline of yoga.
yoga-śālā: Hall for yoga, a place for practising yoga.
yoga-sthāna: Place to experience yoga.
Yoga-Sūtras: Foundational text on yoga, composed in *sūtra* form by the sage Patañjali, consisting of 196 aphorisms, or *sūtra*s, conveying the entire philosophy and methodology of yoga practice. It is the base, source and subject of this very book.
Yoga-Vāsiṣṭha: A classical text on yoga narrated by Sage Vasiṣṭha to Śrī Rāma, the seventh incarnation of Lord Viṣṇu.
yoga-vidyā: Knowledge of yoga, the science of yoga.
yogin: One who lives in yoga.
yukti: Skilfulness, skill to act.

Appendix I

Patañjali's *Yoga Sūtras*

Two versions of each sūtra are provided: the first gives the combined words as they are pronounced in Sanskrit, the second shows their break-up to make it simpler for the new reader to pronounce and understand.

॥ समाधिपादः ॥
SAMĀDHI-PĀDA
(Chapter on Total Absorption)

अथ योगानुशासनम् ॥१॥
I.1 *atha yogānuśāsanam //*
I.1 *atha yoga-anuśāsanam //*

योगश्चित्तवृत्तिनिरोधः ॥२॥
I.2 *yogaścittaḥvṛttinirodhaḥ //*
I.2 *yogaḥ citta-vṛtti-nirodhaḥ //*

तदा द्रष्टुः स्वरूपेऽवस्थानम् ॥३॥
I.3 *tadā draṣṭuḥ svarūpe 'vasthānam //*
I.3 *tadā draṣṭuḥ svarūpe avasthānam //*

वृत्तिसारूप्यमितरत्र ॥४॥
I.4 *vṛttisārūpyamitaratra //*
I.4 *vṛtti-sārūpyam itaratra //*

वृत्तयः पञ्चतय्यः क्लिष्टाक्लिष्टाः ॥५॥

I.5 *vṛttayaḥ pañcatayyaḥ kliṣṭakliṣṭāḥ* //

I.5 *vṛttayaḥ pañcatayyaḥ kliṣṭa-akliṣṭāḥ* //

प्रमाणविपर्ययविकल्पनिद्रास्मृतयः ॥६॥

I.6 *pramāṇaviparyayavikalpanidrāsmṛtayaḥ* //

I.6 *pramāṇa-viparyaya-vikalpa-nidrā-smṛtayaḥ* //

प्रत्यक्षानुमानागमाः प्रमाणानि ॥७॥

I.7 *pratyakṣānumānāgamāḥ pramāṇāni* //

I.7 *pratyakṣa-anumāna-āgamāḥ pramāṇāni* //

विपर्ययो मिथ्याज्ञानमतद्रूपप्रतिष्ठम् ॥८॥

I.8 *viparyayo mithyājñānamatadrūpapratiṣṭham* //

I.8 *viparyayaḥ mithyā-jñānam atad-rūpa pratiṣṭham* //

शब्दज्ञानानुपाती वस्तुशून्यो विकल्पः ॥९॥

I.9 *śabdajñānānupātī vastuśūnyo vikalpaḥ* //

I.9 *śabda-jñāna-anupātī vastu-śūnyaḥ vikalpaḥ* //

अभावप्रत्ययालम्बना वृत्तिर्निद्रा ॥१०॥

I.10 *abhāvapratyayālambanā vṛttirnidrā* //

I.10 *abhāva-pratyaya-ālambanā vṛttiḥ nidrā* //

अनुभूतविषयासंप्रमोषः स्मृतिः ॥११॥

I.11 *anubhūtaviṣayāsaṁpramoṣaḥ smṛtiḥ* //

I.11 *anubhūta-viṣaya-asaṁpramoṣaḥ smṛtiḥ* //

अभ्यासवैराग्याभ्यां तन्निरोधः ॥१२॥

I.12 *abhyāsavairāgyābhyāṁ tannirodhaḥ* //

I.12 *abhyāsa-vairāgyābhyāṁ tad-nirodhaḥ* //

तत्र स्थितौ यत्नोऽभ्यासः ॥१३॥

I.13 *tatra sthitau yatnobhyāsaḥ* //

I.13 *tatra sthitau yatnaḥ abhyāsaḥ* //

स तु दीर्घकालनैरन्तर्यसत्कारासेवितो दृढभूमिः ॥१४॥

I.14 *sa tu dīrghakālanairantaryasatkārāsevitodṛḍhabhūmiḥ* //

I.14 *sa tu dīrgha-kāla-nairantarya-satkāra-āsevitaḥ dṛḍha-bhūmiḥ* //

दृष्टानुश्रविकविषयवितृष्णस्य वशीकारसंज्ञा वैराग्यम् ॥१५॥

I.15 *dṛṣṭānuśravikaviṣayavitṛṣṇasya vaśīkārasaṁjñā vairāgyam //*

I.15 *dṛṣṭa-ānuśravika-viṣaya-vitṛṣṇasya vaśīkārasaṁjñā-*
-vairāgyam //

तत्परं पुरुषख्यातेर्गुणवैतृष्ण्यम् ॥१६॥

I.16 *tatparaṁ puruṣakhyāterguṇavaitṛṣṇyam //*

I.16 *tat-paraṁ puruṣa-khyāteḥ guṇa-vaitṛṣṇyam //*

वितर्कविचारानन्दास्मितारूपानुगमात्संप्रज्ञातः ॥१७॥

I.17 *vitarkavicārānandāsmitārūpānugamātsaṁprajñātaḥ //*

I.17 *vitarka-vicāra-ānanda-asmitārūpa-anugamāt saṁpra-jñātaḥ //*

विरामप्रत्ययाभ्यासपूर्वः संस्कारशेषोऽन्यः ॥१८॥

I.18 *virāmapratyayābhyāsapūrvaḥ saṁskāraśeṣonyaḥ //*

I.18 *virāma-pratyaya-abhyāsa-pūrvaḥ saṁskāra-śeṣaḥ anyaḥ //*

भवप्रत्ययो विदेहप्रकृतिलयानाम् ॥१९॥

I.19 *bhavapratyayo videhaprakṛtilayānām //*

I.19 *bhava-pratyayaḥ videha-prakṛti-layānām //*

श्रद्धावीर्यस्मृतिसमाधिप्रज्ञापूर्वक इतरेषाम् ॥२०॥

I.20 *śraddhāvīryasmṛtisamādhiprajñāpūrvaka itareṣām*

I.20 *śraddhā-vīrya-smṛti-samādhi-prajñā-pūrvakaḥ itareṣām*

तीव्रसंवेगानामासन्नः ॥२१॥

I.21 *tīvrasaṁvegānāmāsannaḥ //*

I.21 *tīvra-saṁvegānām āsannaḥ //*

मृदुमध्याधिमात्रत्वात् ततोऽपि विशेषः ॥२२॥

I.22 *mṛdumadhyādhimātratvāt tato'pi viśeṣaḥ //*

I.22 *mṛdu-madhya-adhimātratvāt tataḥ api viśeṣaḥ //*

ईश्वरप्रणिधानाद्वा ॥२३॥

I.23 *Īśvarapraṇidhānādvā //*

I.23 *Īśvara-praṇidhānāt vā //*

क्लेशकर्मविपाकाशयैरपरामृष्टः पुरुषविशेष ईश्वरः ॥२४॥

I.24 *kleśakarmavipākāśayairaparāmṛṣṭaḥ puruṣaviśeṣa Īśvaraḥ //*

I.24 *kleśa-karma-vipāka-āśayaiḥ aparāmṛṣṭaḥ puruṣa-viśeṣaḥ Īśvaraḥ //*

तत्र निरतिशयं सर्वज्ञबीजम् ॥२५॥

I.25 *tatra niratiśayaṁ sarvajñabījam //*

I.25 *tatra niratiśayaṁ sarvajña-bījam //*

स एष पूर्वेषामपि गुरुः कालेनानवच्छेदात् ॥२६॥

I.26 *sa eṣa pūrveṣāmapi guruḥ kālenānavacchedāt //*

I.26 *sa eṣa pūrveṣām api guruḥ kālena anavacchedāt //*

तस्य वाचकः प्रणवः ॥२७॥

I.27 *tasya vācakaḥ praṇavaḥ //*

I.27 *tasya vācakaḥ praṇavaḥ //*

तज्जपस्तदर्थभावनम् ॥२८॥

I.28 *tajjapastadarthabhāvanam //*

I.28 *taj-japaḥ tad-artha-bhāvanam //*

ततः प्रत्यक्चेतनाधिगमोऽप्यन्तरायाभावश्च ॥२९॥

I.29 *tataḥ pratyakcetanādhigamopyantarāyābhāvaśca //*

I.29 *tataḥ pratyak-cetana adhigamaḥ api antarāya-abhāvaḥ ca //*

व्याधिस्त्यानसंशयप्रमादालस्याविरतिभ्रान्तिदर्शनालब्ध-भूमिकत्वानवस्थितत्वानि चित्तविक्षेपास्तेऽन्तरायाः ॥३०॥

I.30 *vyādhistyānasaṁśayapramādālasyāviratibhrāntidarśanālabdh abhūmikatvānavasthitatvāni cittavikṣepāstentarāyāḥ //*

I.30 *vyādhi-styāna-saṁśaya-pramāda-ālasya-avirati-bhrānti- -darśana-alabdha-bhūmikatva-anavasthitatvāni citta-vikṣepāḥ te antarāyāḥ //*

दुःखदौर्मनस्याङ्गमेजयत्वश्वासप्रश्वासा विक्षेपसहभुवः ॥३१॥

I.31 *duḥkhadaurmanasyāṅgamejayatvaśvāsapraśvāsā vikṣepasahabhuvaḥ //*

I.31 *duḥkha-daurmanasya-aṅgame-jayatva-śvāsa-praśvāsāḥ vikṣepa-sahabhuvaḥ //*

तत्प्रतिषेधार्थमेकतत्त्वाभ्यासः ॥३२॥

I.32 *tatpratiṣedhārthamekatattvābhyāsaḥ //*

I.32 *tat-pratiṣedha-artham eka-tattva-abhyāsaḥ //*

मैत्रीकरुणामुदितोपेक्षाणां सुखदुःखपुण्यापुण्यविषयाणां भावनातश्चित्तप्रसादनम् ॥३३॥

I.33 *maitrīkaruṇāmuditopekṣāṇāṁ sukhaduḥkhapuṇyāpuṇyaviṣayāṇāṁ bhāvanātaścittaprasādanam //*

I.33 *maitrī-karuṇā-muditā-upēkṣāṇāṁ sukha-duḥkha-puṇya--apuṇya-viṣayāṇāṁ bhāva-nātaḥ-citta-prasādanam //*

प्रच्छर्दनविधारणाभ्यां वा प्राणस्य ॥३४॥

I.34 *pracchardanavidhāraṇābhyāṁ vā prāṇasya //*

I.34 *pracchardana-vidhāraṇābhyāṁ vā prāṇasya //*

विषयवती वा प्रवृत्तिरुत्पन्ना मनसः स्थितिनिबन्धनी ॥३५॥

I.35 *viṣayavatī vā pravṛttirutpannā manasaḥ sthitinibandhanī //*

I.35 *viṣayavatī vā pravṛttiḥ utpannā manasaḥ sthiti-nibandhanī //*

विशोका वा ज्योतिष्मती ॥३६॥

I.36 *viśokā vā jyotiṣmatī //*

I.36 *viśokā vā jyotiṣmatī //*

वीतरागविषयं वा चित्तम् ॥३७॥

I.37 *vītarāgaviṣayaṁ vā cittam //*

I.37 *vīta-rāga-viṣayaṁ vā cittam //*

स्वप्ननिद्राज्ञानालम्बनं वा ॥३८॥

I.38 *svapnanidrājñānālambanaṁ vā //*

I.38 *svapna-nidrā-jñāna-ālambanaṁ vā //*

यथाभिमतध्यानाद्वा ॥३९॥

I.39 *yathābhimatadhyānādvā //*

I.39 *yathā-abhimata-dhyānāt vā //*

परमाणुपरममहत्त्वान्तोऽस्य वशीकारः ॥४०॥

I.40 *paramāṇuparamamahattvāntosya vaśīkāraḥ //*

I.40 *parama-aṇu-parama-mahattva-antaḥ asya vaśīkāraḥ //*

क्षीणवृत्तेरभिजातस्येव मणेर्ग्रहीतृग्रहणग्राह्येषु तत्स्थतदञ्जनता समापत्तिः ॥४१॥

I.41 *kṣīṇavṛtterabhijātasyeva maṇergrahītṛgrahaṇagrāhyeṣu tatsthatadañjanatā samāpattiḥ //*

I.41 *kṣīṇa-vṛtteḥ abhijātasya iva maṇeḥ grahītṛ-grahaṇa-grāhyeṣu tat-stha-tad-añjanatā samāpattiḥ //*

तत्र शब्दार्थज्ञानविकल्पैः संकीर्णा सवितर्का समापत्तिः ॥४२॥

I.42 *tatra śabdārthajñānavikalpaiḥ saṅkīrṇā savitarkā samāpattiḥ //*

I.42 *tatra śabda-artha-jñāna-vikalpaiḥ saṅkīrṇā savitarkā samāpattiḥ //*

स्मृतिपरिशुध्दौ स्वरूपशून्येवार्थमात्रनिर्भासा निर्वितर्का ॥४३॥

I.43 *smṛtipariśuddhau svarūpaśūnyevārthamātranirbhāsā nirvitarkā //*

I.43 *smṛti-pariśuddhau sva-rūpa-śūnya iva arthamātra-nirbhāsā nirvitarkā //*

एतयैव सविचारा निर्विचारा च सूक्ष्मविषया व्याख्याता ॥४४॥

I.44 *etayaiva savicārā nirvicārā ca sūkṣmaviṣayā vyākhyātā //*

I.44 *etayā eva savicārā nirvicārā ca sūkṣma-viṣayā vyākhyātā //*

सूक्ष्मविषयत्वं चालिङ्गपर्यवसानम् ॥४५॥

I.45 *sūkṣmaviṣayatvaṁ cāliṅgaparyavasānam //*

I.45 *sūkṣma-viṣayatvaṁ ca aliṅga-paryavasānam //*

ता एव सबीजः समाधिः ॥४६॥

I.46 *tā eva sabījaḥ samādhiḥ //*

I.46 *tā eva sabījaḥ samādhiḥ //*

निर्विचारवैशारद्येऽध्यात्मप्रसादः ॥४७॥

I.47 *nirvicāravaiśāradyedhyātmaprasādaḥ //*

I.47 *nirvicāra-vaiśāradye adhyātma-prasādaḥ //*

ऋतंभरा तत्र प्रज्ञा ॥४८॥

I.48 *ṛtaṁbharā tatra prajñā //*

I.48 *ṛtaṁbharā tatra prajñā //*

श्रुतानुमानप्रज्ञाभ्यामन्यविषया विशेषार्थत्वात् ॥४९॥

I.49 *śrutānumānaprajñābhyāmanyaviṣayā viśeṣārthatvāt //*

I.49 *śruta-anumāna-prajñābhyām anya-viṣayā viśeṣa-arthatvāt //*

तज्जः संस्कारोऽन्यसंस्कारप्रतिबन्धी ॥५०॥

I.50 *tajjaḥ saṁskāro 'nyasaṁskārapratibandhī //*

I.50 *taj-jaḥ saṁskāraḥ anya-saṁskāra-pratibandhī //*

तस्यापि निरोधे सर्वनिरोधान्निर्बीजः समाधिः ॥५१॥

I.51 *tasyāpi nirodhe sarvanirodhānnirbījaḥ samādhiḥ //*

I.51 *tasya āpi nirodhe sarva-nirodhāt nirbījaḥ samādhiḥ //*

इति समाधि पादः॥

// iti samādhi pādaḥ //

॥ साधन पादः ॥
SĀDHANA PĀDA
(Chapter on Practice)

तपःस्वाध्यायेश्वरप्रणिधानानि क्रियायोगः ॥१॥

II.1 *tapaḥsvādhyāyeśvarapraṇidhānāni kriyāyogaḥ //*

II.1 *tapaḥ-svādhyāya-Īśvara-praṇidhānāni kriyā-yogaḥ //*

समाधिभावनार्थः क्लेशतनूकरणार्थश्च ॥२॥

II.2 *samādhibhāvanārthaḥ kleśatanūkaraṇārthaśca //*

II.2 *samādhi-bhāvana-arthaḥ kleśa-tanū-karaṇa-arthaḥ ca //*

अविद्याऽस्मितारागद्वेषाभिनिवेशाः क्लेशाः ॥३॥

II.3 *avidyāsmitārāgadveṣābhiniveśāḥ kleśāḥ //*

II.3 *avidyā-asmitā-rāga-dveṣa-abhiniveśāḥ kleśāḥ //*

अविद्या क्षेत्रमुत्तरेषां प्रसुप्ततनुविच्छिन्नोदाराणाम् ॥४॥

II.4 *avidyā kṣetramuttareṣāṁ prasuptatanuvicchinnodārāṇām //*

II.4 *avidyā kṣetram uttareṣāṁ prasupta-tanu-vicchinna--udārāṇām //*

अनित्याशुचिदुःखानात्मसु नित्यशुचिसुखात्मख्यातिरविद्या ॥५॥

II.5 *anityāśuciduḥkhānātmasu nityaśucisukhātmakhyātiravidyā //*

II.5 *anitya-aśuci-duḥkha-anātmasu nitya-śuci-sukha-ātma-khyātiḥ avidyā //*

दृग्दर्शनशक्त्योरेकात्मतेवास्मिता ॥६॥

II.6 *dṛgdarśanaśaktyorekātmatevāsmitā //*

II.6 *dṛg-darśana-śaktyoḥ eka-ātmatā iva asmitā //*

सुखानुशयी रागः ॥७॥

II.7 *sukhānuśayī rāgaḥ //*

II.7 *sukha-anuśayī rāgaḥ //*

दुःखानुशयी द्वेषः ॥८॥

II.8 *duḥkhānuśayī dveṣaḥ //*

II.8 *duḥkha-anuśayī dveṣaḥ //*

स्वरसवाही विदुषोऽपि तथारूढोऽभिनिवेशः ॥९॥

II.9 *svarasavāhī viduṣo'pi tathārūḍhobhiniveśaḥ //*

II.9 *svarasa-vāhī viduṣaḥ api tathā rūḍhaḥ abhiniveśaḥ //*

ते प्रतिप्रसवहेयाः सूक्ष्माः ॥१०॥

II.10 *te pratiprasavaheyāḥ sūkṣmāḥ //*

II.10 *te pratiprasava-heyāḥ sūkṣmāḥ //*

ध्यानहेयास्तद्वृत्तयः ॥११॥

II.11 *dhyānaheyāstadvṛttayaḥ //*

II.11 *dhyāna-heyāḥ tad-vṛttayaḥ //*

क्लेशमूलः कर्माशयो दृष्टादृष्टजन्मवेदनीयः ॥१२॥

II.12 *kleśamūlaḥ karmāśayo dṛṣṭādṛṣṭajanmavedanīyaḥ //*

II.12 *kleśa-mūlaḥ karma-aśayaḥ dṛṣṭa-adṛṣṭa-janma-vedanīyaḥ //*

सति मूले तद्विपाको जात्यायुर्भोगाः ॥१३॥

II.13 *sati mūle tadvipāko jātyāyurbhogāḥ //*

II.13 *sati mūle tad-vipākaḥ jāti-āyuḥ-bhogāḥ //*

ते ह्लादपरितापफलाः पुण्यापुण्यहेतुत्वात् ॥१४॥

II.14 *te hlādaparitāpaphalāḥ puṇyāpuṇyahetutvāt //*

II.14 *te hlāda-paritāpa-phalāḥ puṇya-apuṇya-hetutvāt //*

परिणामतापसंस्कारदुःखैर्गुणवृत्तिविरोधाच्च दुःखमेव सर्वं विवेकिनः ॥१५॥

II.15 *pariṇāmatāpasaṁskāraduḥkhairguṇavṛtti virodhācca duḥkhameva sarvaṁ vivekinaḥ //*

II.15 *pariṇāma-tāpa-saṁskāra-duḥkhaiḥ guṇa-vṛtti-virodhāt ca duḥkham eva sarvaṁ vivekinaḥ //*

हेयं दुःखमनागतम् ॥१६॥

II.16 *heyaṁ duḥkhamanāgatam //*

II.16 *heyaṁ duḥkham anāgatam //*

द्रष्टृदृश्ययोः संयोगो हेयहेतुः ॥१७॥

II.17 *draṣṭṛdṛśyayoḥ saṁyogo heyahetuḥ //*

II.17 *draṣṭṛ-dṛśyayoḥ saṁyogaḥ heya-hetuḥ //*

प्रकाशक्रियास्थितिशीलं भूतेन्द्रियात्मकं भोगापवर्गार्थं दृश्यम् ॥१८॥

II.18 *prakāśakriyāsthitiśīlaṁ bhūtendriyātmakaṁ bhogāpavargārthaṁ dṛśyam //*

II.18 *prakāśa-kriyā-sthiti-śīlaṁ bhūta-indriya-ātmakaṁ bhoga-apavarga-arthaṁ dṛśyam //*

विशेषाविशेषलिङ्गमात्रालिङ्गानि गुणपर्वाणि ॥१९॥

II.19 *viśeṣāviśeṣaliṅgamātrāliṅgāni guṇaparvāṇi //*

II.19 *viśeṣa-aviśeṣa-liṅga-mātra-aliṅgāni-guṇa-parvāṇi //*

द्रष्टा दृशिमात्रः शुद्धोऽपि प्रत्ययानुपश्यः ॥२०॥

II.20 *draṣṭā dṛśimātraḥ śuddho' pi pratyayānupaśyaḥ //*

II.20 *draṣṭā dṛśi-mātraḥ śuddhaḥ api pratyaya-anupaśyaḥ //*

तदर्थ एव दृश्यस्याऽत्मा ॥२१॥

II.21 *tadartha eva dṛśyasyātmā //*

II.21 *tad-arthaḥ eva dṛśyasya ātmā //*

कृतार्थं प्रति नष्टमप्यनष्टं तदन्यसाधारणत्वात् ॥२२॥

II.22 *kṛtārthaṁ prati naṣṭamapyanaṣṭaṁ tadanyasādhāraṇatvāt //*

II.22 *kṛta-arthaṁ prati naṣṭam api anaṣṭaṁ tad-anya--sādhāraṇatvāt //*

स्वस्वामिशक्त्योः स्वरूपोपलब्धिहेतुः संयोगः ॥२३॥

II.23 *svasvāmiśaktyoḥ svarūpopalabdhihetuḥ saṁyogaḥ //*

II.23 *sva-svāmi-śaktyoḥ sva-rūpa-upalabdhi-hetuḥ saṁyogaḥ //*

तस्य हेतुरविद्या ॥२४॥

II.24 *tasya heturavidyā //*

II.24 *tasya hetuḥ avidyā //*

तदभावात्संयोगाभावो हानं तद्दृशेः कैवल्यम् ॥२५॥

II.25 *tadabhāvātsaṁyogābhāvo hānaṁ taddṛśeḥ kaivalyam //*

II.25 *tad-abhāvāt saṁyoga-abhāvaḥ hānaṁ tad-dṛśeḥ kaivalyam //*

विवेकख्यातिरविप्लवा हानोपायः ॥२६॥

II.26 *vivekakhyātiraviplavā hānopāyaḥ //*

II.26 *viveka-khyātiḥ aviplavā hāna-upāyaḥ //*

तस्य सप्तधा प्रान्तभूमिः प्रज्ञा ॥२७॥

II.27 *tasya saptadhā prāntabhūmiḥ prajñā //*

II.27 *tasya saptadhā prānta-bhūmiḥ prajñā //*

योगाङ्गानुष्ठानादशुद्धिक्षये ज्ञानदीप्तिराविवेकख्यातेः ॥२८॥

II.28 *yogāṅgānuṣṭhānādaśuddhikṣaye jñānadīptirāvivekakhyāteḥ //*

II.28 *yoga-aṅga-anuṣṭhānāt aśuddhi-kṣaye jñāna-dīptiḥ aviveka-khyāteḥ //*

यमनियमासनप्राणायामप्रत्याहारधारणाध्यानसमाधयोऽष्टावङ्गानि ॥२९॥

II.29 *yamaniyamāsanaprāṇāyāmapratyāhāradhāraṇādhyāna samādhayo 'ṣṭāv aṅgāni //*

II.29 *yama-niyama-āsana-prāṇāyāma-pratyāhāra-dhāraṇā--dhyāna-samādhayaḥ aṣṭau aṅgāni //*

अहिंसासत्यास्तेयब्रह्मचर्यापरिग्रहा यमाः ॥३०॥

II.30 *ahiṁsāsatyāsteyabrahmacaryāparigrahā yamāḥ //*

II.30 *ahiṁsā-satya-asteya-brahmacarya-aparigrahāḥ yamāḥ //*

जातिदेशकालसमयानवच्छिन्नाः सार्वभौमा महाव्रतम् ॥३१॥

II.31 *jātideśakālasamayānavacchinnāḥ sārvabhaumā mahāvratam //*

II.31 *jāti-deśa-kāla-samaya-anavacchinnāḥ sārva-bhaumāḥ mahāvratam //*

शौचसंतोषतपःस्वाध्यायेश्वरप्रणिधानानि नियमाः ॥३२॥

II.32 *śaucasaṅtoṣatapaḥ svādhyāyeśvarapraṇidhānāni niyamāḥ //*

II.32 *śauca-saṅtoṣa-tapaḥ-svādhyāya-Īśvara-praṇidhānāni niyamāḥ //*

वितर्कबाधने प्रतिपक्षभावनम् ॥३३॥

II.33 *vitarkabādhane pratipakṣabhāvanam //*

II.33 *vitarka-bādhane pratipakṣa-bhāvanam //*

वितर्का हिंसादयः कृतकारितानुमोदिता लोभक्रोधमोहपूर्वका मृद मध्याधिमात्रा दुःखाज्ञानानन्तफला इति प्रतिपक्षभावनम् ॥३४॥

II.34 *vitarkā hiṁsādayaḥ kṛtakāritānumoditā lobhakrodhamohapūrvakā mṛdu madhyādhimātrā duḥkhājñānānantaphalā iti pratipakṣabhāvanam //*

II.34 *vitarkāḥ hiṁsā-ādayaḥ kṛta-kārita-anumoditāḥ lobha--krodha-moha-pūrvakāḥ-mṛdu-madhya-adhimātrāḥ duḥkha--ajñāna-ananta-phalāḥ iti pratipakṣa-bhāvanam //*

अहिंसाप्रतिष्ठायां तत्संनिधौ वैरत्यागः ॥३५॥

II.35 *ahiṁsāpratiṣṭhāyāṁ tatsannidhau vairatyāgaḥ //*

II.35 *ahiṁsā-pratiṣṭhāyāṁ tat-sannidhau vaira-tyāgaḥ //*

सत्यप्रतिष्ठायां क्रियाफलाश्रयत्वम् ॥३६॥

II.36 *satyapratiṣṭhāyāṁ kriyāphalāśrayatvam //*

II.36 *satya-pratiṣṭhāyāṁ kriyā-phala-āśrayatvam //*

अस्तेयप्रतिष्ठायां सर्वरत्नोपस्थानम् ॥३७॥

II.37 *asteyapratiṣṭhāyāṁ sarvaratnopasthānam //*

II.37 *asteya-pratiṣṭhāyāṁ sarva-ratna-upasthānam //*

ब्रह्मचर्यप्रतिष्ठायां वीर्यलाभः ॥३८॥

II.38 *brahmacaryapratiṣṭhāyāṁ vīryalābhaḥ //*

II.38 *brahmacarya-pratiṣṭhāyāṁ vīrya-lābhaḥ //*

अपरिग्रहस्थैर्ये जन्मकथंतासंबोधः ॥३९॥

II.39 *aparigrahasthairye janmakathaṁtāsaṁbodhaḥ //*

II.39 *aparigraha-sthairye janma-kathaṁtā saṁbodhaḥ //*

शौचात्स्वाङ्गजुगुप्सा परैरसंसर्गः ॥४०॥

II.40 *śaucāt svāṅgajugupsā parairasaṁsargaḥ //*

II.40 *śaucāt sva-aṅga-jugupsā paraiḥ asaṁsargaḥ //*

सत्त्वशुद्धिसौमनस्यैकाग्र्येन्द्रियजयात्मदर्शनयोग्यत्वानि च ॥४१॥

II.41 *sattvaśuddhisaumanasyaikāgryendriyajayātmadarśana yogyatvāni ca //*

II.41 *sattva-śuddhi-saumanasya-eka-agrya-indriya-jaya--ātma-darśana yogyatvāni ca //*

संतोषादनुत्तमः सुखलाभः ॥४२॥

II.42 *saṅtoṣādanuttamaḥ sukhalābhaḥ //*

II.42 *saṅtoṣāt anuttamaḥ sukha-lābhaḥ //*

कायेन्द्रियसिध्दिरशुद्धिक्षयात्तपसः ॥४३॥

II.43 *kāyendriyasiddhiraśuddhikṣayāttapasaḥ //*

II.43 *kāya-indriya-siddhiḥ aśuddhi-kṣayāt tapasaḥ //*

स्वाध्यायादिष्टदेवतासंप्रयोगः ॥४४॥

II.44 *svādhyāyādiṣṭadevatāsaṁprayogaḥ //*

II.44 *svādhyāyāt iṣṭa-devatā-saṁprayogaḥ //*

समाधिसिध्दिरीश्वरप्रणिधानात् ॥४५॥

II.45 *samādhisiddhirīśvarapraṇidhānāt //*

II.45 *samādhi-siddhiḥ Īśvara-praṇidhānāt //*

स्थिरसुखमासनम् ॥४६॥

II.46 *sthirasukhamāsanam //*

II.46 *sthira-sukhaṁ āsanam //*

प्रयत्नशैथिल्यानन्तसमापत्तिभ्याम्॥४७॥

II.47 *prayatnaśaithilyānantasamāpattibhyām //*

II.47 *prayatna-śaithilya-ananta-samāpattibhyām //*

ततो द्वंद्वानभिघातः ॥४८॥

II.48 *tato dvandvānabhighātāḥ //*

II.48 *tataḥ dvandva-anabhighātaḥ //*

तस्मिन्सति श्वासप्रश्वासयोर्गतिविच्छेदः प्राणायामः ॥४९॥

II.49 *tasminsati śvāsapraśvāsayorgativicchedaḥ prāṇāyāmaḥ //*

II.49 *tasmin sati śvāsa-praśvāsayoḥ gati-vicchedaḥ prāṇāyāmaḥ //*

बाह्याभ्यन्तरस्तम्भवृत्तिर्देशकालसंख्याभिः परिदृष्टो दीर्घसूक्ष्मः ॥५०॥

II.50 *bāhyābhyantarastambhavṛttirdeśakālasaṁkhyābhiḥ paridṛṣṭo dīrghasūkṣmaḥ //*

II.50 *bāhya-abhyantara-staṃbha-vṛttiḥ deśa-kāla-saṁkhyābhiḥ paridṛṣṭaḥ dīrgha-sūkṣmaḥ //*

बाह्याभ्यन्तरविषयाक्षेपी चतुर्थः ॥५१॥

II.51 *bāhyābhyantaraviṣayākṣepī caturthaḥ //*

II.51 *bāhya-abhyantara-viṣaya-ākṣepī caturthaḥ //*

ततः क्षीयते प्रकाशावरणम् ॥५२॥

II.52 *tataḥ kṣīyate prakāśāvaraṇam //*

II.52 *tataḥ kṣīyate prakāśa-āvaraṇam //*

धारणासु च योग्यता मनसः ॥५३॥

II.53 *dhāraṇāsu ca yogyatā manasaḥ //*

II.53 *dhāraṇāsu ca yogyatā manasaḥ //*

स्वविषयासंप्रयोगे चित्तस्यस्वरूपानुकार इवेन्द्रियाणां प्रत्याहारः ॥५४॥

II.54 *svaviṣayāsaṁprayoge cittasyasvarūpānukāra ivendriyāṇāṁ pratyāhāraḥ //*

II.54 *sva-viṣaya-asaṁprayoge cittasya sva-rūpa-anukāraḥ iva indriyāṇāṁ pratyāhāraḥ //*

ततः परमा वश्यतेन्द्रियाणाम् ॥५५॥

II.55 *tataḥ paramā vaśyatendriyāṇām //*

II.55 *tataḥ paramā vaśyatā indriyāṇām //*

इति साधनपादः॥

// iti sādhanapādaḥ //

॥ विभूतिपादः॥
VIBHŪTI-PĀDA
(Chapter on Attainments)

देशबन्धश्चित्तस्य धारणा ॥१॥
III.1 *deśabandhaścittasya dhāraṇā //*
III.1 *deśa-bandhaḥ cittasya dhāraṇā //*

तत्र प्रत्ययैकतानता ध्यानम् ॥२॥
III.2 *tatra pratyayaikatānatā dhyānam //*
III.2 *tatra pratyaya-eka-tānatā dhyānam //*

तदेवार्थमात्रनिर्भासं स्वरूपशून्यमिव समाधिः ॥३॥
III.3 *tadevārthamātranirbhāsaṁ svarūpaśūnyamiva samādhiḥ //*
III.3 *tad eva artha-mātra-nirbhāsaṁ svarūpa-śūnyam iva samādhiḥ //*

त्रयमेकत्रसंयमः ॥४॥
III.4 *trayamekatra saṁyamaḥ //*
III.4 *trayam ekatra saṁyamaḥ //*

तज्जयात् प्रज्ञालोकः ॥५॥
III.5 *tajjayāt prajñālokaḥ //*
III.5 *taj-jayāt prajñā-ālokaḥ //*

तस्य भूमिषु विनियोगः ॥६॥
III.6 *tasya bhūmiṣu viniyogaḥ //*
III.6 *tasya bhūmiṣu viniyogaḥ //*

त्रयमन्तरङ्गं पूर्वेभ्यः ॥७॥
III.7 *trayamantaraṅgaṁ pūrvebhyaḥ //*
III.7 *trayam-antar-aṅgaṁ pūrvebhyaḥ //*

तदपि बहिरङ्गं निर्बीजस्य ॥८॥
III.8 *tadapi bahiraṅgaṁ nirbījasya //*
III.8 *tadapi bahir-aṅgaṁ nirbījasya //*

व्युत्थाननिरोधसंस्कारयोरभिभवप्रादुर्भावौ निरोधक्षणचित्तान्वयो निरोधपरिणामः ॥९॥

III.9 *vyutthānanirodhasaṁskārayorabhibhavaprādurbhāvau nirodhakṣaṇacittānvayo nirodhapariṇāmaḥ //*

III.9 *vyutthāna-nirodha-saṁskārayoḥ abhibhava-prādurbhāvau nirodha-kṣaṇa-citta-anvayaḥ nirodha-pariṇāmaḥ //*

तस्य प्रशान्तवाहिता संस्कारात् ॥१०॥

III.10 *tasya praśāntavāhitā saṁskārāt //*

III.10 *tasya praśānta-vāhitā saṁskārāt //*

सर्वार्थतैकाग्रतयोः क्षयोदयौ चित्तस्य समाधिपरिणामः ॥११॥

III.11 *sarvārthataikāgratayoḥ kṣayodayau cittasya samādhipariṇāmaḥ //*

III.11 *sarva-arthatā-ekāgratayoḥ kṣaya-udayau cittasya samādhi--pariṇāmaḥ //*

ततः पुनः शान्तोदितौ तुल्यप्रत्ययौ चित्तस्यैकाग्रतापरिणामः ॥१२॥

III.12 *tataḥ punaḥ śāntoditau tulyapratyayau cittasyaikāgratāpariṇāmaḥ //*

III.12 *tataḥ punaḥ śānta-uditau tulya-pratyayau cittasya ekāgratā--pariṇāmaḥ //*

एतेन भूतेन्द्रियेषु धर्मलक्षणावस्थापरिणामा व्याख्याताः ॥१३॥

III.13 *etena bhūtendriyeṣu dharmalakṣaṇāvasthāpariṇāmā vyākhyātāḥ //*

III.13 *etena bhūta-indriyeṣu dharma-lakṣaṇa-avasthā-pariṇāmāḥ vyākhyātāḥ //*

शान्तोदिताव्यपदेश्यधर्मानुपाती धर्मी ॥१४॥

III.14 *śāntoditāvyapadeśyadharmānupātī dharmī //*

III.14 *śānta-udita-avyapadeśya-dharma-anupātī dharmī //*

क्रमान्यत्वं परिणामान्यत्वे हेतुः ॥१५॥

III.15 *kramānyatvaṁ pariṇāmānyatve hetuḥ //*

III.15 *krama-anyatvaṁ pariṇāma-anyatve hetuḥ //*

परिणामत्रयसंयमादतीतानागतज्ञानम् ॥१६॥

III.16 *pariṇāmatrayasaṁyamādatītānāgatajñānam //*

III.16 *pariṇāma-traya-saṁyamāt atīta-anāgata-jñānam //*

शब्दार्थप्रत्ययानामितरेतराध्यासात् संकरस्तत्प्रविभागसंयमात् सर्वभूतरुतज्ञानम् ॥१७॥

III.17 *śabdārthapratyayānāmitaretarādhyāsāt saṅkarastatpravibhāga saṁyamāt sarvabhūtarutajñānam //*

III.17 *śabda-artha-pratyayānām itara-itara-adhyāsāt saṅkaraḥ tat-pravibhāga-saṁyamāt sarva-bhūta-rūta-jñānam //*

संस्कारसाक्षात्करणात् पूर्वजातिज्ञानम् ॥१८॥

III.18 *saṁskārasākṣātkaraṇāt pūrvajātijñānam //*

III.18 *saṁskāra-sākṣāt-karaṇāt pūrva-jā-ti-jñānam //*

प्रत्ययस्य परचित्तज्ञानम् ॥१९॥

III.19 *pratyayasya paracittajñānam //*

III.19 *pratyayasya para-citta-jñānam //*

न च तत्सालम्बनं तस्याविषयीभूतत्वात् ॥२०॥

III.20 *na ca tatsālambanaṁ tasyāviṣayībhūtatvāt //*

III.20 *na ca tat sālambanaṁ tasya aviṣayī bhūtatvāt //*

कायरूपसंयमात् तद्ग्राह्यशक्तिस्तम्भे चक्षुष्प्रकाशासंप्रयोगेऽन्तर्धानम् ॥२१॥

III.21 *kāyarūpasaṁyamāt tadgrāhyaśaktistambhe cakṣuṣprakāśāsa ṁprayogentardhānam //*

III.21 *kāya-rūpa-saṁyamāt tad-grāhya-śakti-stambhe cakṣuḥ prakāśa-asaṁprayoge antardhānam //*

एतेन शब्दाद्यन्तर्धानमुक्तम् ॥२२॥

III.22 *etena śabdādyantardhānamuktam //*

III.22 *etena śabda-ādi antardhānam uktam //*

सोपक्रमं निरुपक्रमं च कर्म तत्संयमादपरान्तज्ञानमरिष्टेभ्यो वा ॥२३॥

III.23 *sopakramaṁ nirupakramaṁ ca karma tatsaṁyamādaparān tajñānamariṣṭebhyo vā //*

III.23 *sa-upakramaṁ-nirupakramaṁ ca karma tat-saṁyamāt aparānta-jñānam ariṣṭebhyaḥ vā //*

मैत्र्यादिषु बलानि ॥२४॥

III.24 *maitryādiṣu balāni //*

III.24 *maitrī-ādiṣu balāni //*

बलेषु हस्तिबलादीनि ॥२५॥

III.25 *baleṣu hastibalādīni //*

III.25 *baleṣu hasti-bala-ādīni //*

प्रवृत्त्यालोकन्यासात् सूक्ष्मव्यवहितविप्रकृष्टज्ञानम् ॥२६॥

III.26 *pravṛttyālokanyāsāt sūkṣmavyavahitaviprakṛṣṭajñānam //*

III.26 *pravṛtti-āloka-nyāsāt sūkṣma-vyavahita-viprakṛṣṭa-jñānam //*

भुवनज्ञानं सूर्ये संयमात् ॥२७॥

III.27 *bhuvanajñānaṁ sūrye saṁyamāt //*

III.27 *bhuvana-jñānaṁ sūrye saṁyamāt //*

चन्द्रे ताराव्यूहज्ञानम् ॥२८॥

III.28 *candre tārāvyūhajñānam //*

III.28 *candre tārā-vyūha-jñānam //*

ध्रुवे तद्गतिज्ञानम् ॥२९॥

III.29 *dhruve tadgatijñānam //*

III.29 *dhruve tad-gati-jñānam //*

नाभिचक्रे कायव्यूहज्ञानम् ॥३०॥

III.30 *nābhicakre kāyavyūhajñānam //*

III.30 *nābhi-cakre kāya-vyūha-jñānam //*

कण्ठकूपे क्षुत्पिपासानिवृत्तिः ॥३१॥

III.31 *kaṇṭhakūpe kṣutpipāsānivṛttiḥ //*

III.31 *kaṇṭha-kūpe kṣut-pipāsā-nivṛttiḥ //*

कूर्मनाड्यां स्थैर्यम् ॥३२॥

III.32 *kūrmanāḍyāṁ sthairyam //*

III.32 *kūrma-nāḍyāṁ sthairyam //*

मूर्धज्योतिषि सिद्धदर्शनम् ॥३३॥

III.33 *mūrdhajyotiṣi siddhadarśanam //*

III.33 *mūrdha-jyotiṣi siddha-darśanam //*

प्रातिभाद्वा सर्वम् ॥३४॥

III.34 *prātibhādvā sarvam //*

III.34 *prātibhāt vā sarvam //*

हृदये चित्तसंवित् ॥३५॥

III.35 *hṛdaye cittasaṁvit //*

III.35 *hṛdaye citta-saṁvit //*

सत्त्वपुरुषयोरत्यन्तासंकीर्णयोः प्रत्ययाविशेषो भोगः परार्थत्त्वात् स्वार्थसंयमात् पुरुषज्ञानम् ॥३६॥

III.36 *sattvapuruṣayoratyantāsaṁkīrṇayoḥ pratyayāviśeṣo bhogaḥ parārthatvāt svārthasaṁyamāt puruṣajñānam //*

III.36 *sattva-puruṣayoḥ atyanta-asaṁkīrṇayoḥ pratyaya-aviśeṣaḥ bhogaḥ para-arthatvāt sva-artha-saṁyamāt puruṣa-jñānam //*

ततः प्रातिभश्रावणवेदनादर्शास्वादवार्ता जायन्ते ॥३७॥

III.37 *tataḥ prātibhaśrāvaṇavedanādarśāsvādavārtā jāyante //*

III.37 *tataḥ prātibha-śrāvaṇa-vedanā-ādarśa-āsvāda-vārtāḥ jāyante //*

ते समाधावुपसर्गा व्युत्थाने सिद्धयः ॥३८॥

III.38 *te samādhāvupasargā vyutthāne siddhayaḥ //*

III.38 *te samādhau upasargāḥ vyutthāne siddhayaḥ //*

बन्धकारणशैथिल्यात् प्रचारसंवेदनाच्च चित्तस्य परशरीरावेशः ॥३९॥

III.39 *bandhakāraṇaśaithilyāt pracārasaṁvedanācca cittasya paraśarīrāveśaḥ //*

III.39 *bandha-kāraṇa-śaithilyāt pracāra-saṁvedanāt ca cittasya para-śarīra-āveśaḥ //*

उदानजयाज्जलपङ्ककण्टकादिष्वसङ्ग उत्क्रान्तिश्च ॥४०॥

III.40 *udānajayājjalapaṇka kaṇṭakādiṣvasaṅga utkrāntiśca //*

III.40 *udāna-jayāt jala-paṅka-kaṇṭaka-ādiṣu asaṅgaḥ utkrāntiḥ ca //*

समानजयाज्ज्वलनम् ॥४१॥

III.41 *samānajayājjvalanam //*

III.41 *samāna-jayāt jvalanam //*

श्रोत्राकाशयोः संबन्धसंयमाद्दिव्यं श्रोत्रम् ॥४२॥

III.42 *śrotrākāśayoḥ saṁbandhasaṁyamāddivyaṁ śrotram //*

III.42 *śrotra-ākāśayoḥ saṁbandha-saṁyamāt divyaṁ śrotram //*

कायाकाशयोः संबन्धसंयमाल्लघुतूलसमापत्तेश्चाऽऽकाशगमनम् ॥४३॥

III.43 *kāyākāśayoḥ saṁbandhasaṁyamāllaghutūla samāpatteścākāśagamanam //*

III.43 *kāya-ākāśayoḥ saṁbandha-saṁyamāt laghu-tūla--samāpatteḥ ca ākāśa-gamanam //*

बहिरकल्पिता वृत्तिर्महाविदेहा ततः प्रकाशावरणक्षयः ॥४४॥

III.44 *bahirakalpitā vṛttirmahāvideha tataḥ prakāśāvaraṇakṣayaḥ //*

III.44 *bahiḥ akalpitā vṛttiḥ mahāvideha tataḥ prakāśa-āvaraṇa--kṣayaḥ //*

स्थूलस्वरूपसूक्ष्मान्वयार्थवत्त्वसंयमात् भूतजयः ॥४५॥

III.45 *sthūlasvarūpasūkṣmānvayārthavatvasaṁyamātbhūtajayaḥ //*

III.45 *sthūla-svarūpa-sūkṣma-anvaya-arthavattva-saṁyamāt bhūta-jayaḥ //*

ततोऽणिमादिप्रादुर्भावः कायसंपत् तद्धर्मानभिघातश्च ॥४६॥

III.46 *tato'ṇimādi prādurbhāvaḥ kāyasaṁpat taddharmānabhighātaśca //*

III.46 *tato' ṇima-ādi-prādur-bhāvaḥ kāya-saṁpat tad-dharma--anabhighātaḥ ca //*

रूपलावण्यबलवज्रसंहननत्वानि कायसंपत् ॥४७॥

III.47 *rūpalāvaṇyabalavajrasaṁhananatvāni kāyasaṁpat //*

III.47 *rūpa-lāvaṇya-bala-vajra-saṁhananatvāni kāya-saṁpat //*

ग्रहणस्वरूपास्मितान्वयार्थवत्त्वसंयमादिन्द्रियजयः ॥४८॥

III.48 *grahaṇasvarūpāsmitānvayārthavattvasaṁyamādindriyajyaḥ //*

III.48 *grahaṇa-svarūpa-asmitā-anvaya-arthavattva-saṁyamāt indriya-jayaḥ //*

ततो मनोजवित्वं विकरणभावः प्रधानजयश्च ॥४९॥

III.49 *tato manojavitvaṁ vikaraṇabhāvaḥ pradhānajayaśca //*

III.49 *tataḥ mano-javitvaṁ vikaraṇa-bhāvaḥ pradhāna-jayaḥ ca //*

सत्त्वपुरुषान्यताख्यातिमात्रस्य सर्वभावाधिष्ठातृत्वं सर्वज्ञातृत्वं च ॥५०॥

III.50 *sattva puruṣānyatākhyātimātrasya sarvabhāvādhiṣṭhātṛtvaṁ sarvajñātṛtvaṁ ca //*

III.50 *sattva-puruṣa-anyatā-khyāti-mātrasya sarva-bhāva--adhiṣṭhātṛtvaṁ sarva-jñātṛtvaṁ ca //*

तद्वैराग्यादपि दोषबीजक्षये कैवल्यम् ॥५१॥

III.51 *tadvairāgyādapi doṣabījakṣaye kaivalyam //*

III.51 *tad-vairāgyāt api doṣa-bīja-kṣaye kaivalyam //*

स्थान्युपनिमन्त्रणे सङ्गस्मयाकरणं पुनरनिष्टप्रसङ्गात् ॥५२॥

III.52 *sthānyupanimantraṇe saṅgasmayākaraṇaṁ punaraniṣṭa prasaṅgāt //*

III.52 *sthāni-upanimantraṇe saṅga-smaya-akaraṇam punar--aniṣṭa-prasaṅgāt //*

क्षणतत्क्रमयोः संयमाद्विवेकजं ज्ञानम् ॥५३॥

III.53 *kṣaṇatatkramayoḥ saṁyamādvivekajaṁ jñānam //*

III.53 *kṣaṇa-tat-kramayoḥ saṁyamāt viveka-jaṁ jñānam //*

जातिलक्षणदेशैरन्यतानवच्छेदात् तुल्ययोस्ततः प्रतिपत्तिः ॥५४॥

III.54 *jātilakṣaṇadeśairanyatānavacchedāt tulyayostataḥ pratipattiḥ //*

III.54 *jāti-lakṣaṇa deśaiḥ anyatā anavacchedāt tulyayoḥ tataḥ pratipattiḥ //*

तारकं सर्वविषयं सर्वथाविषयमक्रमं चेति विवेकजं ज्ञानम् ॥५५॥

III.55 *tārakaṁ sarvaviṣayaṁ sarvathāviṣayamakramaṁ ceti vivekajaṁ jñānam //*

III.55 *tārakaṁ sarva-viṣayaṁ sarvathā viṣayaṁ akramaṁ ca iti viveka-jaṁ jñānam //*

सत्त्वपुरुषयोः शुद्धिसाम्ये कैवल्यमिति ॥५६॥

III.56 *sattvapuruṣayoḥ śuddhisāmye kaivalyamiti //*

III.56 *sattva-puruṣayoḥ śuddhi-sāmye kaivalyam iti //*

॥ इति विभूति पादः ॥

// iti vibhūti-pādaḥ //

॥ कैवल्यपादः ॥

KAIVALYA-PĀDA

(Chapter on Absolute Liberation)

जन्मौषधिमन्त्रतपःसमाधिजाः सिद्धयः ॥१॥

IV.1 *janmauṣadhimantratapaḥ samādhijāḥ siddhayaḥ //*

IV.1 *janma-auṣadhi-mantra-tapaḥ-samādhi-jāḥ siddhayaḥ //*

जात्यन्तरपरिणामः प्रकृत्यापूरात् ॥२॥

IV.2 *jātyantarapariṇāmaḥ prakṛtyāpūrāt //*

IV.2 *jāti-antara-pariṇāmaḥ prakṛti-āpūrāt //*

निमित्तमप्रयोजकं प्रकृतीनां वरणभेदस्तु ततः क्षेत्रिकवत् ॥३॥

IV.3 *nimittamaprayojakaṁ prakṛtīnāṁ varaṇabhedastu tataḥ kṣetrikavat //*

IV.3 *nimittaṁ aprayojakaṁ prakṛtīnāṁ varaṇa-bhedaḥ tu tataḥ kṣetrikavat //*

निर्माणचित्तान्यस्मितामात्रात् ॥४॥

IV.4 *nirmāṇacittānyasmitāmātrāt //*

IV.4 *nirmāṇa-cittāni asmitā-mātrāt //*

प्रवृत्तिभेदे प्रयोजकं चित्तमेकमनेकेषाम् ॥५॥

IV.5 *pravṛttibhede prayojakaṁ cittaṁekamanekeṣām //*

IV.5 *pravṛtti-bhede prayojakaṁ cittaṁ ekam anekeṣām //*

तत्र ध्यानजमनाशयम् ॥६॥

IV.6 *tatra dhyānajamanāśayam //*

IV.6 *tatra dhyāna-jam anāśayam //*

कर्माशुक्लाकृष्णं योगिनस्त्रिविधमितरेषाम् ॥७॥

IV.7 *karmāśuklākṛṣṇaṁ yoginastrividhamitareṣām //*

IV.7 *karma aśukla-akṛṣṇaṁ yoginaḥ trividham itareṣām //*

ततस्तद्विपाकानुगुणानामेवाभिव्यक्तिर्वासनानाम् ॥८॥

IV.8 *tatastadvipākānuguṇānāmevābhivyaktirvāsanānām //*

IV.8 *tataḥ tad-vipāka-anuguṇānām eva abhivyaktiḥ vāsanānām //*

जातिदेशकालव्यवहितानामप्यानन्तर्यं स्मृतिसंस्कारयोरेकरूपत्वात् ॥९॥

IV.9 *jātideśakālavyavahitānāmapyānantaryaṁ smṛtisaṁskārayorekarūpatvāt //*

IV.9 *jāti-deśa-kāla-vyavahitānām api ānantaryaṁ smṛti--saṁskārayoḥ eka-rūpatvāt //*

तासामनादित्वं चाशिषो नित्यत्वात् ॥१०॥

IV.10 *tāsāmanāditvaṁ cāśiṣo nityatvāt //*

IV.10 *tāsām anāditvaṁ ca āśiṣaḥ nityatvāt //*

हेतुफलाश्रयालम्बनैः संगृहीतत्वादेषामभावे तदभावः ॥११॥

IV.11 *hetuphalāśrayālambanaiḥ saṅgṛhītatvādeṣāmabhāve tadabhāvaḥ //*

IV.11 *hetu-phala-āśraya-ālambanaiḥ saṅgṛhītatvāt eṣām abhāve tad-abhāvaḥ //*

अतीतानागतं स्वरूपतोऽस्त्यध्वभेदाद्धर्माणाम् ॥१२॥

IV.12 *atītānāgataṁ sarvarūpatostyadhvabhedātdharmāṇām //*

IV.12 *atīta-anāgataṁ-sarva-rūpataḥ asti adhva-bhedāt dharmāṇām //*

ते व्यक्तसूक्ष्मा गुणात्मानः ॥१३॥

IV.13 *te vyaktasūkṣmā guṇātmānaḥ //*

IV.13 *te vyakta sūkṣmāḥ guṇa-ātmānaḥ //*

परिणामैकत्वाद्वस्तुतत्त्वम् ॥१४॥

IV.14 *pariṇāmaikatvādvastutattvam //*

IV.14 *pariṇāma-ekatvāt-vastu-tattvam //*

वस्तुसाम्ये चित्तभेदात् तयोर्विभक्तः पन्थाः ॥१५॥

IV.15 *vastusāmye cittabhedāttayorvibhaktaḥ panthāḥ //*

IV.15 *vastu-sāmye citta-bhedāt tayoḥ vibhaktaḥ panthāḥ //*

न चैकचित्ततन्त्रं चेद्वस्तु तदप्रमाणकं तदा किं स्यात् ॥१६॥

IV.16 *na caikacittatantraṁ ced vastu tadapramāṇakaṁ tadā kiṁ syāt //*

IV.16 *na ca eka-citta-tantraṁ ced vastu tat-apramāṇakaṁ tadā kiṁ syāt //*

तदुपरागापेक्षित्वाच्चित्तस्य वस्तु ज्ञाताज्ञातम् ॥१७॥

IV.17 *taduparāgāpekṣitvātcittasya vastu jñātājñātam //*

IV.17 *tad-uparāga-apekṣitvāt cittasya vastu jñāta-ajñātam //*

सदा ज्ञाताश्चित्तवृत्तयस्तत्प्रभोः पुरुषस्यापरिणामित्वात् ॥१८॥

IV.18 *sadā jñātāścittavṛttayastatprabhoḥ puruṣasyāpariṇāmitvāt //*

IV.18 *sadā jñātāḥ citta-vṛttayaḥ tat-prabhoḥ puruṣasya apariṇāmitvāt //*

न तत् स्वाभासं दृश्यत्वात् ॥१९॥

IV.19 *na tatsvābhāsaṁ dṛśyatvāt //*

IV.19 *na tat-svābhāsaṁ dṛśyatvāt //*

एकसमये चोभयानवधारणम् ॥२०॥

IV.20 *ekasamaye cobhayānavadhāraṇam //*

IV.20 *eka-samaye ca ubhaya-anava-dhāraṇam //*

चित्तान्तरदृश्ये बुद्धिबुद्धेरतिप्रसङ्गः स्मृतिसंकरश्च ॥२१॥

IV.21 *cittāntaradṛśye buddhibuddheratiprasaṇgaḥ smṛtisaṇkaraśca //*

IV.21 *citta-antara-dṛśye buddhi-buddheḥ atiprasaṇgaḥ smṛti--saṇkaraḥ ca //*

चितेरप्रतिसंक्रमायास्तदाकारापत्तौ स्वबुद्धिसंवेदनम् ॥२२॥

IV.22 *citerapratisaṁkramāyāstadākārāpattau svabuddhisaṁvedanam //*

IV.22 *citeḥ apratisaṁkramāyāḥ tad-ākāra-āpattau sva-buddhi-saṁvedanam //*

द्रष्टृदृश्योपरक्तं चित्तं सर्वार्थम् ॥२३॥

IV.23 *draṣṭṛdṛśyoparaktaṁ cittaṁ sarvārthaṁ //*

IV.23 *draṣṭṛ-dṛśya-uparaktaṁ cittaṁ sarva-arthaṁ //*

तदसंख्येयवासनाभिश्चित्रमपि परार्थं संहत्यकारित्वात् ॥२४॥

IV.24 *tadasaṇkhyeyavāsanābhiścitramapi parārthaṁ saṁhatyakāritvāt //*

IV.24 *tat-asaṇkhyeya-vāsanābhiḥ citram api para-arthaṁ saṁhatya-kāritvāt //*

विशेषदर्शिन आत्मभावभावनानिवृत्तिः ॥२५॥

IV.25 *viśeṣadarśina ātmabhāvabhāvanānivṛttiḥ //*

IV.25 *viśeṣa-darśinaḥ ātma-bhāva-bhāvanā-nivṛttiḥ //*

तदा विवेकनिम्नं कैवल्यप्राग्भारं चित्तम् ॥२६॥

IV.26 *tadā vivekanimnaṁ kaivalyaprāgbhāraṁ cittam //*

IV.26 *tadā viveka-nimnaṁ kaivalya-prāgbhāraṁ cittam //*

तच्छिद्रेषु प्रत्ययान्तराणि संस्कारेभ्यः ॥२७॥

IV.27 *tacchidreṣu pratyayāntarāṇi saṁskārebhyaḥ //*

IV.27 *tat-chidreṣu pratyaya-antarāṇi saṁskārebhyaḥ //*

हानमेषां क्लेशवदुक्तम् ॥२८॥

IV.28 *hānameṣāṁ kleśavaduktam //*

IV.28 *hānam eṣāṁ kleśavat uktam //*

प्रसंख्यानेऽप्यकुसीदस्य सर्वथा विवेकख्यातेर्धर्ममेघः समाधिः ॥२९॥

IV.29 *prasaṁkhyāne'pyakusīdasya sarvathā vivekakhyāterdharmameghaḥ samādhiḥ //*

IV.29 *prasaṁkhyāne api akusīdasya sarvathā viveka-khyāteḥ dharma-meghaḥ samādhiḥ //*

ततः क्लेशकर्मनिवृत्तिः ॥३०॥

IV.30 *tataḥ kleśakarmanivṛttiḥ //*

IV.30 *tataḥ kleśa-karma-nivṛttiḥ //*

तदा सर्वावरणमलापेतस्य ज्ञानस्याऽऽनन्त्याज्ज्ञेयमल्पम् ॥३१॥

IV.31 *tadā sarvāvaraṇamalāpetasya jñānasyānantyātjñeyamalpam //*

IV.31 *tadā sarva-āvaraṇa-mala-apetasya jñānasya ānantyāt--jñeyam alpam //*

ततः कृतार्थानां परिणामक्रमसमाप्तिर्गुणानाम् ॥३२॥

IV.32 *tataḥ kṛtārthānāṁ pariṇāmakrama samāptirguṇānāṁ //*

IV.32 *tataḥ kṛtā-arthānāṁ pariṇāma-krama-samāptiḥ guṇānāṁ //*

क्षणप्रतियोगी परिणामापरान्तनिर्ग्राह्यः क्रमः ॥३३॥

IV.33 *kṣaṇapratiyogī pariṇāmāparāntanirgrāhyaḥ kramaḥ //*

IV.33 *kṣaṇa-pratiyogī pariṇāma-aparānta-nirgrāhyaḥ kramaḥ //*

पुरुषार्थशून्यानां गुणानां प्रतिप्रसवः कैवल्यं स्वरुपप्रतिष्ठा वा चितिशक्तिरिति ॥३४॥

IV.34 *puruṣārthaśūnyānāṁ guṇānāṁ pratiprasavaḥ kaivalyaṁ svarūpapratiṣṭhā vā citiśaktiriti //*

IV.34 *puruṣa-artha-śūnyānāṁ guṇānāṁ pratiprasavaḥ kaivalyaṁ sva-rūpa-pratiṣṭhā vā citi-śaktiḥ iti //*

॥ इति कैवल्यपादः ॥

// iti kaivalya-pādaḥ //

Appendix II

Alphabetical Index of the *Sūtras*

abhāva-pratyaya-ālambanā vṛttiḥ nidrā (I.10) 85

abhyāsa-vairāgyābhyāṁ tad-nirodhaḥ (I.12) 120

ahiṁsā-pratiṣṭhāyāṁ tat-sannidhau vaira-tyāgaḥ (II.35) 145

ahiṁsā-satya-asteya-brahmacarya-aparigrahāḥ yamāḥ (II.30) 144

anitya-aśuci-duḥkha-anātmasu nitya-śuci-sukha-ātma-khyātiḥ avidyā (II.5) 80

anubhūta-viṣaya-asaṁpramoṣaḥ smṛtiḥ (I.11) 85

aparigraha-sthairye janma-kathaṅtā saṁbodhaḥ (II.39) 146

asteya-pratiṣṭhāyāṁ sarva-ratna-upasthānam (II.37) 146

atha yoga-anuśāsanam (I.1) 15,168

atīta-anāgataṁ-sarva-rūpataḥ asti adhva-bhedāt dharmāṇām (IV.12) 25

avidyā-asmitā-rāga-dveṣa-abhiniveśāḥ kleśāḥ (II.3) 80

avidyā kṣetram uttareṣāṁ prasupta-tanu-vicchinna--udārāṇām (II.4) 97

bahiḥ akalpitā vṛttiḥ mahāvidehā tataḥ prakāśa--āvaraṇakṣayaḥ (III.44) 41

bāhya-abhyantara-staṃbha-vṛttiḥ deśa-kāla-saṁkhyābhiḥ paridṛṣṭaḥ dīrgha-sūkṣmaḥ (II.50) 74, 156

bāhya-abhyantara-viṣaya-ākṣepī caturthaḥ (II.51) 157

baleṣu hasti-bala-ādīni (III.25) 89, 145

bandha-kāraṇa-śaithilyāt pracāra-saṁvedanāt ca cittasya para-śarīra-āveśaḥ (III.39) 41

bhava-pratyayaḥ videha-prakṛti-layānām (I.19) 25, 122–3, 175
bhuvana-jñānaṁ sūrye saṁyamāt (III.27) 46, 47, 180
brahmacarya-pratiṣṭhāyāṁ vīrya-lābhaḥ (II.38) 146
candre tārā-vyūha-jñānam (III.28) 47, 68
citeḥ apratisaṁkramāyāḥ tad-ākāra-āpattau sva-buddhi-saṁvedanam (IV.22) 48, 71, 103, 170
citta-antara-dṛśye buddhi-buddheḥ atiprasaṇgaḥ smṛti--saṇkaraḥ ca (IV.21) 65, 75
deśa-bandhaḥ cittasya dhāraṇā (III.1) 91, 167
dhāraṇāsu ca yogyatā manasaḥ (II.53) 59, 158
dhruve tad-gati-jñānam (III.29) 47, 55, 68
dhyāna-heyāḥ tad-vṛttayaḥ (II.11) 169
draṣṭā dṛśi-mātraḥ śuddhaḥ api pratyaya-anupaśyaḥ (II.20) 40, 45
draṣṭṛ-dṛśyayoḥ saṁyogaḥ heya-hetuḥ (II.17) 39, 125
draṣṭṛ-dṛśya-uparaktaṁ cittaṁ sarva-arthaṁ (IV.23) 71, 81, 103
dṛg-darśana-śaktyoḥ eka-ātmatā iva asmitā (II.6) 52, 81, 123, 180
dṛṣṭa-ānuśravika-viṣaya-vitṛṣṇasya vaśīkārasaṁjñā--vairāgyam (I.15) 29
duḥkha-daurmanasya-aṅgame-jayatva-śvāsa-praśvāsāḥ vikṣepa-sahabhuvaḥ (I.31) 96
duḥkha-anuśayī dveṣaḥ (II.8) 81
eka-samaye ca ubhaya-anava-dhāraṇam (IV.20) 64, 70
etayā eva savicārā nirvicārā ca sūkṣma-viṣayā vyākhyātā (I.44) 173
etena bhūta-indriyeṣu dharma-lakṣaṇa-avasthā-pariṇāmāḥ vyākhyātāḥ (III.13) 41, 116
etena śabda-ādi antardhānam uktam (III.22) 141
grahaṇa-svarūpa-asmitā-anvaya-arthavattva-saṁyamāt indriya-jayaḥ (III.48) 58, 101, 166, 182
hānam eṣāṁ kleśavat uktam (IV.28) 65, 76, 126
hetu-phala-āśraya-ālambanaiḥ saṅgṛhītatvāt eṣām abhāve tad-abhāvaḥ (IV.11) 24, 87
heyaṁ duḥkham anāgatam (II.16) 178
hṛdaye citta-saṁvit (III.35) 68, 119, 163

Īśvara-praṇidhānāt vā (I.23) 111,187
janma-auṣadhi-mantra-tapaḥ-samādhi-jāḥ siddhayaḥ (IV.1) 17
jāti-deśa-kāla-samaya-anavacchinnāḥ sārva-bhaumāḥ mahāvratam (II.31) 145
jāti-deśa-kāla-vyavahitānām api ānantaryaṁ smṛti--saṁskārayoḥ eka-rūpatvāt (IV.9) 24
jāti-lakṣaṇa deśaiḥ anyatā anavacchedāt tulyayoḥ tataḥ pratipattiḥ (III.54) 150
jāti-antara-pariṇāmaḥ prakṛti-āpūrāt (IV.2) 17, 63, 103
kaṇṭha-kūpe kṣut-pipāsā-nivṛttiḥ (III.31) 163
karma aśukla-akṛṣṇaṁ yoginaḥ trividham itareṣām (IV.7) 24, 95
kāya-ākāśayoḥ saṁbandha-saṁyamāt laghu-tūla--samāpatteḥ ca ākāśa-gamanam (III.43) 141
kāya-rūpa-saṁyamāt tad-grāhya-śakti-stambhe cakṣuḥ prakāśa-asaṁprayoge antardhānam (III.21) 140
kāya-indriya-siddhiḥ aśuddhi-kṣayāt tapasaḥ (II.43) 147
kleśa-karma-vipāka-āśayaiḥ aparāmṛṣṭaḥ puruṣa-viśeṣaḥ Īśvaraḥ (I.24) 29,82
kleśa-mūlaḥ karma-aśayaḥ dṛṣṭa-adṛṣṭa-janma-vedanīyaḥ (II.12) 23
krama-anyatvaṁ pariṇāma-anyatve hetuḥ (III.15) 13
kṛta-arthaṁ prati naṣṭam api anaṣṭaṁ tad-anya--sādhāraṇatvāt (II.22) 39
kṣaṇa pratiyogī pariṇāma aparānta nirgrāhyaḥ kramaḥ (IV.33)
kṣaṇa-tat-kramayoḥ saṁyamāt viveka-jaṁ jñānam (III.53) 55, 141
kṣīṇa-vṛtteḥ abhijātasya iva maṇeḥ grahītṛ-grahaṇa-grāhyeṣu tat-stha-tad-añjanatā samāpattiḥ (I.41) 173
kūrma-nāḍyāṁ sthairyam (III.32) 153, 163
maitrī-karuṇā-muditā-upēkṣāṇāṁ sukha-duḥkha-puṇya--apuṇya-viṣayāṇāṁ bhāva-nātaḥ-citta-prasādanam (I.33) 3, 16, 89
maitrī-ādiṣu balāni (III.24) 89, 145
mṛdu-madhya-adhimātratvāt tataḥ api viśeṣaḥ (I.22) 17

mūrdha-jyotiṣi siddha-darśanam (III.33) 120, 163
nābhi-cakre kāya-vyūha-jñānam (III.30) 120, 163
na ca eka-citta-tantraṁ ced vastu tat-apramāṇakaṁ tadā kiṁ syāt (IV.16) 64–5
na ca tat sālambanaṁ tasya aviṣayī bhūtatvāt (III.20) 140
na tat-svābhāsaṁ dṛśyatvāt (IV.19) 65, 70
nimittaṁ aprayojakaṁ prakṛtīnāṁ varaṇa-bhedaḥ tu tataḥ kṣetrikavat (IV.3) 5
nirmāṇa-cittāni asmitā-mātrāt (IV.4) 52, 60, 76, 117, 123
nirvicāra-vaiśāradye adhyātma-prasādaḥ (I.47) 18, 173–4
parama-aṇu-parama-mahattva-antaḥ asya vaśīkāraḥ (I.40) 153
pariṇāma-ekatvāt-vastu-tattvam (IV.14) 37
pariṇāma-tāpa-saṁskāra-duḥkhaiḥ guṇa-vṛtti-virodhāt ca duḥkham eva sarvaṁ vivekinaḥ (II.15) 53
pariṇāma-traya-saṁyamāt atīta-anāgata-jñānam (III.16) 140
pracchardana-vidhāraṇābhyāṁ vā prāṇasya (I.34) 59, 90,156
prakāśa-kriyā-sthiti-śīlaṁ bhūta-indriya-ātmakaṁ bhoga--apavargarthaṁ dṛśyam (II.18) 36, 124, 179
pramāṇa-viparyaya-vikalpa-nidrā -smṛtayaḥ (I.6) 74
prasaṁkhyāne api akusīdasya sarvathā viveka-khyāteḥ dharma-meghaḥ samādhiḥ (IV.29) 73
prātibhāt vā sarvam (III.34) 119, 163
pratyakṣa-anumāna-āgamāḥ pramāṇāni (I.7) 84
pratyayasya para-citta-jñānam (III.19) 140
pravṛtti-bhede prayojakaṁ cittam ekam anekeṣām (IV.5) 64, 70
pravṛtti-āloka-nyāsāt sūkṣma-vyavahita-viprakṛṣṭa-jñānam (III.26) 150
prayatna-śaithilya-ananta-samāpattibhyām (II.47) 151, 174, 179
puruṣa-artha-śūnyānāṁ guṇānāṁ pratiprasavaḥ kaivalyaṁ sva--rūpa-pratiṣṭhā vā citi-śaktiḥ iti (IV.34) 48, 77, 177, 183, 187
ṛtaṁbharā tatra prajñā (I.48) 177, 180
rūpa-lāvaṇya-bala-vajra-saṁhananatvāni kāya-saṁpat (III.47) 101, 153, 162, 182
śabda-jñāna-anupātī vastu-śūnyaḥ vikalpaḥ (I.9) 85

śabda-artha-pratyayānām itara-itara adhyāsāt saṇkaraḥ tat-pravibhāga-saṁyamāt sarva-bhūta-rūta-jñānam (III.17) 94, 140
sadā jñātāḥ citta-vṛttayaḥ tat-prabhoḥ puruṣasya apariṇāmitvāt (IV.18) 47, 65, 70
sa eṣa pūrveṣām api guruḥ kālena anavacchedāt (I.26) 29–30
samādhi-bhāvanā-arthaḥ kleśa-tanū-karaṇa-arthaḥ ca (II.2) 172, 185
samādhi-siddhiḥ Īśvara-praṇidhānāt (II.45) 115, 147, 174, 186
samāna-jayāt jvalanam (III.41) 161
saṁskāra-sākṣāt-karaṇāt pūrva-jā-ti-jñānam (III.18) 20, 25, 86, 146
śānta-udita-avyapadeśya-dharma-anupātī dharmī (III.14) 31
saṅtoṣāt anuttamaḥ sukha-lābhaḥ (II.42) 147
sarva-arthatā-ekāgratayoḥ kṣaya-udayau cittasya samādhi--pariṇāmaḥ (III.11) 174
sati mūle tad-vipākaḥ jāti-āyuḥ-bhogāḥ (II.13) 23
sattva-puruṣa-anyatā-khyāti-mātrasya sarva-bhāva--adhiṣṭhātṛtvaṁ sarva-jñātṛtvaṁ ca (III.50) 47, 55, 102, 176, 183
sattva-puruṣayoḥ śuddhi-sāmye kaivalyam iti (III.56) 41, 56, 116, 126, 186
sattva-puruṣayoḥ atyanta-asaṁkīrṇayoḥ pratyaya-aviśeṣaḥ bhogaḥ para-arthatvāt sva-artha-saṁyamāt puruṣa-jñānam (III.36) 40, 48, 120, 141
sattva-śuddhi-saumanasya-eka-agrya-indriya-jaya-ātma--darśana yogyatvāni ca (II.41) 58, 147
sa tu dīrgha-kāla-nairantarya-satkāra-āsevitaḥ dṛḍha-bhūmiḥ (I.14) 4, 113
satya-pratiṣṭhāyāṁ kriyā-phala-āśrayatvam (II.36) 146
śauca-saṅtoṣa-tapaḥ-svādhyāya-Īśvara-praṇidhānāni niyamāḥ (II.32) 146
śaucāt sva-aṅga-jugupsā paraiḥ asaṁsargaḥ (II.40) 147
smṛti-pariśuddhau sva-rūpa-śūnya iva arthamātra-nirbhāsā nirvitarkā (I.43) 173

sa-upakramaṁ-nirupakramaṁ ca karma tat-saṁyamāt aparānta-jñānam ariṣṭebhyaḥ vā (III.23) 119
śraddhā-vīrya-smṛti-samādhi-prajñā-pūrvakaḥ itareṣām (I.20) 120
śrotra-ākāśayoḥ saṁbandha-saṁyamāt divyaṁ śrotram (III.42) 141, 161
śruta-anumāna-prajñābhyām anya-viṣayā viśeṣa-arthatvāt (I.49) 93, 117, 177
sthāni-upanimantraṇe saṅga-smaya-akaraṇam punar-aniṣṭa--prasaṅgāt (III.52) 102, 123, 176
sthira-sukhaṁ āsanam (II.46) 148
sthūla-svarūpa-sūkṣma-anvaya-arthavattva-saṁyamāt bhūta-jayaḥ (III.45) 99, 181
sukha-anuśayī rāgaḥ (II.7) 81
sūkṣma-viṣayatvaṁ ca aliṅga-paryavasānam (I.45) 123, 174, 178–9
svādhyāyāt iṣṭa-devatā-saṁprayogaḥ (II.44) 147
svapna-nidrā-jñāna-ālambanaṁ vā (I.38) 92,169
svarasa-vāhī viduṣaḥ api tathā rūḍhaḥ abhiniveśaḥ (II.9) 81
sva-svāmi-śaktyoḥ sva-rūpa-upalabdhi-hetuḥ saṁyogaḥ (II.23) 40, 46, 126, 179
sva-viṣaya-asaṁprayoge cittasya sva-rūpa-anukāraḥ iva indriyāṇāṁ pratyāhāraḥ (II.54) 165–6
tad-abhāvāt saṁyoga-abhāvaḥ hānaṁ tad-dṛśeḥ kaivalyam (II.25) 40, 125, 186
tadā draṣṭuḥ svarūpe avasthānam (I.3) 45
tadapi bahir-aṅgaṁ nirbījasya (III.8) 138–9
tad-arthaḥ eva dṛśyasya ātmā (II.21) 38, 45–6
tadā sarva-āvaraṇa-mala-apetasya jñānasya ānantyāt-jñeyam alpam (IV.31) 77, 104
tadā vivekan-imnaṁ kaivalya-prāgbhāraṁ cittam (IV.26) 56, 186–7
tad eva artha-mātra-nirbhāsaṁ svarūpa-śūnyam iva samādhiḥ (III.3) 174, 185
tad-uparāga-apekṣitvāt cittasya vastu jñāta-ajñātam (IV.17) 65

tad-vairāgyāt api doṣa-bīja-kṣaye kaivalyam (III.51) 102, 126, 176, 186
tā eva sabījaḥ samādhiḥ (I.46) 138, 175–6
taj-japaḥ tad-artha-bhāvanam (I.28) 30
taj-jayāt prajñā-ālokaḥ (III.5) 139
tapaḥ-svādhyāya-Īśvara-praṇidhānāni kriyā-yogaḥ (II.1) 46, 111
tārakaṁ sarva-viṣayaṁ sarvathā viṣayaṁ akramaṁ ca iti viveka-jaṁ jñānam (III.55) 55, 141
tāsām anāditvaṁ ca āśiṣaḥ nityatvāt (IV.10) 25, 87, 125
tasmin sati śvāsa-praśvāsayoḥ gati-vicchedaḥ prāṇāyāmaḥ (II.49) 155
tasya bhūmiṣu viniyogaḥ (III.6) 139, 180
tasya hetuḥ avidyā (II.24) 93
tasya praśānta-vāhitā saṁskārāt (III.10) 73, 75, 114
tasya āpi nirodhe sarva-nirodhāt nirbījaḥ samādhiḥ (I.51) 117, 139, 177
tasya saptadhā prānta-bhūmiḥ prajñā (II.27) 72, 139, 181
tataḥ dvandvāḥa-anabhighātaḥ (II.48) 62, 152
tataḥ kleśa-karma-nivṛttiḥ (IV.30) 104, 180–1
tataḥ kṛtā-arthānāṁ pariṇāma-krama samāptiḥ guṇānāṁ (IV.32) 37, 71, 104
tataḥ kṣīyate prakāśa-āvaraṇam (II.52) 58, 158
tataḥ paramā vaśyatā indriyāṇām (II.55) 166
tataḥ prātibha-śrāvaṇa-vedanā-ādarśa-āsvāda-vārtāḥ jāyante (III.37) 163
tataḥ pratyak-cetana adhigamaḥ api antarāya-abhāvaḥ ca (I.29) 30
tataḥ punaḥ śānta-uditau tulya-pratyayau cittasya ekāgratā-pariṇāmaḥ (III.12) 73, 75, 114, 126
tataḥ tad-vipāka-anuguṇānām eva abhivyaktiḥ vāsanānām (IV.8) 24, 97
tataḥ mano-javitvaṁ vikaraṇa-bhāvaḥ pradhāna-jayaḥ ca (III.49) 59, 101–2, 123, 166, 182
tat-asaṇkhyeya-vāsanābhiḥ citram api para-arthaṁ saṁhatya-kāritvāt (IV.24) 46, 103

tat-chidreṣu pratyaya-antarāṇi saṁskārebhyaḥ (IV.27) 73, 75, 126
tato' ṇima-ādi-prādur-bhāvaḥ kāya-saṁpat tad-dharma--anabhighātaḥ ca (III.46) 99–100, 182
tat-paraṁ puruṣa-khyāteḥ guṇa-vaitṛṣṇyam (I.16) 36
tat-pratiṣedha-artham eka-tattva-abhyāsaḥ (I.32) 109, 114
tatra dhyāna-jam anāśayam (IV.6) 103, 169–70
tatra niratiśayaṁ sarvajña-bījam (I.25) 29
tatra pratyaya-eka-tānatā dhyānam (III.2) 169
tatra śabda-artha-jñāna-vikalpaiḥ saṅkīrṇā savitarkā samāpattiḥ (I.42) 173
tatra sthitau yatnaḥ abhyāsaḥ (I.13) 29, 113
te hlāda-paritāpa-phalāḥ puṇya-apuṇya-hetutvāt (II.14) 23
te pratiprasava-heyāḥ sūkṣmāḥ (II.10) 82
te samādhau upasargāḥ vyutthāne siddhayaḥ (III.38) 123, 176
te vyakta sūkṣmāḥ guṇa-ātmānaḥ (IV.13) 37
tīvra-saṁvegānām āsannaḥ (I.21) 17
tadapi bahir-aṅgaṁ nirbījasya (III.8) 117, 138
trayam-antar-aṅgaṁ pūrvebhyah (III.7) 118, 139
trayam ekatra saṁyamaḥ (III.4) 116, 135
udāna-jayāt jala-paṅka-kaṇṭaka-ādiṣu asaṅgaḥ utkrāntiḥ ca (III.40) 161
vastu-sāmye citta-bhedāt tayoḥ vibhaktaḥ panthāḥ (IV.15) 64
viparyayaḥ mithyā-jñānam atad-rūpa pratiṣṭham (I.8) 84
virāma-pratyaya-abhyāsa-pūrvaḥ saṁskāra-śeṣaḥ anyaḥ (I.18) 25, 86, 122
viṣayavatī vā pravṛttiḥ utpannā manasaḥ sthiti-nibandhanī (I.35) 91, 165
viśeṣa-darśinaḥ ātma-bhāva-bhāvanā-nivṛttiḥ (IV.25) 103, 157
viśeṣa-aviśeṣa-liṅga-mātra-aliṅgāni-guṇa-parvāṇi (II.19) 38
viśokā vā jyotiṣmatī (I.36) 91–2, 168
vīta-rāga-viṣayaṁ vā cittam (I.37) 92, 168
vitarkāḥ hiṁsā-ādayaḥ kṛta-kārita-anumoditāḥ lobha-krodha--moha-pūrvakāḥ-mṛdu-madhya-adhimātrāḥ duḥkha-ajñāna--ananta-phalāḥ iti pratipakṣa-bhāvanam (II.34) 22, 125

vitarka-vicāra-ānanda-asmitārūpa-anugamāt saṁpra-jñātaḥ (I.17) 16, 76
viveka-khyātiḥ aviplavā hāna-upāyaḥ (II.26) 54
vṛttayaḥ pañcatayyaḥ kliṣṭā-akliṣṭāḥ (I.5) 83
vṛtti-sārūpyam itaratra (I.4) 60, 122
vyādhi-styāna-saṁśaya-pramāda-ālasya-avirati-bhrānti-darśana-alabdha-bhūmikatva-anavasthitatvāni citta-vikṣepāḥ te antarāyāḥ (I.30) 52, 96
vyutthāna-nirodha-saṁskārayoḥ-abhibhava-prādurbhāvau nirodha-kṣaṇa-citta-anvayaḥ nirodha-pariṇāmaḥ (III.9) 73, 113
yama-niyama-āsana-prāṇāyāma-pratyāhāra-dhāraṇā-dhyāna-samādhayaḥ aṣṭau aṅgāni (II.29) 143
yathā-abhimata-dhyānāt vā (I.39) 92, 169
yoga-aṅga-anuṣṭhānāt aśuddhi-kṣaye jñāna-dīptiḥ aviveka-khyāteḥ (II.28) 58, 144, 181
yogaḥ citta-vṛtti-nirodhaḥ (I.2) 15, 74

Index

Page numbers in italics refer to charts and tables.

absorption (*samādhi*), 25, 86, 114, 115, 116–17, 119–20, 135–6, *136*, 137–8, 143, 147, 186
  cautions to, 123, 164, 176
  effects of, 172–6
  four types of, 3
  and liberation (*kaivalya*), 185–7
  pause in (*virāma-pratyaya*), 86, 122, 164–5, 167, 171, 172, *173*, 175
  effects of, 175–6
  stages of awareness:
    seeded (*sabīja-samādhi*), 24, 86, 122, 138, 167, 171–3, 175–6, 185
    seedless (*nirbīja-samādhi*), 24, 77, 86, 104, 117, 122, 136, 138–9, 167, 171–3, 176–7, 185
actions:
  five organs of action (*karmendiyas*), 2, 33, 37, 182
  path of (*karma-mārga*), 2, 94, 142
  qualities of (*guṇa-karma*), 4
  and reactions, 22–6
  right (*puṇya*) and wrong (*apuṇya*), 95
  ripe action (*paripakva-karma*), 8
  types of (*karma*, *vikarma*, *sukarma* and *akarma*), 7, *8*, 23, 24, 180–1
  see also cause and effect (*karma*)
afflictions (*kleśas*), 1–2, 28, 78–9, 95, 97, 125, 171
  attachment (*rāga*), 80
  aversion (*dveṣa*), 80
  egoism (*asmitā*), 81
  fear of death (*abhiniveśa*), 1, 80, 81–2
  ignorance (*avidyā*), 80, 97, 104
  involution/cessation of (*kleśa-nivṛtti*), 2
aims of life (*puruṣa-artha*): duty (*dharma*), livelihood (*artha*), emancipation (*mokṣa*), enjoyment (*kāma*), 4, 6, 7, 9, 48, 104, 187
  see also individual entries
air (*vāyu*), 160–2

art of living (*kalā*), 116, 117, 137
attachment (*rāga*), 80, 81, 171
awareness (*prajñā*), 47, 55, 114, 116, 166, 169
  stages/states of, 72–7, 136, 138–9, 167, 171–3, 177, 181

Bhagavad Gītā, 11, 13–15, 22, 26, 29, 30, 53, 89, 101, 118, 122, 124
bliss (*ānanda*), 3, 12, 16, 50, 76
  sheaths of (*ānandamaya kośa*), *34*, 100, 129
body (*śārīra*), 101, 127, 106–9, 167
  anatomical (*annamaya*), 50, 115
  causal (*kāraṁa*), 1, 107, 127, *131*, *134*, 135, 162
  evolution and involution of three facets, 129, *130–1*, *132–3*, 143
  inner/subtle (*antaraṅga/sūkṣma*) and gross (*kārya/sthūla*), 1, 3, 4, 99, 107, 129, *132*, *133*, 162, 181
  mastery over (*śārīra-jaya*), 101, 182
  and mind, 142
  physiological (*prāṇamaya*), 50, 99, 112, 115, *131*, *132*, *161*
  sheaths of (*kośas*), 128–9
  and universal energy, 33–4
Brahmā, 11–12, 159
Brahmānanda, 158
Brahmā Sūtra, 29
brain (*mastiṣka*), 14, 16
  analytical (*vitarka*), 16
  silencing of (*pratyāhāra*), 164–6
breath control (*prāṇāyāma*), 13, 58–9, 60–2, 74–5, 89, 90–1, 117, 120, 143, 155–7, 166, 182
  effects of, 157–60
  and air (*vāyu*), 160–2
  and the self/seer, 170–1
breath of life (*prāṇa*), 3, 33–4, 47, 74–5, 110, 114, 119, 170

cause and effect (*karma*), 7, 14, 20–6, 97, 180–1
  and rebirth, 20, 22–3
  types of, 7, 23, 24, 180–1
  see also actions
concentration (*dhāraṇa*), 59, 91, 116–17, 119, 126, 134–6, *136*, 143, 166–7
  definition (aspects of), 167–8
  effects of, 168
consciousness (*citta*), 4, 14, 15, 42–3, 45, *51*, *67*, 121
  absolute/universal (*kūṭastha/nirmana*) (Big 'I'), 3, 42–3, 59, 60–2, 70, 117, 170, 187
  alternating/individual (*pariṇāma/nirmita*) (small 'I'), 3, 42–3, 45, 59–63, 70, 117, 170
  characteristics/qualities of (*citta-lakṣaṇa*), 66, 69–71
  cosmic/universal consciousness (*mahat*), 37, 59, 66, *67*, 101–2, 122–3, 166, 178–9, 182
  divine/pure (*divya*), 77
  and duty (*dharma*) 12, 13, 116, 118
  facets of (mind, intelligence, ego), 42–3, 49, 53–6
  and I-maker (*ahaṁkāra*), 51–3, 117, 119
  as integration (*saṁyama)* of head and heart
  mature/fully ripened (*paripakva-citta*), 77, 118–19
  movement/fluctuations (*vṛttis*) of, 1–2, 78–80, 83–6, *88*, 93, 121–2, 171, 184

five types of, 83–4
helpful (*anukūla*) 87–93, *88*
imprints/latent impressions (*saṁskāra*), 86–7, 170
mixed imprints/impressions (*saṅkara*), 170
restraint/control of (*vṛtti nirodha*), 2, 14, 15, 74, 83, 129, 157
unfavourable (*pratikūla*), 87, *88*, 93–4, 97
quality of actions according to (*guṇa karma citta*), 4–5
representation or definition of (*citta-nirūpaṇa*) of, 64–5
and Self, 116
seven provinces of, *73*
states of (*citta-bhūmi*), 68–9
steady state of (*citta-stambha-vṛtti*), 13, 14, 74
and wisdom (*buddhi*), 53–6, 119–20, 122
and yoga, 13
contemplation *see* absorption (*samādhi*)

dharma see duty
death, fear of (*abhiniveśa*), 1, 80, 81–2
desires (*vāsanā*), 125, 134
devotion (*parābhakti*), 97
disease/pain/suffering (*roga*), types of, 178
duty (*dharma*), 12, 13, 116, 118

ego, 37, 52, 80, 171
Big 'I' (*kūṭastha-citta*) and small 'I' (*pariṇāma-citta*), 59–63
egoism (*asmitā*), 81
I-ness (*ahaṁ-ākāra*), 32–3, 40, 44, 50, 51, 52, 59, 117, 128
I-maker (*ahaṁkāra*), 2, 25, 33, 35, 37, 38, 42, 44, 50–3, 59, *68*, 117, 119, 128, 142, 165, 169, 176
see also consciousness
elements (*mahābhūta*) of nature (*prakṛti*), 34, 99–100, 181
mastery over (*bhūta-jaya*), 181
emancipation (freedom from attachment) (*mokṣa*) 7, 36, 102, 125, 127, 157
see also aims of life, liberation (*kaivalya*)
ethical disciplines (*yama*), 116, 117, 120, 136–7
effects of, 145–6
three aspects of, 144–5
see also personal discipline (*niyama*)
energy centres (*cakras*), 143, 162–3
energy, universal (*viśva-caitanya-śakti*), 33–4
enlightenment, paths for, 26
evolution and involution of body, 129, *130–1*, *132–3*

fluctuations (*vṛtti*) *see* consciousness

God (*Ādi-puruṣa*/*Īśvara*/*Sṛṣṭikartā*), 2, 27–31, 95, 110, 115, 171
attributes and qualities, 28–31
cosmic intellignce (*mahat*), 37, 66, *67*, 101–2, 122–3, 166, 178–9, 182
and nature/humans, 12, 32–3
power (*śakti*) of, 33–4
sight of (*paramātma-darśana*/*viśva-cetana-śakti*), 95, 159
supreme being (*Viśva Cetana Puruṣa*), 32, 159

surrender to (*Īśvara-pranidhāna*), 6, 7, 9, 110–11, 112, 115–20
and universal energy, 33–4

Haṭhayoga Pradīpikā, 17, *18*, 158
humans:
and God, 12, 32–3
and the universal energy 34

ignorance (*avidyā*), 80, 97, 104, 124–5, 134
causes of, 143–4
impediments (*antarāya*), 78–9, 169–70
nine types of (*nava-antarāya*), 94–7, 121
impressions, subliminal (*saṁskāra*), 24, 25, 71, 73, 76, 86–7, 94, 113, 139, 170
imprints *see* memory (*smrti*)
individuality *see* ego; self
integration (*saṁyama*), 166
effects of, 139–41
of external practices (*bahiraṅga saṁyama*), 117, 119, 135, 136, 137, 138, 164–5
of head and heart, 15
of internal practices (concentration, meditation and absorption) (*antaraṅga saṁyama*), 117, 134–6, 137–8, 164–5
pause in (*pratyāhāra*), 164–5
intelligence (*buddhi*), 12, 14, 37, 44, 48, 50, 53–6, *67*, 81, 119–20, *131*, *133*, 142, 166, 167
evolution of, 69
integration with heart, 15
mature/ripened, 181

karma, *see* cause and effect
knowledge (*jñāna*), 55, 104–5
of awareness, 139
and consciousness (*vṛtti*), 85, 97, 117
path of (*jñāna-mārga*), 94, 142
scientific enquiry (*vijñāna*), *8*, 116, 136–7
types of, *8*
see also awareness (*prajñā*); ignorance (*avidyā*); Self-study/knowledge (*svādhyāya*)
Krishna, Lord, 11, 13–14, 26, 53, 101
see also Bhagavad Gītā

liberation, emancipation and freedom (*kaivalya*), 21, 26, 62, 102, 126, 152, 157, 175, 176, 185–7
life force (*prāṇa*) *see* breath
love, path of spiritual (*bhakti-mārga*), 94, 115, 142

Mahābhārata (Vyāsa), 11, 55
Maheśvara, 159
matter, 24
principles of, 33
meditation (*dhyāna*), 134–6, *136*, 143, 155, 166
aspects of, 168–9
effects of, 169–71, 174
memory (*smṛti*), 85, 87, 120
Menakā, 165
mind (*manas*), 14, 55, 56, *67*, 123
facets of, 56–7
internal (*antarendriya*) and external (*bāhyendriya*), 50, 101, 107, 166
mastery of (*manojaya*), 59, 101, 122, 175, 182

states of, 165, 174, 179
Muṇḍakopaniṣad, 42

nature (*prakṛti*):
elements (*mahābhūta*) of (earth, water, fire, air, ether), 27, 34, 99–100, 181
mastery of, 99, 100, 181–4
organs of action, 37
power (*śakti*) of, 103
principles (*tattvas*) of, 98, 174, 179, 183
qualities (*guṇas*) of, *32*, 34–7, 177, 179
and self, 38–9, 103, 179–80
senses of perception (*jñānendriyas*), 33, 37, 101
subtle elements (*panca- tanmatras*), 37
and universal energy, 33–4

Patañjali, Lord, 9, 11, 23, 25, 63, 74, 79, 88–9, 102, 110, 116–17, 137–8, 143, 144, 152, 155–6, 168, 171, 183
perception:
five senses of (*jñānendriyas*), 2, 33, 37, 101
mastery over (*indriya-jaya*), 101, 182
personal disciplines (*niyama*), 112, 116, 117, 120, 136–7, 138, 143, 146, 164, 167
effects of, 147
see also ethical disciplines (*yama*)
postures (*āsanas*), 61–2, 108, 116, 136, 143, 153, 153, 182
effects of, 153–4, 174, 176
and meditation (*dhyāna*), 155, 170
practice of, 89, 106, 148–52, 165–6
practice (*sādhanā*), 2, 15, 17–18, 21, 25, 63, 86–7, 95, 96, 98, 104, 106, 109–17, 134–5, 180
actions of (*sādhanā-kriyā*), 111–13
ascetic/effort (*tapas*), 2, 63, 112, 113–14, 115, 116, 165
divisions of, *18*, 134
external (*antaraṅga*) and internal (*bahiraṅga*), 134, 142, 165
innermost level/final state (*antarātma*), 77, 111, 112, 117, 134, 138, 142, 145, 153
method of (*sādhanā-krama*), 109–11, *112*, 113, 116, 120
obstacles to, 178; *see also* impediments
pillars of (*sādhanā-stambha*), 111, 120
and self-study (*svādhyāya*), 2, 112, 114–15, 116
see also practitioner (*sādhaka*); yoga
practitioner (*sādhaka*), 5, 8, 27–8, 30, 47, 64, 82, 84, 91, 102, 104–5, 110–14, 117–20, 121–4, 127, 134, 136, 137, 142, 149, 151, 155, 165, 178–9, 187
classification/levels of, 17–18, *18*, 120
see also practice (*sādhanā*); yoga

self (seer, soul) (*ātman*), 3, 14, 16, 50, 81, 85, 95, 98, 99, 129, 142, 151, 177, 178, 179–80, 183
expansion/diffusion of (*ātma-prasāda*), 95, 126, 176, 187
and meditation (*dhyāna*), 170–1
and nature (*prakṛti*), 38–9, 103
seat of soul (*citta-prasādanam*), 15
and Self, 7–8, 13–14, 51, 122, 136

sheaths of, 99–100, 181
sight of (*ātmajaya*), 183
Self (Seer, Soul) (*puruṣa*), 2–3, 5, 8, 32–3, 44, 46, 49, 94–5, 106, 107, 110, 116, 124, 174, 186
awareness of (*asmitā-rūpa prajnā*), 110, 186
forms of (*nirākāra* and *sākāra*), 2–3
and God, 8
heart of (*ātma-sākṣātkāra*), 77, 137
and I-maker (*ahaṁkāra*), 51–3, 186
and self, 7–8, 13–14, 51, 122, 136
sheaths (*kośa*) of, 99–100, 112–13, 115
sight of (*ātma-darśana*), 5, 8, 58, 94–5, 97, 137
self-gratification (*avirati*), 52, 96, 164
Self-realisation, 30, 87, *88*, 110, 140
Self-study/knowledge (*svādhyāya*), 2, 114–15, 116, 147
sense withdrawal (*pratyāhāra*), 91, 115, 116–17, 135, 137, 143, 164–6
effects of, 166
sensual pleasures (*bhoga*), 36, 95, 127
sheaths (*kośa*), *34*, 112–13, 115
of bliss (*ānandamaya kośa*), *34*, 100, 129
of body, 127–9
of conscience (*dharmendriya*), 129
intellectual (*vijñānamaya*), 99, 112, 128, 161
of investigation (*anveṣaṇa*), 164
physical/anatomical (*annamaya*), *34*, 99, 128, 162
physiological/organic (*prāṇāmāya*), *34*, 99, 112, 128
of self/Self, 99–100, 112–13, 115, 181
Śiva Saṁhitā, 17, *18*
sleep (*nidrā*), 85, 94
spiritual pursuit, obstacles (*antārayas*) to, 52
Śrī Rāmakrishna, 119
Śrī Rāmaṇa, 119
Śrī Rāmānujācārya, 9
supernatural powers (*siddhis*), 6, 100–1, 182
Śvetaśvtara Upaniṣad, 29

thought waves *see* consciousness, movement (*vrtti*) of
trust (*śraddhā*), 91, 95, 120

universal energy *see* energy, universal
universe, 25, 47, 48
and God, 27–8
structure of, 32–43
see also nature (*prakṛti*); God
Upaniṣad, 42

Vaśiṣta, Sage, 165, 181
vigour/will-power (*virya*), 91, 120
Viṣṇu, 11, 12, 159
Viśvāmitra, King, 165
void (*śūnya*), 25, 122, 158
Vyāsa, Sage, 69, 92, 139, 148, 167, 172, 175, 181

wisdom, *see* intelligence (*buddhi*)

yoga:
of action (*kriyā yoga*), 111–13, 185
application of, 143–4
concept/duty of (*yoga dharma*), 13–19
and consciousness, 13
definition, 1, 13–15, 83
eightfold path of (*aṣṭāṅga yoga*),

115, 116–17, 127–9, 136–7, 140, 142, 143–62, 164
effects of, 178–81
three parts, 136–7
see also breath control (*prāṇāyāma*); ethical disciplines (*yama*); personal disciplines (*niyama*); postures (*āsanas*); sense withdrawal (*pratyāhāra*)
fall from the grace of, 121–6
and God, 27–8
importance of, 97–8
innermost aspect of (*antarātma*), 117, 144, 171
as lifestyle, 127–9
and mastery of mind (*manojaya*), 59, 122, 175, 182
origins and evolution of, 11–12, 13
path of (*yoga-mārga*), 84, 94, 134, 187
three aspects, 134
power/wealth (*vibhūti*) of, 7, *8*
practice of, 4, 14–15, 121, 178–81
states of, 122
supernatural powers (*siddhis*), 6, 100–1, 182
teaching of, 183
universal, 12
see also practice (*sādhanā*)
Yoga Sūtras of Patañjali, four chapters of, 6–8
Yoga Vāsiṣṭha, 140, 181
yogis, 14, 20, 25, 41, 47, 51, 55, 63, 65, 73, 77, 94, 140, 177
actions of, 9, 16, 24
five classes of, 63